Universal Newborn
Hearing Screening

Universal Newborn Hearing Screening

edited by
Lynn G. Spivak, Ph.D.

Director, Hearing & Speech Center
Long Island Jewish Medical Center
New Hyde Park, New York

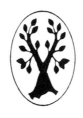

1998
Thieme
New York · Stuttgart

Thieme
381 Park Avenue South
New York, NY 10016

UNIVERSAL NEWBORN HEARING SCREENING
Lynn G. Spivak

Library of Congress Cataloging-in-Publication Data

Universal newborn hearing screening / edited by Lynn G. Spivak.
    p.   cm.
    Includes bibliographical references and index.
    ISBN 0-86577-699-7 (alk. paper)—ISBN 3-13-108081-7
    1. Hearing disorders in infants—Diagnosis.   2. Infants (Newborn)-
-Medical examinations. I. Spivak, Lynn G.
    RF291.5.C45U55   1997   97-22870
    618.92'0978075—DC21   CIP

This book is dedicated to the members of The Long Island Hearing and Speech Society in recognition of their generous, enthusiastic, and consistent support of universal new-born hearing screening,

and

to Steven, Joshua, and Mitchell, my personal support group.

Contents

Preface ix

Acknowledgments xi

Contributors xiii

1. Setting the Stage for Universal Newborn
   Hearing Screening 1
   Judith S. Gravel and Laura L. Tocci

2. Preparing the Groundwork: Planning the Universal
   Newborn Hearing Screening Program 28
   Lynn G. Spivak and Tina Jupiter

3. Models for Universal Newborn Hearing
   Screening Programs 50
   Beth A. Prieve and Mark S. Orlando

4. Personnel and Supervisory Options for Universal Newborn
   Hearing Screening 67
   Mark S. Orlando and Heidi Sokol

5. Instrumentation for Newborn Hearing Screening 87
   Barbara Kurman and Lynn G. Spivak

6. The Normal Newborn Nursery 120
   Grace Rowan

7. The Neonatal Intensive Care Unit 132
   Kathi Smillie

8. Practical Medical Issues When Screening Normal Nursery
   and Neonatal Intensive Care Unit (NICU) Infants 145
   Betty R. Vohr

9. Data and Quality Management for a Universal Newborn
   Hearing Screening Program 167
   Patricia Moore

10. **Follow-Up** 187
  Larry E. Dalzell and Matthew S. MacDonald

11. **Newborn Hearing Screening in the United States:
  Is it Becoming the Standard of Care?** 225
  *Karl R. White, Gary W. Mauk, N. Brandt Culpepper,
  and Yusnita Weirather*

  Index 257

Preface

In 1993, the National Institutes of Health (NIH) issued a consensus statement recommending hearing screenings for all infants within the first 3 months of life, but preferably before discharge from the newborn nursery. This statement represented a significant departure from the more common practice of screening only those newborns who were at risk for hearing loss and, thus, initiated a heated debate among professionals concerning the pros and cons of universal newborn screening. Although few disagreed with the need for early identification and habilitation of hearing loss in infants, many argued that the practice of screening all newborns for hearing loss would be impractical, and not cost-effective. Since 1993, however, the number of hospitals that have acted on the NIH recommendations and started universal newborn hearing screening programs has been growing. Now with four states that mandate universal newborn hearing screening (UNHS) and more than 100 hospitals throughout the country that have successfully implemented programs, we have compelling data to support the practice of UNHS.

In addition to fueling a nationwide debate, the NIH consensus statement also provided the impetus for many hospitals to begin UNHS. As a result, a growing number of audiologists are faced with the challenge of implementing these programs. Audiologists, by virtue of their expertise in electrophysiological assessment of hearing and management of hearing-impaired infants, are the most appropriate professionals to organize, implement, and supervise neonatal hearing screening programs. On the other hand, many skills not ordinarily taught in graduate audiology programs will be required of the audiologist who coordinates a newborn hearing screening program. Audiologists may find that they are ill prepared to apply their testing skills within the context of the newborn nursery or neonatal intensive care unit (NICU). Audiologists who are expert in the administration and interpretation of the auditory brainstem response and otoacoustic emissions tests, will need to adapt their skills to work in a less than optimal test environment. They will be called upon to teach and supervise technical staff, oversee the compilation and analysis of statistical data, and develop systems for quality management. Audiologists who's primary concern and focus may have been the diagnosis and habilitation of hearing loss, must now balance these concerns with those related to test efficiency and cost-effectiveness. This will require the acquisition of good management skills in addition to already acquired clinical skills. Finally, the audiologist will quickly discover that s/he cannot implement a program alone. A successful neonatal screening program requires a multidisciplinary effort at every stage of the process.

At the time of this writing, there were 120 hospitals in the United States that had UNHS programs in operation. The professionals who were involved in developing these programs were, in many cases, pioneers who had little in the way of published reports, prior experience, or advice from established screening programs from which to draw. To a greater or lesser extent, each had to start from scratch, negotiating with hospital administrations, designing protocols, selecting equipment, hiring and training staff, devising systems for data and quality management, and finding ways to ensure effective follow-up. Conversations with individuals around the country who have been involved in starting newborn hearing screening programs revealed a remarkable number of common experiences, successes, failures, mistakes, and solutions. The shared experiences of professionals who have "been there" are the foundation of this book. By compiling this wealth of information into one volume, it was hoped that developers of future hearing screening programs could avoid "reinventing the wheel."

The chapter authors are all experienced and actively involved, in various capacities, in UNHS programs. They represent a broad range of disciplines including audiology, medicine, nursing, industry, and administration and each brings to the subject his or her unique expertise and perspective. The information that they present in the following pages ranges from the theoretical to the practical. This book is not intended to be an instruction manual in test procedures and interpretation; those topics are covered in numerous other publications available to audiologists. Instead, the book provides in-depth discussion of topics that may be unfamiliar to the audiologist including an inside look at the organization and operation of newborn nurseries, tips on proper handling of newborns, procedures for infant tracking and data management, and issues concerning management and supervision. Thus, in addition to presenting the background, rationale, and controversies surrounding neonatal hearing screening, this book will serve as a practical, "how to" guide for the audiologist who is faced with the complex task of implementing UNHS.

It was not intended for this book to be a prescription for a single "correct" model for newborn hearing screening. There are many screening models that have been successfully implemented and there are, at this time, no conclusive data to support the superiority of any one. The authors, therefore, attempted to present available information in as unbiased a way as possible so that the reader could make informed decisions about how best to create his or her own program. Finally, it should be stressed that, although the target audience for this book is audiologists, the information provided would be useful to any professional faced with organizing and implementing a newborn hearing screening program.

Lynn G. Spivak

Acknowledgments

In addition to the professionals who have contributed chapters to this book, there were many other individuals who have generously shared their experiences, frustrations, problems, and successes in implementing and managing universal newborn hearing screening programs. I wish to thank the individuals listed below for their invaluable contributions to this book and to universal newborn hearing screening.

Judith Marlowe, Ph.D., Natus Medical Inc.; Winter Park Memorial Hospital, Florida

Lisa Barsky, Ph.D., St. Barnabas Hospital, New Jersey

Barbara Wendt Harris, Masonic Medical Center, Illinois

Joachim Pinnherio, M.D., Albany Medical Center, New York

Mary Bradley, Stony Brook University Hospital, New York

Douglas Divello, Long Island Jewish Medical Center, New York

Susan Morgan, Georgetown Hospital, Washington, DC

Diana Hill Homer, Memorial Hospital, Louisiana

Melanie Sisson, Lawrence and Memorial Hospital, Connecticut

Vicki Thompson, Boulder Community Hospital, Colorado

Stacey Tregeagle, Boulder Community Hospital, Colorado

Abbey Berg, Ph.D., Columbia Presbyterian Hospital, New York

Finally, I would like to acknowledge the hard work and dedication of Fran Stevens, Director of the New York State Department of Health Disability Prevention Program, who organized the New York State Universal Hearing Screening Project and contributed immeasurably to the promotion of universal newborn hearing screening.

Contributors

N. Brandt Culpepper, Ph.D.
Associate Professor, Gallaudet
University, Washington, D.C.

Larry E. Dalzell, Ph.D.
Strong Memorial Hospital,
University of Rochester
Medical Center, Rochester,
New York

Judith S. Gravel, Ph.D.
Albert Einstein College of
Medicine, Bronx, New York

Tina Jupiter, Ph.D.
Speech and Hearing Center,
St. John's University, Jamaica,
New York

Barbara Kurman, M.S., CCC/A
Northeastern Technologies
Group, Glen Cove, New York

Matthew S. MacDonald, M.A.
Strong Memorial Hospital,
University of Rochester
Medical Center, Rochester,
New York

Gary W. Mauk, Ph.D.
Utah State University, Logan,
Utah

Patricia E. Moore, R.N., MBA
Rhode Island Hearing
Assessment Program, Women
and Infants Hospital,
Providence, Rhode Island

Mark S. Orlando, Ph.D.
Strong Memorial Hospital,
University of Rochester
Medical Center, Rochester,
New York

Beth A. Prieve, Ph.D.
Communication Sciences,
Syracuse University, Syracuse,
New York

Grace Rowan, R.N., M.S.
Long Island Jewish Medical
Center, Newborn Nursery,
New Hyde Park, New York

Kathi Smillie, R.N., M.P.A.
Long Island Jewish Medical
    Center, Neonatal Intensive
    Care Unit, New Hyde Park,
    New York

Heidi Sokol, M.A., CCC/A
Long Island Jewish Medical
    Center, New Hyde Park,
    New York

Lynn G. Spivak, Ph.D.
Director, Hearing and Speech
    Center, Long Island Jewish
    Medical Center, New Hyde
    Park, New York

Laura L. Tocci, M.A., CCC/A
Jacobi Medical Center, Bronx,
    New York

Betty R. Vohr, M.D.
Department of Pediatrics, Women
    and Infants Hospital,
    Providence, Rhode Island

Yusnita Weirather, M.A.
Utah State University, Logan,
    Utah

Karl R. White, Ph.D.
Department of Psychology, Utah
    State University, Logan, Utah

Setting the Stage for Universal Newborn Hearing Screening

Judith S. Gravel
Laura L. Tocci

Introduction

Throughout the past three decades, the field of audiology has been challenged in achieving its long-held goal of identifying hearing loss at the earliest age possible. In the late 1990s, our vision of reliably detecting hearing loss in infants within the first few months of life appears realizable. Our attempts to deliver available local, state, and federal services as well as to apply ever-expanding assessment and amplification technologies, however, continue to be frustrated by the delays that are encountered by the lack of early identification programs. In this chapter we set the stage for this text on the practical aspects of universal neonatal hearing screening. We will review the history of mass newborn screening, identify some of the critical issues surrounding its implementation, relate how consensus building has impacted its past, and how it will continue to impact its future. The ultimate view society has for audiology will, in part, be based on the ability of our profession to provide timely and efficacious identification of the youngest consumers: infants with hearing loss who will ultimately benefit most from our services and available technologies.

Rationale for the Identification of Neonatal Hearing Loss

Normal hearing is a prerequisite for the development of optimum aural/oral communication[1-3]. Speech production and perception are negatively affected by the lack of a normal input model and an intact auditory feedback loop.[2,4] The communication consequences of bilateral congenital deafness of severe to profound degree have been well documented, literally, for centuries.[5] Profound congenital cochlear hearing loss deprives the individual of essentially all exposure to the acoustic cues of spoken language and results in the lack of development of aural/oral communication. Congenital mild and moderate hearing loss does not totally preclude speech and language development because some speech cues are available even without amplification. However, depending upon the degree and configuration of the deficit, varying effects on aural/oral language are evident beginning very early in life.[3]

Children with hearing loss frequently experience speech–language deficits, difficulties in listening in competitive background noise, and, on average, lower academic achievement and poorer social-emotional development than their peers with normal hearing.[6,7] There is also a relationship between congenital severe-to-profound hearing loss and vocational outcomes.[2]

Adequate sensory experience is critical to the developing nervous system for the expression and maintenance of certain sensory functions.[8] Much of our knowledge regarding the effects of sound deprivation on the developing auditory system has been gained through animal models. Adverse anatomical, physiological, and behavioral sequelae have been shown to result from various forms of auditory deprivation, particularly when the impairments are imposed at or before birth, or very early in life. Indeed, through animal research an important period in the auditory development of several species has been delineated, during which time access to normal auditory input (experience) is crucial for the later development of optimal auditory function. This time interval, occurring before the complete maturation of the organism, is referred to as the "critical" period. When sound deprivation was imposed before or during this time period, the resulting sequelae were not completely reversed by subsequent experience with sound.[5] It was generally held that if auditory deprivation was imposed after the critical period, no effects on the neural system would be evident. Recent studies of plasticity and neural reorganization, however, suggest that the mature auditory system may be susceptible to late onset auditory deprivation (e.g., ref. 9).

While it is tempting to directly apply the animal literature on auditory deprivation and the critical period to humans, there are numerous reasons that preclude their direct application. Animal studies serve as valuable models and notable parallels among the species do exist (see ref. 10 for a review). Variables such as the quantity, quality, duration, timing, and reversibility of auditory deprivation, controllable in animal research, are not amenable to systematic study in humans.

Clinical researchers may have means of studying the influence of restoring "typical" auditory experiences in the child with hearing loss, however. For example, the effects of "reversing auditory deprivation" can be studied indirectly by examining outcome relative to the timing of prosthetic device acquisition, surgery, or changes/enhancements in the acoustic environment. Whether partial or complete reversal of any sequelae can be achieved after the restoration or provision of auditory input is a question that has scientific and clinical ramifications for the timing of screening, assessment, and intervention strategies.

Our clinical practice, as well as some empirical evidence, does support the importance of auditory input early in infancy. The intelligibility of spoken (expressive) language appears enhanced in children who experienced some period of normal hearing before the onset of deafness.[11,12] As clinicians, we have all assessed young children with late onset or progressive cochlear hearing loss who experienced a brief period of normal hearing during infancy. Often, such children seem to acquire aural/oral communication more rapidly than children without early auditory experiences (i.e., the congenitally deaf). Typically, children who receive cochlear implants following acquired profound hearing loss (as after meningitis), tend to make greater clinical improvement in aural/oral communication acquisition than do those who have never heard spoken language (e.g., refs. 11 and 12). Although more research is needed, children with congenital deafness who receive their cochlear implants early in life (minimal age is 24 months) often achieve greater aural/oral communication competency than do those implanted later in childhood or adolescence.[12]

The consequences of the moderate to moderate-severe conductive hearing loss resulting from congenital cranio-facial malformations, such as complete bilateral atresia, are undisputed. Still debated, however, are the questions of whether there are long-term adverse developmental consequences (language delays, behavior and attention deficits, and academic problems) that result from the milder, temporary conductive hearing loss frequently associated with otitis media with effusion (e.g., ref. 13). Of interest, recent studies that used psychoacoustic and electrophysiological test techniques found that atypical auditory indicators (increased absolute and interwave intervals, interaural interwave asymmetries, and reduced binaural interaction on auditory brainstem response (ABR) measures and smaller-than-typical masking level differences) are related to early histories of chronic mild conductive hearing loss.[14–17]

The animal literature demonstrates that more dramatic reorganization of the auditory system (particularly at the level of the brainstem) occurs in unilateral than bilateral auditory deprivation (e.g., refs. 18 and 19). Interestingly, early onset unilateral hearing loss (once considered of little consequence[20]), appears to put some children at risk for auditory, communication, academic, and behavioral problems at school age.[21,22]

Recent evidence supports the concept that the age at which early intervention (e.g., provision of hearing aids and therapeutic programs) is initiated is related to speech and language outcome. Levitt and his colleagues[23] found that children with severe and profound hearing loss who received special education services before the age of 3 years had better expressive communication outcomes (more intelligible speech) than those who began receiving remediation at older ages. Recently, Yoshinaga-Itano and Apuzzo[24] reported that infants with hearing loss who were identified and provided with amplification/intervention before the age of 6 months were at age level on language tasks measured at 40 months of age compared to infants who were identified and received remediation after 12 months of age.

Based on the available literature, as well as clinical experiences, advocates of infant hearing screening programs stress the need for early identification of hearing loss and the initiation of remediation strategies well within the first year of life. Proponents maintain that sufficient evidence exists supporting a relationship between the age of detection and intervention, and later communication competence. In truth, empirical evidence for the delineation of one or more "critical" or "sensitive" period(s) for audition in early childhood is still minimal. While it is held that the first 3 years of life are particularly important for language development (see, for example, ref. 25), systematic studies of any specific developmental periods that are critical for language acquisition are lacking.

It was the lack of research on these and other important issues that caused Bess and Paradise[26] to question the recent call from the National Institutes of Health for mass hearing screening of all newborns.[27] These authors contended that the relationship between age of onset, degree and type of hearing loss, and intervention efficacy had not been established. Moreover, other critical programmatic issues, they suggested, needed to be addressed before such universal screening programs should be advocated (see discussion that follows). Bess and Paradise[26] argued that large randomized, case-control, double-blind studies would be necessary to fully address these topics. Some have questioned, however, whether such studies are feasible or justifiable.[28,29]

Thus, the recent debate regarding universal neonatal screening has been heated and, at times, divisive. We would contend, however, that in numerous ways the controversy has been extremely positive. The points raised by Bess and Paradise[26] have challenged neonatal screening advocates to directly address the criticisms leveled and to thoughtfully consider all of the ramifications resulting from neonatal screening initiatives. Some issues, such as Bess and Paradise's[26] concern over the impact of false-positive screening results on the family, were perhaps not fully appreciated previously in the enthusiasm to establish newborn hearing screening programs. However, all of the concerns raised by these authors are critical to the ultimate establishment of efficacious early identification programs.

In summary, there is evidence that permanent, congenital, and early onset hearing loss can negatively affect all areas of child development, in particular spoken language. Resulting sequelae are related to the degree, configuration, type, symmetry, and persistence of the auditory disability. Moreover, the age at which the hearing loss is identified and intervention initiated also appears to impact outcome. While some of these statements may appear intuitively obvious to readers, the systematic study of these issues are important topics for ongoing clinical research. In today's health-care delivery/reimbursement climate, support for universal neonatal hearing screening programs will be predicated on the availability of outcome data that support the efficacy, as well as the ultimate cost-benefit of newborn hearing screening programs.

Average Age of Detection

A continuing concern often expressed by advocates of universal newborn hearing screening is the average age at which hearing loss is first detected in children living in the United States. Traditionally, the average age of identification has generally been considered to be about two and one-half years (e.g., refs. 30 and 31). The age of detection appears related to the degree of the hearing loss[32,33] with lesser degrees of impairment going undetected longest, often not until the child's entry into the public schools. In several reports, the age of identification for severe and profound hearing loss has been reported to be between 11 and 17 months of age.[32–36] These studies suggest that there may be a decrease in the age of identification, at least for severe and profound hearing losses.

Figure 1–1 presents data from Harrison and Roush,[33] thus far the only data that have been obtained through a nationwide survey. Importantly, their report extends beyond data on the "age of identification" to the time of other critical follow-up and management provisions. Displayed are the ages (in months) at which children were first suspected of having hearing loss, the age at which hearing loss was confirmed, the age at which amplification was fit, and the age at which intervention/habilitation programs were initiated. The data are displayed according to whether the child was considered to have been at risk for hearing loss or whether no risk factors were present. Finally, the degree of hearing impairment is presented according to two general categories: mild-to-moderate and severe-to-profound. Note the relationship between degree of hearing loss and age of identification. Also observe that children with mild-to-moderate hearing loss considered at risk (high risk [HR]: $N = 39$) tended to be identified sooner than children with no risk factors and an equal degree of impairment ($N = 42$). With severe-to-profound hearing loss, risk category (no risk: $N = 118$; HR: $N = 132$) does not appear to impact service provision.

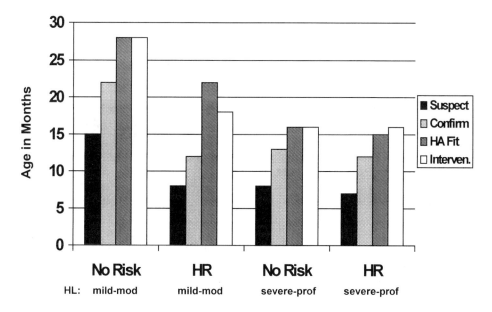

Figure 1–1. Data from Harrison and Roush[33] demonstrating age of identification in months as a function of both risk status (HR = high risk; No Risk = no risk factors for hearing loss) and degree of diagnosed hearing loss (mild-to-moderate loss versus severe and profound impairments). Bars represent the age at which the hearing loss was first suspected (Suspect), the age of diagnosis (Confirm), the age at which hearing aids (HA) were provided (HA Fit) and the age at which intervention was begun (Interven.).

These data are somewhat encouraging in that there may be a heightened awareness among parents and professionals regarding the early indicators of hearing loss in young children. Programs that deliver services to children with disabilities may be more sensitive to the possibility of coexisting hearing loss in children with developmental disabilities.[37]

Still startling in the Harrison and Roush[33] report, however, are the lengthy delays between suspicion of the loss, confirmation of the impairment, and the initiation of habilitation. These delays in the follow-up process defeat the purpose of universal screening. As will be emphasized below, the program components of: (1) prompt comprehensive assessment after screening failure, and (2) the provision of timely and appropriate intervention (including the fitting of personal amplification) are critical services that must be integral to all neonatal hearing screening initiatives. Screening without prompt and appropriate follow-up services for infants referred means that the program is inadequate. Under such circumstances, fundamental changes must be made or the screening program should be discontinued.

In sum, although there appears to be some progress in the lowering of the age of identification of hearing loss in young children in the United States, it is apparent that the goal of detecting all congenital hearing loss before the age of 12 months has not been attained. This goal was voiced by former Surgeon General Dr. C. Everett Koop[38] and the challenge echoed in the recommendations set forth in the Public Health initiative, *Healthy People 2000*.[39] It is stressed that even if identification of all babies having hearing loss at birth could be universally lowered to 12 months, without diagnosis and intervention our efforts will have been futile.

Prevalence and Cost-Effectiveness Considerations

There has been ongoing interest in determining the prevalence of hearing loss in infancy. Prevalence (the number of cases of hearing loss within the population during a specific time period) estimates are required for valid program analyses to be completed, including the critical estimate of cost-effectiveness. In general, it is difficult to make comparisons among reports on the prevalence of hearing loss in the newborn population.[40] Those studies that have examined prevalence are variable or non-specific with regard to the population considered. In addition, in most reports, the program failed to follow both screening passes as well as screening failures so that hit rates and false alarm rates could be determined accurately.[40]

Prevalence estimates vary widely depending upon whether the general population (all babies born), the well-baby nursery (WBN), or the intensive care nursery (ICN) populations are considered. This information is critical when evaluating and comparing the accuracy (positive and negative predictive values) of newborn hearing screening programs.[40] Prevalence data are also important when the efficacy (sensitivity and specificity) of screening test protocols must be evaluated (see subsequent chapters in this text for in-depth discussions). Factual information on the prevalence of hearing loss in newborns is also mandatory in determining the cost-effectiveness of newborn screening initiatives.

Cost-effectiveness is determined by computing the cost per hearing loss (CPHL) identified: the greater the CPHL the less cost effective the screening program.[40] Turner and Cone-Wesson[40] have provided an excellent review of this issue. Suffice it to say that CPHL is determined based on the prevalence of hearing loss in the population, the costs incurred in delivering the screening test, the hit and false alarm rates for the screening protocol, and the cost of follow-up (diagnostic) assessment. (Readers are encouraged to read other discussions by Turner[41,42] for valuable information on modeling the cost and performance of newborn hearing screening protocols.)

As Turner and Cone-Wesson[40] reported, estimates of hearing loss in neonates do vary widely, ranging from 0.9 per 1000[43,44] to 2.4 of 1000.[45–47] In 1993, the NIH Consensus Statement[27] estimated the prevalence of profound congenital loss to be 1 per 1000. White, Vohr, and Behrens[48] estimated the prevalence of all degrees of cochlear hearing loss in neonates to be 5.9 per 1000. Recently, White[49] revised his 1993 estimate, suggesting the median prevalence of cochlear hearing loss was about 3 per 1000. Presumably all the aforementioned estimates refer to the general population of newborns, which includes WBN and ICN.

Actually, we know little about prevalence of hearing loss in the largest population of newborns; that is the WBN.[40] Depending on the demographics of the population served by a local hospital, WBN may account for varying percentages of infants born to the facility. For example, in two of the hospitals in which we conduct universal screening in the Bronx, NY, 12–14% of the newborn population are in the ICN. Prevalence of hearing loss in the ICN population is markedly higher than that estimated for the WBN. Estimates of hearing loss in the ICN ranges from 2 to 4 per 100 (e.g., refs. 26 and 50).

It is also important for clinicians to clearly delineate a priori, the types of auditory impairments that are the targets of their individual screening program. This includes decisions of what degrees (mild, moderate, severe, and profound), configurations (flat, sloping, and rising), types (cochlear, neural, and conductive), and symmetries (bilateral and unilateral) of auditory deficits the program considers significant, conditions for which the program is prepared to provide timely and appropriate follow-up.

Consider the following caveat. Recently, Stein and his colleagues[51] have reported on neonates in the ICN who display absent or abnormal ABRs and present EOAEs. Of concern is whether infants displaying this "paradoxical" screening outcome are at high risk for communication deficits. There are reports of older children and adults with similar findings (termed auditory neuropathy; e.g., ref. 52) who frequently display severe deficits in speech recognition. Clinicians conducting neonatal screening programs must consider whether the detection of babies at risk for this type of auditory deficit should be targets of their individual initiative. If so, then screening tests selected and the protocol adopted must be designed to specifically detect those at risk for the condition. Figure 1–2 (A and B) depicts a traditional screening protocol (A: suggested by the NIH[27] and used for screening in our WBN in the Bronx), and a second protocol (B) that we use only in our ICN. Note that for both protocols two types of screening technology (transient evoked otoacoustic emissions [TEOAE] and ABR) are used. However, the tests were selected and ordered to accomplish two distinct purposes.

A

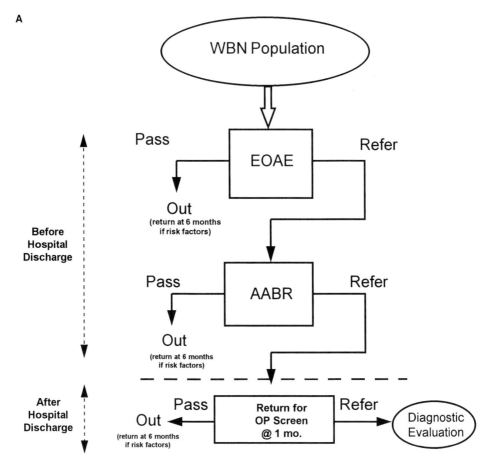

Figure 1–2 (A and B).   Figure 2A represents the protocol used to screen in the well-baby nursery (WBN) at one of our facilities. EOAE refers to evoked otoacoustic emissions, AABR refers to automated ABR (ALGO-II), OP = out patient. Figure 2B represents the protocol used for screening in our intensive care nursery (ICN).

Protocol A was instituted to: (1) identify newborns at risk for cochlear hearing loss (our primary target condition in WBN, and unlikely to be identified through use of only the high-risk register[40]); and (2) lower the failure rate (FR) obtained when we used TEOAE screening alone. In one of our hospitals, screening must be completed in an extremely noisy WBN. Even when the infant is tested in a nonfunctioning isolette, frequently high ambient noise levels have resulted in unacceptable FRs on TEOAE tests. Immediate rescreening (using automated ABR) of these TEOAE "fails" dramatically lowers our in-hospital FR from 25 to 3%. The second protocol (B) is used in our ICN, specifically to detect infants at risk for the auditory deficits described by Stein and colleagues.[51] In addition, protocol B identifies babies at risk for the more prevalent cochlear types of impairments in the ICN.

B

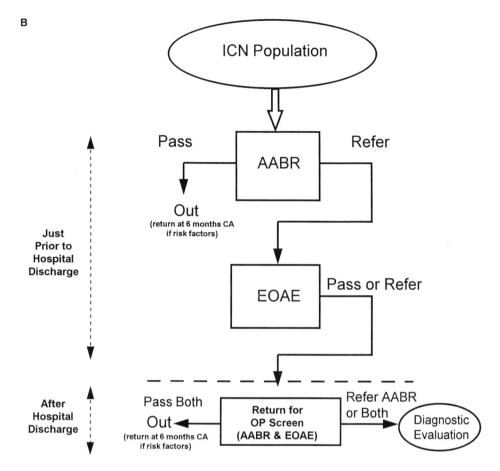

Figure 1–2. (*Continued*)

In sum, wide differences in prevalence estimates are attributable to several factors including the population tested (e.g., WBN vs. ICN), the condition targeted for identification (e.g., the degree, symmetry, and type of auditory impairment the program desires to detect), and the age at which the hearing loss is finally confirmed.[26] Moreover, without specific information based on the follow-up of large numbers of WBN and ICN babies targeted as at risk based on their in-hospital screening result, determining the prevalence of hearing loss will continue to be problematic.[40] These data will remain confounded due to the fact that nearly 25 to 50% of babies who fail newborn screening subsequently fail to return for follow-up testing.[26]

Principles of Screening: Building the Foundation

The purpose of any screening initiative is to "separate from among apparently healthy individuals those for whom there is a greater probability of having a disease (condition) and to refer those individuals for appropriate diagnostic testing."[53] As such, newborn screening must be considered from the public health perspective. Therefore, early identification programs should adhere to the well-established principles of screening, tenants that are valid regardless of the targeted condition or disease.[26,54] As developers of newborn hearing screening programs, we are further obligated by these principles to periodically review our screening initiatives to affirm their compliance with these guidelines. The principles of screening, first proffered by the World Health Organization[55] have been delineated in numerous other reports (e.g., refs. 26,53,54, and 56). In summary, they are as follows.

- The disease/condition must be significant. That is, the disease/condition must result in significant consequences for the individual and to society at large.
- The screening test must be appropriate, easy to administer, comfortable for the patient, short in duration, and inexpensive. Importantly, the performance of the screening instrument must be determined for the particular setting. The test must be precise and accurate (have high sensitivity and specificity).
- Diagnostic criteria for the condition must be available and acceptable. There must be a clear and measurable definition of the condition.
- Treatment must be available for the condition. Early intervention for the condition must be demonstrated to provide better outcomes than delay of intervention until sequelae are obvious. Therefore, treatment must be well established.
- Costs of the screening program must be estimated before the program is undertaken, including the costs incurred in screening, diagnosis of the condition, and treatment. Program costs should be periodically evaluated.
- Mechanisms should be established and sufficient resources available to ensure that implementation of the program and compliance with follow-up recommendations are realized.

It was the point-by-point examination of the NIH Consensus Statement[27] recommendation for universal newborn screening against the screening principles outlined above that prompted Bess and Paradise's[26] criticism in 1994. These authors did agree that bilateral cochlear hearing losses of moderate to profound degree met the criterion of being of significant consequence for the individual and for society. However, Bess and Paradise[26] contended that universal newborn hearing screening did not sufficiently meet the requirements of the remainder of the screening principles. Others took issue with their conclusions (e.g., refs. 29 and 49). Parenthetically, it should be remembered that in some areas (e.g., the demonstrated performance of available screening test instruments), rapid changes have been made in the 3 years since Bess and Paradise's[26] concerns were raised.

Overview of Early Newborn Screening Initiatives

Figure 1–3 presents a timeline that depicts the course of the movement toward universal newborn screening in this country. (Notably, individuals and initia-

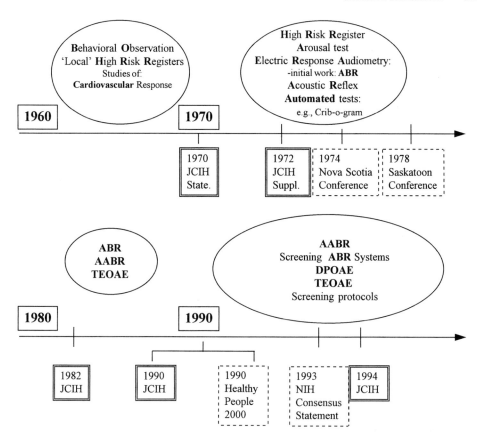

Figure 1–3. Timeline representing key conferences, consensus statements and screening technology (see text for details).

tives outside of the United States contributed to this synopsis.) In the next sections of this chapter, we will address some of those events, in particular the consensus statements, scientific conferences, and screening technology development that shaped the course of early identification efforts. Our purpose in presenting the course of newborn screening in this manner is to visually demonstrate how clinical programs, available technology, the outcomes of conferences, and the actions of committees have shaped the current state of newborn screening. Readers may be struck by the similarity of some of the issues raised in the 1970s to those still being debated over 25 years later. On the one hand, we can applaud remarkable progress in our early identification efforts; on the other hand, we are struck by how far we still must go.

Joint Committee on Infant Hearing

Perhaps one of the most important developments in our efforts to achieve early identification of hearing loss was the formation of what is now known as the

Table 1–1.   Joint Committee on Infant Screening 1970: ASHA, AAP AAOO

- Recognized need to identify hearing loss as early in life as possible.
- Determined results of neonatal mass screening programs were inconsistent and misleading.
- Urged further investigation of screening variables including stimuli, response patterns, environmental factors, infant states, and behavior of observers.
- Suggested follow-up studies were needed to confirm screening results.
- Discouraged routine screening unless completed for research purposes.

Joint Committee on Infant Hearing (JCIH). JCIH was formed, in part, in response to the reports coming from several universal behavioral newborn hearing screening initiatives (e.g., refs. 57 and 58). A need for direction for the growing number of newborn screening programs was perceived by the American Speech and Hearing Association (ASHA). As such, representatives from ASHA, the then American Academy of Ophthalmology and Otolaryngology (AAOO), and the American Academy of Pediatrics met as a "National Joint Committee on Infant Hearing Screening" in 1970 to discuss the state of newborn hearing screening.

Based on available clinical reports and the limited research on the topic, the Joint Committee issued a Statement[59] in 1970 (Table 1–1). The Joint Committee recognized the need to identify hearing loss early in life, but concluded that mass hearing screening for other than research purposes could not be justified. This was due to the lack of an appropriate test procedure for identifying hearing loss in newborns.

In 1972, the Joint Committee issued a supplement[60] to their 1970 statement (Table 1–2). At that time, many hospitals were using "locally compiled" high-risk indicators to identify or register those babies who were considered to be at particular risk for hearing loss.[20] The 1972 Joint Committee statement delineated

Table 1–2.   JCIH 1972

- History of hereditary childhood hearing impairment.
- Rubella or other nonbacterial intrauterine fetal infections (e.g., cytomegalovirus infections and herpes infection).
- Defects of the ear, nose, or throat. Malformed, low-set or absent pinnae; cleft lip or palate (including submucous cleft); and residual abnormality of the otorhinolaryngeal system.
- Birthweight <1500 g.
- Bilirubin level
  >20 mg/100 mL serum.

Developed as a Supplement to 1970 Statement. Added High-Risk Factors. Infants falling into these categories should be referred for in-depth audiological evaluation within the first 2 months of life. Even if hearing appears to be normal, suggested baby should receive regular hearing evaluations thereafter at office or well-baby clinics. Familial hearing impairment not necessarily present at birth may develop at an uncertain period of time later.

Table 1–3.   JCIH 1982

- Family history of hearing impairment.
- Congenital perinatal infection (e.g., CMV, rubella, herpes, toxoplasmosis, syphilis-TORCH).
- Anatomical malformations involving the head or neck.
- Birthweight <1500 g.
- Hyperbilirubinnemia at level exceeding indications for exchange transfusions.
- Bacterial meningitis, especially Haemophilus influenzae.
- Severe asphyxia including infants with Apgar scores of 0–3 or infants who fail to institute spontaneous respiration by 10 min and infants with hypotonia persisting to 2 h of age.

Screen at-risk infants under supervision of audiologist prior to 3 months of age but no later than 6 months after birth.
Initial screening should include BOA or electrophysiology.
Equivocal result: refer for diagnostic testing.
Diagnostic: includes physical exam and history, audiological and communication evaluation, acoustic immittance, developmental tests, audiological testing for parents and siblings, complete medical and lab work.
Management: ongoing otological, audiological, educational and mental health support services.

---

five high-risk factors for hearing loss that were subsequently referred to as the *High Risk Register* (HRR). Importantly, the 1972 Joint Committee supplement also made recommendations regarding the need for follow-up of high-risk infants for late onset hearing loss.

Other statements[61–63] in 1984, 1990, and most recently, 1994, of the JCIH (member organizations have expanded from the original three) have resulted in several additions to the list of high-risk factors (now termed "indicators"). Moreover, the statements have become more explicit with regard to the minimal requirements for screening tests, the appropriate members of the screening team, recommendations for follow-up, and the extension of identification efforts into early childhood (see Tables 1–3, 1–4, and 1–5).

While universal direct *screening* of babies has yet to be advocated by the JCIH, universal *detection* of hearing loss is recommended. Despite the availability of screening technology that is demonstrably more sensitive and specific than the HRR, the JCIH's risk indicators still serve an important function in our early identification efforts. The education of primary-care providers, educators, parents and, others with regard to children at risk for hearing loss remains important as is the JCIH's unified advocacy for early identification of hearing loss in children. The JCIH is still actively meeting today.

Conferences and Consensus Statements

Historically, several scientific and professional meetings and consensus development conferences have been particularly prominent in focusing attention on early identification of hearing loss in children. We highlight several of these below.

Table 1–4.   JCIH 1990

Neonates: Birth–28 days

- Family history of congenital or delayed onset childhood sensorineural hearing loss.
- Congenital infection known or suspected to be associated with sensorineural hearing impairment (TORCH).
- Craniofacial anomalies.
- Birthweight < 1500 g.
- Hyperbilirubinnemia at level exceeding indications for exchange transfusions.
- Ototoxic medication including but not limited to the aminoglycosides used for > 5 days and loop diuretics used in combination with aminoglycosides.
- Bacterial meningitis.
- Severe depression at birth, which may include infants with Apgar scores of 0–3 at 5 min, or those who fail to institute spontaneous respiration by 10 min, or those with hypotonia persisting to 2 h of age.
- Prolonged mechanical ventilation ≥ 10 days (e.g., persistent pulmonary hypertension).
- Stigmata or other findings associated with a syndrome known to include sensorineural hearing loss (e.g., Waardenburg's or Usher's Syndrome).

Provides risk criteria for infants 29 days–2 years.
Recommended screening be completed prior to discharge but no later than 3 months of age.
Specifies audiologists to supervise screening.
ABR recommended as screening procedure.
Early intervention recommendations for hearing-impaired infants and their families.
Future considerations for risk criteria.

Nova Scotia Conference 1974

Held in Halifax, the Nova Scotia Conference was the first meeting held to specifically focus on the detection of hearing loss in infancy. The presentations and discussions from that conference were published as the *Proceedings of the Nova Scotia Conference on Early Identification of Hearing Loss.*[64] Specific resolutions were adopted at the conclusion of the conference including: (1) implementation of HRR as recommended in the 1972 Joint Committee supplement; (2) behavioral screening to be used as a supplement to the HRR; (3) provision of periodic hearing screening throughout childhood as part of public health–well-baby-care programs; (4) evaluation of every child at age 2 years for language, hearing, and speech abilities; and (5) continued research into the causes, prevention, and early detection of hearing loss.

Saskatoon Conference 1978

The Saskatoon Conference on the Early Diagnosis of Hearing Loss was planned as a follow-up to the Nova Scotia Conference. As a result of the recommendations of the Nova Scotia Conference, a need was identified to determine if reliable and valid assessment of hearing was possible in young infants identified through screening as being at high risk. Thus, the focus of this meeting was to address important issues on the evaluation of hearing in infants and young chil-

Table 1–5.   JCIH 1994

Indicators: For Use with Neonates When Universal Screening is not Available

- Family history of hereditary childhood sensorineural hearing loss.
- In utero infection (e.g., TORCH).
- Craniofacial anomalies.
- Birthweight < 1500 g.
- Hyperbilirubinnemia at serum level requiring exchange transfusion.
- Ototoxic medications including but not limited to the aminoglycosides used in multiple courses or in combination with loop diuretics.
- Bacterial meningitis.
- Apgar scores of 0–4 at 1 min or 0–6 at 5 min.
- Mechanical ventilation ≥ 5 days.
- Stigmata or other findings associated with a syndrome known to include sensorineural and/or conductive hearing loss.

> *Endorsed universal detection of infants with hearing loss.*
> *Includes indicators for infants 29 days–2 years.*
> *Includes indicators for children 29 days–3 years who require periodic monitoring of hearing.*
> *Early intervention recommendations in accordance with IDEA.*
> *Provides future directions and considerations.*
> *Specifies audiologist should supervise screening program.*
> *Recognizes the adverse effects of fluctuating conductive hearing loss (otitis media).*
> *Recommended screening be completed prior to discharge*
> *but no later than 3 months of age.*
> *Recommends ABR or EOAE as screening tools; specifically excludes*
> *behavioral screening for use with infants < 6 months of age.*
> *Maintains a role for Risk Indicators in screening initiatives.*

dren. The organizers recognized the need to address this critical component of early identification initiatives.

Healthy People 2000

In 1990, the U.S. Department of Health and Human Services (HHS) issued a report entitled *Healthy People 2000*.[39] The purpose of the document was to set goals directed at improving the health of the citizens of this country by the beginning of the new millennium. Important to bolstering newborn hearing screening efforts was the explicit recommendations to reduce the age of identification of children with hearing loss to 12 months or less.[39] Moreover, the explanation provided for the goal included mention of the consequences of undetected hearing loss on child development and academic achievement, and also called for the provision of early and appropriate intervention services. HHS's inclusion of the early detection goal was welcomed by early identification advocates.

NIH Consensus Conference 1993

Nearly 20 years after the *Nova Scotia Conference*, the problem of early identification of hearing loss in young children was once again addressed in March of 1993. The National Institutes of Health (NIH) convened a Consensus Development Conference. The tradition of NIH Consensus Development Conferences has been to evaluate available scientific information on the safety and efficacy of a particular technology or issue and to develop a statement on the subject that would be useful to professionals and to the public. The specific issues to be addressed by the 1993 Consensus Conference (titled *The Early Identification of Hearing Impairment in Infants and Young Children*) were: (1) the advantages and consequences of early and late identification of hearing loss, respectively; (2) which children should be screened and when; (3) the advantages and disadvantages of available screening tools; (4) which screening model was most appropriate; and (5) future directions for research.

Investigators in the fields of audiology, otology, pediatrics, speech–language pathology, child development, epidemiology, and other related areas presented pertinent data. After hearing these reports, statements from conference attendees, and following a day and one-half of deliberations, a panel consisting of experts and the public developed the 1993 NIH Consensus Statement,[27] outlined in Table 1–6. While other recommendations were delineated, the single most discussed was the endorsement of universal newborn hearing screening. This recommendation from the prestigious NIH had been long awaited by newborn screening advocates. It is safe to say that the NIH Consensus Statement[27] and the subsequent response to the statement by Bess and Paradise[26] have served as cat-

---

Table 1–6.   NIH Consensus Statement (1993)

- Recommended that all infants admitted to the NICU be screened for hearing loss prior to discharge from the hospital.
- Recommended universal screening be implemented for all infants within the first 3 months of life.
  - the disadvantages of hospital well-baby screening outweighed by the accessibility of all newborns.
- Recommended screening techniques that are rapid, reliable, highly sensitive, specific, and easy to administer by trained and supervised personnel.
- Recommended a two-stage screening process: an initial screen by EOAE. All babies who pass the screen are discharged; babies who fail are rescreened by ABR. Those passing ABR rescreen should return for rescreen at 3–6 months.
- Babies failing ABR rescreen are referred for diagnostic evaluation to: (1) verify the existence of loss and to determine the type and severity of the impairment; and (2) to initiate remediation program for child and family.
- Recognized critical component of any screening program is a database system: for tracking infants and for monitoring performance aspects of the program.

Parental concern should be sufficient reason to prompt formal hearing evaluation.
Emphasized other risk factors for hearing loss that should result in audiological evaluation.
Sites using successful screening models other than that recommended should continue the program.
Detection of late onset or progressive losses requires pluralistic approach.
Recognized that comprehensive intervention and management programs were integral to universal screening.
Outlined important directions for future research.

alysts for the expanding universal screening movement we are experiencing today.

The Search for Sensitive and Specific Tools

One of the principles of screening is that the tests used to screen individuals must be thoroughly evaluated. That is, that the validity and predictive accuracy of the test instrument should be established.[26] In subsequent chapters of this text, considerable detail will be provided regarding the performance characteristics of currently available test methods, in particular, otoacoustic emissions and auditory brainstem response procedures. As suggested earlier, the lack of valid and reliable screening instruments has been the primary obstacle to the development of large-scale screening efforts. Below, we review some of the techniques that have been used previously in newborn detection programs along with data that support why such procedures were unsuitable for newborn screening purposes.

The High-Risk Register

As discussed previously, the HRR was developed to identify infants who because of family histories or pre- and perinatal birth complications were considered at risk for hearing loss (see Tables 1–1 to 1–5 for examples). As a screening tool, the performance of the HRR has been evaluated by Turner and Cone-Wesson[40] who completed a detailed analysis of each factor. They examined the indicators found in the 1990 JCIH position statement[62] against other screening strategies, including no screening at all. Turner and Cone-Wesson[40] concluded that the use of the HRR in the ICN performed fairly comparably to other screening measures in terms of its efficiency in identifying infants at risk for hearing loss. Interestingly, the HRR screen was not significantly more cost-effective in the ICN when compared to other screening instruments (ABR). In the WBN, the performance of the HRR was quite different. While the use of the HRR for screening had a lower cost than other methods, its hit rate was relatively poor (<60%). Turner and Cone-Wesson[40] concluded that despite its low cost, the HRR misses significant numbers of infants with hearing loss in the WBN, making it an unacceptable tool for identification purposes.

Indeed, studies that have retrospectively examined for the presence of risk indicators in infants with diagnosed hearing loss found that only about 50% of children who have cochlear impairments have any of the high-risk factors (e.g., refs. 65–68). As suggested previously, the high-risk indicators may be useful for educational purposes and to maintain awareness among professionals regarding late-onset, progressive, and/or acquired hearing loss in early childhood. However, as a screening tool the HRR has not been demonstrated to be sufficiently sensitive or specific for universal screening purposes.

Behavioral Observation/Arousal Techniques

In the 1950s and 1960s, numerous centers in this and other countries relied on the behavioral observation or "arousal" method for the direct screening of hearing in newborns (see refs. 20 and 69). Indeed, detailed reports of how to conduct newborn screening using the behavioral/arousal method were proffered (e.g., ref. 70).

The advantages of the behavioral observation or arousal method included its ease and brevity of administration (generally by trained volunteers), low-cost, and the opportunity to observe an infant's overt response to sound. The disadvantages of the method were the use of a high-intensity screening stimulus (generally 90 dB SPL or higher using a high-frequency weighted noise, rapid response habituation, use of biased observers, acceptance of numerous less-than-specific responses consisting of reflexive and more subtle general body, eye, and facial movements, and the critical dependence of the behavioral response on infant state.

Through application of the behavioral/arousal method, Marion Downs and her colleagues, [56–58] in the mid- and late 1960s, pioneered universal screening in this country. (Indeed Dr. Downs has served as our conscience for well over 30 years, advocating for the early detection of hearing loss in children.) In 1969, Downs and Hemenway[58] described the behavioral screening of 17,000 newborns; 17 were identified with profound hearing loss. In 1974 at the Nova Scotia Conference, Downs[71] reported on the application of the HRR and behavioral screening of 3681 newborns. Approximately 8% (n = 288) were identified as at risk for hearing loss based on the HRR, 0.6% (n = 23) failed behavioral screening, and 6 infants were confirmed to have hearing loss.

Feinmesser and Tell[72,73] reported on data collected in Israel. Eighty-five percent of the babies in the study were followed prospectively and given hearing tests at age 3 years. Sensitivity of the behavioral observation method was 27% and specificity was 97% for the particular procedure used. Finally, Jacobson and Moorehouse[74] compared a similar arousal technique with ABR screening. Sensitivity was 87% and specificity was 13%. Thus, the variability in performance values suggested that behavioral observation methods were not efficient tools for application in universal newborn hearing screening initiatives.

Automated Behavioral Tests

The introduction of the Crib-o-gram by Simmons[75] at Stanford University and later the Auditory Response Cradle (ARC) by Bennett[76] in the mid 1970s provided an automated method for behavioral hearing screening. The advantages of these techniques were the elimination of biased observer judgments (the protocol included control trials), increased testing opportunities in the nursery due to automation of the screening, and a hard copy of movement responses for later scoring. The disadvantages of the method continued to be the use of high-level stimuli, the length of time required to complete a test, and the continued dependence on infant state.

While McFarland and colleagues[77] reported acceptable sensitivity and specificity of the Crib-o-gram in well-baby and high-risk nurseries, comparisons of the Crib-o-gram screening with the ABR screening on the same newborns by Durieux-Smith and colleagues[78] were not encouraging. These investigators demonstrated that approximately 50% of the infants who passed the ABR screening procedure failed the Crib-o-gram, while 30% of infants with moderate losses by ABR passed the Crib-o-gram behavioral screen. Moreover, when the reliability of the automated screener was examined, over 30% of neonates changed pass–fail categories from screen 1 to screen 2.

Thus, available data on neonatal behavioral screening procedures (observational and automated) indicated that these techniques were not sufficiently sensitive or reliable, and that false-negative and false-positive rates were unacceptably high to warrant their use in newborn hearing screening programs. However, a recent review of data obtained from a Universal Neonatal Screening Program in Great Britain suggests a high detection rate and low false-positive rate for the ARC.[79]

Cardiovascular Response Audiometry

Numerous researchers in the late 1960s and early 1970s investigated changes in heart rate in response to auditory stimulation in newborns (e.g., refs. 80–84). Gerber and colleagues,[85] at the Nova Scotia Conference, reported data that demonstrated significant variability in the cardiovascular response in neonates. While initially receiving a great deal of attention in the developmental psychoacoustic literature, this early physiological measure was not applied on any large-scale basis for the purposes of neonatal screening.

Acoustic Reflex Screening

A report at the 1978 Saskatoon Conference[86] examined acoustic reflexes (AR) in a small group of WBN neonates. The authors concluded that with the use of existing methods, the acoustic reflex could not be used for the purposes of detecting hearing impairment. This was the result of the elevation or absence of the acoustic reflex to tonal and noise elicitors using a 220-Hz probe frequency. They suggested that neonatal acoustic reflex assessment required a different method for predicting hearing loss and called for a longitudinal study of the AR in hearing-impaired infants. In 1978, McCandless and Allred[87] evaluated the acoustic reflex of 53 neonates from birth to 48 hours of life. They then tested the infants weekly after discharge from the hospital. They found 89% of infants showed acoustic reflexes using the 660-Hz probe tone and a 500-Hz stimulus. Only 4% of the infants tested showed an acoustic reflex using the 220-Hz probe tone and 500-Hz stimulus. The infants' acoustic reflexes showed no significant change during the first 6 weeks of life.

In general, however, because of the variability in obtaining the AR in neonates, studies needed to address the question of the efficacy of using AR for universal hearing screening purposes were not completed. Moreover, the development of electric response audiometry procedures impacted further work on the use of the AR for neonatal screening purposes.

Auditory Brainstem Response (ABR)

Critical to the implementation of sensitive and specific tools for neonatal screening was the report in 1974 of Hecox and Galambos[88] on the recording of brainstem auditory evoked responses in infants. Subsequently, Galambos and colleagues' 1984 report[89] as well as numerous other studies (e.g., ref. 90) demonstrated the validity and reliability of ABR for screening auditory sensitivity in high-risk infants. The use of auditory evoked potentials literally revolutionized hearing screening and the assessment of auditory sensitivity in the newborn period and early childhood.

In the late 1980s an automated ABR procedure (ALGO-I) served to reduce costs, and did not require a trained observer. This first commercially available automated ABR screening tool involved internal template matching. The unit provided only a "pass-refer" outcome (specifically designed to be used in screening programs). The performance characteristics of the ALGO-I were similar to that of conventional ABR.[91,92] Currently the ALGO-II, the second generation of AABR (automated ABR) equipment provides greater screening flexibility and better control of myogenic artefact. Other automated screening systems are available for use in the newborn nurseries. (See Kurman and Spivak in this text for more detailed descriptions of these and other currently available screening tools.)

Evoked Otoacoustic Emissions

Kemp's[93] description of the presence of evoked otoacoustic emmissions in normally hearing, healthy individuals was soon recognized for its utility as a tool for neonatal screening. The development of evoked otoacoustic emissions technology (transient and distortion product) has provided screening advocates with another important physiologic for neonatal screening. EOAEs are quick, reliable, safe, efficient, cost-effective, and demonstrate excellent performance characteristics. Subsequent chapters of this text will provide detailed information regarding the evolution and current use of this technique.

Recent Efforts in Implementing Newborn Hearing Screening

The following are brief descriptions of three programs that typify current efforts in universal newborn hearing screening.

Rhode Island

The universal newborn screening program in Rhode Island (RI) has served as the model for the implementation of many local and statewide newborn hearing screening initiatives. The initiative developed out of a 1988 RI legislative mandate to screen every newborn at risk for hearing impairment. In 1990, the Rhode Island Hearing Assessment Project (RIHAP) was funded by the Office of Special Education, U.S. Department of Education and the Bureau of Maternal and Child Health (U.S. Public Health Service). RIHAP began as a study to examine the feasibility, validity, and cost effectiveness of using TEOAE for the universal screening program at the Women and Infants Hospital in Providence.[48,94]

The protocol of the investigation initially called for TEOAE and ABR screening to be completed on every infant (WBN and ICN). In fact, both tests were completed on 404 babies. Based on the results of this phase of the project, only TEOAE screening was used thereafter with ABR completed only on those babies who failed TEOAE screening. Subsequently, RIHAP has continued to use this protocol with some modification of their original pass–fail criteria. Well over 30,000 babies have been screened since the inception of the program.[94] Based on the success of the program, RI mandated statewide universal newborn hearing screening in 1992.

Colorado

The Colorado Newborn Hearing Screening project began in 1992 with a small-grant through the Colorado Department of Public Health. The purpose of the initiative was to promote and provide professional assistance toward the development of universal neonatal hearing screening by interested programs throughout the state. Further incentives (in the way of financial and technological support) were provided by an equipment manufacturer and the Marion Downs Foundation.

Of the 54,000 annual births in the state, 88% are born in 30 of Colorado's 80 hospitals. Currently, there are 27 hospitals (urban and rural) participating in the Colorado Newborn Hearing Screening Project, accounting for approximately 56% of the state's births annually. The goal was to achieve 80% of all births screened by the end of 1996.[95] Data from Colorado (from 2/92–9/96) indicate that in 26 hospitals that were participating during the period, an average of 70% (mode: 85%) of all births were screened, and a 6% (range: 2–7%) refer rate was achieved. Unfortunately, similar to most programs, only 48% of babies who referred in the hospital returned as outpatients for rescreening.

Many of the specifics of the screening program (e.g., technology, screening personnel, and hospital support systems) are left up to the decisions made by the individual facility. Presently, there is no state mandate for mass newborn screening. However, an active multidisciplinary State Advisory Board for Newborn Hearing Screening, as well as a newly formed coalition of state professional organizations is promoting, supporting, and providing guidance for the passage of a legislative mandate in Colorado.[95]

In the fall of 1996, the University of Colorado in collaboration with the Colorado Department of Public Health and Environment received a Maternal and Child Health grant to pursue the development of comprehensive early identification programs (including hospital-based universal neonatal screening, assessment, and intervention components) in 17 other states.[95]

New York

In 1994, the New York State (NYS) Department of Health received funding through the Department of Education (IDEA-Part H) to conduct an examination of the feasibility of implementing universal newborn hearing screening as an interface with the NYS Early Identification system. A Request for Proposals was issued to all regional perinatal centers in NYS advising of funds available for 3-year demonstration projects. Seven centers, geographically dispersed across the state were selected. The birth rate at the seven sites (approximately 27,000 babies annually) accounts for about 10% of the births in NYS each year.

Implementation of universal screening began at six sites between February and June of 1995. The screening protocol varies somewhat among the facilities.

TEOAE screening is used in all programs as the first-stage screen in WBN. At all but one site, TEOAE screening failure is followed by immediate ABR (in most cases automated) screening. ICN screening protocols vary among the sites (e.g., see Figure 1–2B). Outpatient follow-up protocols vary, but are included in the cost of the screening program.

At the end of the start-up year (1995), the average number of infants screened was 94.7% (range: 88–99%). Data for the first 6 months of 1996 demonstrate that 97% (range: 91.6–99.6%) of neonates were screened prior to discharge. Importantly for follow-up considerations, the failure rate has been lowered significantly over the course of the project. Figure 1–4 presents the failure rates by hospital for 1995 and for the first 6 months of 1996. Average refer rates dropped to 2.6% in the first half of 1996, compared to the average rate in 1995 of 4.4%.

The constraints and problems associated with implementing universal programs in urban and suburban regions of NYS, as well as the constraints associated with providing seamless follow-up services are currently being examined. By midyear of 1996, approximately 30,000 babies were screened in NYS with

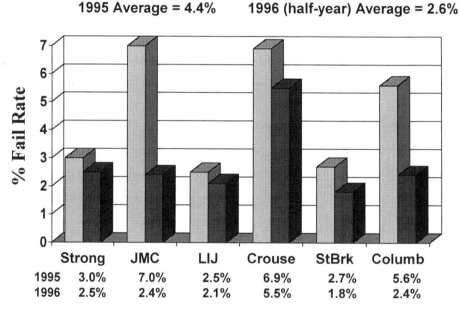

Figure 1–4. Data from the New York State Hearing Demonstration Project for the years 1995 and the first half of 1996. Data depicted are from six sites that had fully active universal programs in the first year of the initiative. Presented are the in-hospital failure rates for each site during the period as well as the average fail rate for each year. (Strong = Strong Memorial Hospital, Rochester; JMC = Jacobi Medical Center, Bronx; LIJ = Long Island Jewish Medical Center, Crouse = Crouse Irving Memorial Hospital, Syracuse; StBrk = New York State University Medical Center at Stony Brook; Columb = Columbia-Presbyterian Medical Center, Manhattan).

over 20 babies with confirmed cochlear impairments identified and others involved in diagnostic testing.

Data from programs such as those in Rhode Island, Colorado, and New York are important for demonstrating the feasibility and cost-effectiveness of universal newborn hearing screening. They are useful in engendering support of physicians and legislators on the need for universal newborn hearing screening programs.

Current International Experiences

The 48th World Health Assembly met in May of 1995. Part of the agenda centered around the prevention of hearing impairment. The assembly urged members to prepare national plans for the prevention and control of avoidable hearing loss, including the early detection of hearing loss in babies. It requested assistance in bringing the assessment of hearing loss to the forefront as a public health concern. It also requested support for planning, implementation, monitoring, and evaluation of hearing loss, as well support for research in this area.

According to Grandori and Lutman,[96] large universal neonatal hearing screening trials have been funded in Austria, France, Denmark, Germany, Italy, Netherlands, Spain, Sweden, Turkey, and the United Kingdom. In addition to these 10 European countries, there are 6 (CIS, Hungary, Lithuania, Poland, Romania, and Slovenia) central and eastern European countries that have begun pilot projects. Over 100,000 babies have been screened since 1995.[96] With the advent of OAEs and the 1993 NIH Consensus Statement,[26] the European community has been moving toward creating a hearing screening data base and developing testing protocols. In mid-1997, Advancement of Hearing Testing Methods and Devices (AHEAD) will sponsor a meeting for the European consensus development conference on universal newborn hearing screening to develop a European statement on the early identification of hearing loss.

Conclusions

This chapter supports the following concepts: (1) undetected and unremediated hearing loss will adversely affect oral/aural communication development and later academic achievement, (2) while useful for public and professional awareness of risk indicators for congenital hearing loss and for identifying children at risk for late-onset and progressive hearing loss, the HRR is not an efficient or cost-effective screening procedure particularly for WBN newborns, (3) direct screening for hearing loss in the neonatal period is critical for the identification of all infants with congenital impairments within the first 12 months of life, (4) models for hearing screening programs will be dictated by the prevalence of hearing loss in various newborn populations, and the specific circumstances within individual nursery environments, and (5) application of current screening technology currently affords us an opportunity to achieve the goal of detecting congenital hearing loss before the age of 12 months.

We emphasize that early identification programs must consider screening beyond the newborn period. This is critical if we are to identify all infants and children including those who will acquire late onset/progressive hearing loss after the newborn period. Our challenge for the remainder of this century and into the new millennium is to develop comprehensive, cost-effective, efficacious, and accessible screening programs designed to identify babies with hearing loss at the earliest age possible. This will provide audiologists the opportunity to provide appropriate and timely intervention. We must accomplish our goal while always being cognizant of the tremendous impact our efforts will have. Our mission is to make our identification programs positive for infants and their families. Finally, early identification initiatives must go beyond testing in newborn nurseries. Newborn screening, by definition, must extend to the full provision of comprehensive evaluation and management services.

References

1. Skinner MW. The hearing of speech during language acquisition. *Otolaryngol Clin North Am* 1978;11:631–50
2. Boothroyd A. *Hearing Impairments in Young Children*. Washington DC, Alexander Graham Bell Assoc Deaf, 1988
3. Oller DK, Eilers RE. The role of audition in infant babbling. *Child Devel* 1988;59:441–9
4. Carney AE. Audition and the development of oral communication competency. In Bess FH, Gravel JS, Tharpe AM (eds): *Amplification for Children with Auditory Deficits*. Nashville, Bill Wilkerson Press, 1996, pp 29–53
5. Ruben RJ, Rapin I. Plasticity of the developing auditory system. *Ann Otol Rhinol Laryngol* 1980;89:303–11
6. Davis JM, Elfenbein J, Schum R, Bentler R. Effects of mild and moderate hearing impairments on language, educational, and psychosocial behavior of children. *J Speech Hear Res* 1986;51:53–62
7. Crandell C. Speech recognition in noise by children with minimal hearing loss. *Ear Hear* 1993;14:210–16
8. Knudsen EI. Experience alters the spatial tuning of auditory units in the optic tectum during a sensitive period in the barn owl. *J Neurosci* 1985;5:3094–109
9. Moore DR. Plasticity of binaural hearing and some possible mechanisms following late-onset deprivation. *J Am Acad Audiol* 1993;4:277–83
10. Gravel JS, Ruben RJ. Auditory deprivation and its consequences: from animal models to humans. In Van De Water TR, Popper AN, Fay RR (eds): *Clinical Aspects of Hearing* Springer Handbook of Auditory Research. New York, NY, Springer-Verlag, 1996, pp 86–115
11. Boothroyd A, Eran O, Hanin L. Speech perception and production in children with hearing impairment. In Bess FH, Gravel JS, Tharpe AM (eds): *Amplification for Children with Auditory Disorders*. Nashville, Bill Wilkerson Press, 1996, pp 55–74
12. Tobey EA. Speech Production. In Tyler R (ed): *Cochlear Implants*. San Diego, CA, Singular Publishing Group, 1993, pp 257–316
13. Stool SE, Berg AO, Berman S, *et al*. Otitis media with effusion in young children. *Clinical Practice Guidelines*. Number 12, AHCPR Publication No. 94–0622. Rockville, MD, U.S. Department of Health and Human Services, 1994
14. Hall JW, Grose JH, Pillsbury HC. Long-term effects of chronic otitis media on binaural hearing in children. *Arch Otolaryngol* 1994;37:1441–9
15. Moore DR, Hutchings ME, Meyer SE. Binaural masking level differences in children with a history of otitis media. *Audiology* 1993,30:91–101
16. Gunnarson AD, Finitzo T. Conductive hearing loss during infancy: Effects on later auditory brain stem electrophysiology. *J Speech Hear Res* 1991;34:1207–15
17. Hall JW, Grose JH. The effect of otitis media with effusion on the masking-level difference and the auditory brainstem response. *J Speech Hear Res* 1993;36:210–17
18. Trahiotis C. Developmental considerarions in binaural hearing experiments. In Werner LA, Rubel EW (eds): *Developmental Psychoacoustics*. Washington, DC, American Psychological Association, 1992, pp 281–92
19. Moore DR, Hutchings ME, King AJ, Kowalchuk NE. Auditory brainstem of the ferret: Some effects of the rearing with a unilateral earplug on the cochlea, cochlear nucleus, and projections to the inferior colliculus. *J Neurosci* 1989;9:1213–22

20. Northern JL, Downs MP. *Hearing in Children*. Baltimore, Williams & Wilkins, 1984
21. Bess FH, Tharpe AM. Unilateral hearing impairment in children. *Pediatrics* 1984;74:206–16
22. Oyler RF, Oyler AL, Matkin ND. Unilateral hearing loss: Demographics and educational impact. *Lang Speech Hear in Schools* 1988;19:201–10
23. Levitt H, McGarr NS, Geffner D. Development of language and communication skills in hearing impaired children. *ASHA Monographs* 1987;26. Rockville, MD, American Speech–Language–Hearing Association
24. Yoshinaga-Itano C, Apuzzo ML. Early identification of infants with significant hearing loss and the Minnesota Child Development Inventory. *Semin Hear* 1995;16(2):124–39
25. Menyuk P. Predicting speech and language problems with persistent otitis media. In Kavanagh J (ed): *Otitis Media and Child Development*. York Press, Parkton MD, 1986, pp 83–96
26. Bess FH, and Paradise JL. Universal screening for infant hearing impairment: Not simple, not risk-free, not necessarily beneficial, and not presently justified. Pediatrics 1994;98: 330–4
27. NIH Consensus Statement. *Early Identification of Hearing Impairment in Infants and Young Children*. March 1–3, 1993, Rockville, MD, Author, pp 1–24
28. Gravel JS, Diefendorf AO, Matkin ND. Letter to the editor. Pediatrics 1994;6:957–9
29. Northern JL, Hayes D. Universal screening for infant hearing impairment: Necessary, beneficial and justifiable. *Audiology Today* 1994;6(2)
30. Coplan J. Deafness: Ever heard of it? Delayed recognition of permanent hearing loss. Pediatrics 1987;79:206–13
31. Stein L, Clark S, Kraus N, *et al.* The hearing-impaired infant: Patterns of identification and habilitation. *Ear Hear* 1983;4:232–6
32. Stein L, Jabaley T, Spitz R, *et al.* The hearing-impaired infant: Patterns of identification and habilitation revisited. *Ear hear* 1990;11:201–5
33. Harrison M, Roush J. Age of suspicion, identification, and intervention for infants and young children with hearing loss: A national study. *Ear Hear* 1996;17:55–62
34. Mahoney TM, Eichwald JG. The ups and "downs" of high-risk screening: The Utah statewide program. *Semin Hear* 1987;8:155–63
35. Mace AL, Wallace KL, Whan MA, Stelmachowitz PG. Relevant factors in the identification of hearing loss. *Ear Hear* 1991;12;287–93
36. Bess FH, Paradise JL. Reply. Pediatrics 1994;6:959–63
37. Roush J, Gravel JS: Acoustic amplification and sensory devices for infants and toddlers. In Roush J, Matkin N (eds): *Infants and Toddlers with Hearing Loss: Family Centered Assessment and Intervention*. Baltimore, MD, York Press, 1994, pp 65–79
38. Koop CE. We can identify children with hearing impairment before their first birthday. *Semin Hear* 1993;14(1): Foreword
39. U.S. Department of Health and Human Services, Public health Service. *Healthy People 2000: National Health Promotion and Disease Prevention Objectives*. Washington, D.C, U.S. Government Printing Office, 1990
40. Turner RG, Cone-Wesson BK. Prevalence rates and cost-effectiveness of risk factors. In Bess FH, Hall JW (eds): *Screening Children for Auditory Function*. Nashville, Bill Wilkerson Press, 1992, pp 79–104
41. Turner RG. Modeling the cost and performance of early identification protocols. *J Amer Acad Audiol* 1991;2;195–205
42. Turner RG. Factors that determine the cost and performance of early identification protocols. *J Amer Acad Audiol* 1992;3:233–241
43. Barr 1980. In: Mauk GW, Behrens TR. Historical, political and technological context associatied with early identification of hearing loss. *Semin Hear* 1993;14:2
44. Martin 1982. In: Mauk GW, Behrens TR. Historical, political and technological context associatied with early identification of hearing loss. *Semin Hear* 1993;14:2
45. Sehlin et al. 1990. In: Mauk GW, Behrens TR. Historical, political and technological context associatied with early identification of hearing loss. *Semin Hear* 1993;14:2
46. Feinmesser et al. 1986. In: Mauk GW, Behrens TR. Historical, political and technological context associatied with early identification of hearing loss. *Semin Hear* 1993;14:2
47. Davis, Wood 1992. In: Mauk GW, Behrens TR: Historical, political and technological context associatied with early identification of hearing loss. *Semin Hear* 1993;14:2
48. White KR, Vohr BR, Behrens TR. Universal newborn hearing screening using transient otoacoustic emissions: Results of the Rhode Island Hearing Assessment Project. *Semin Hear* 1993;14;18–29
49. White KR. Universal newborn hearing screening using transient evoked otoacosutic emissions: Past, present, and future. *Semin Hear* 1996;17:171–83

50. American Speech–Language–Hearing Association: Guidelines for audiologic screening of newborn infants who are at risk for hearing impairment. *ASHA* 1989;31:89–92
51. Stein L, Trembly K, Pasternak J, *et al.* Brainstem abnormalities in neonates with normal otoacoustic emissions. *Semin Hear* 1996;17:197–213
52. Sininger Y, Hood L, Starr A, *et al.* Hearing loss due to auditory neuropathy. *Audiol Today* 1995; 7:10–13
53. ASHA Ad-Hoc Committee on Screening for Hearing Loss. *Middle Ear Disorder and Disability,* 1993
54. Feightner JW. Screening in the 1990s: Some principles and guidelines. In Bess FH, Hall JW (eds): *Screening Children for Auditory Function,* Nashville, Bill Wilkerson Press, 1992, pp 1–16
55. World Health Orgainzation. Public Health Papers no. 45: Mass Health Examinations Geneva, Author, 1982, pp 81–2
56. Northern JL, Downs MP. *Hearing in Children.* Baltimore, Williams & Wilkins, 1991
57. Downs MP, Sterritt GM. Identification audiometry for neonates: A preliminary report. *J Audit Res* 1964;4:69–80
58. Downs MP, Hemenway WG. Report on the hearing screening of 17,000 neonates. *Int Audiol* 1969;8:72–6
59. Joint Committee. 1970 statement on neonatal screening for hearing impairment. In Mencher G (ed): *Early Identification of Hearing Loss,* Basel, Karger, 1976, p 5
60. Joint Committee on Infant Screening. 1972 supplementary statement. In Mencher G (ed): *Early Identification of Hearing Loss,* Basel, Karger, 1976, p 4
61. Joint Committee on Infant Hearing. 1982 Position statement. *Pediatrics* 1982;70:496–7
62. Joint Committee on Infant Hearing. 1990 Position statement. ASHA 1991;33(Suppl. 5):3–6
63. Joint Committee on Infant Hearing. 1994 Position statement. *Pediatrics* 1995;100:152–6
64. Mencher G (ed). *Proceedings of the Nova Scotia Conference on Early Identification of Hearing Loss,* 1976
65. Shimizu H, Walters RJ, Proctor LR, *et al.* Identification of hearing impairment in the neonatal intensive care unit population: Outcome of a five-ear project at the Johns Hopkins Hospital. *Semin Hear* 1990;11:150–60
66. Elssmann SF, Matkin ND, Sabo MP. Early identification of congenital sensorineural hearing impairment. Hear J 1987;40:13–17
67. Epstein S, Reilly JS. Sensorineural hearing loss. *Pediatr Clin North Am* 1989;36:1501–20
68. Mauk GW, White KR, Mortensen LB, *et al.* The effectiveness of screening programs based on high-risk characteristics in early identification of hearing impairment. *Ear Hear* 1991;12:312–19
69. Gerber SE, Mencher GT. *Early Diagnosis of Hearing Loss.* New York, Grune & Stratton, 1978
70. Mencher GT. *Early Identification of Hearing Loss.* Basel, Karger, 1976
71. Downs MP. Early identification of hearing loss: Where are we? Where do we go from here? In Mencher G (ed): *Early Identification of Hearing Loss.* Basel, Karger, 1976, pp 14–22
72. Feinmesser M, Tell L. Evaluation of methods for detecting hearing impairment in infancy and early childhood. In Mencher G (ed): *Early Identification of Hearing Loss.* Basel, Karger, 1976, pp 102–13
73. Feinmesser M, Tell L. Neonatal screening for detecting deafness. *Arch Otolaryngol* 1976;102: 297–9
74. Jacobson JT, Moorehouse CR. A comparison of auditory brainstem response and behavioral screening in high-risk and normal newborn infants. *Ear Hear* 1984;5:247–53
75. Simmons FB. Automated hearing screening test for newborns: The Crib-o-gram. In Mencher G (ed): *Early Identification of Hearing Loss,* Basel, Karger, 1976, pp 171–80
76. Bennett MJ. Trials with the auditory response cradle: I. Neonatal responses to auditory stimuli. *Br J Audiol* 1979;13:125
77. McFarland WH, Simmons FB, Jones FR. An automated hearing screening technique for newborns. *J Speech Hear Disord* 1980;45:495
78. Durieux-Smith A, Picton T, Edwards C, *et al.* The Crib-o-gram in the NICU: An evaluation based on brain stem electric response audiometry. *Ear Hear* 1985;6:20–4
79. Tucker SM, Bhattacharya J. Screening of hearing impairment in the newborn, using the auditory response cradle. *Arch Dis Child* 1992;67:911–919
80. Bartoshuk AK. Human neonatal cardiac accleration to sound: habituation and dishabituation. *Percept Mot Skills* 1962;15:15–27
81. Graham FK, Clifton RK, Hatton HM. Habituation of heart rate response to repeated auditory stimulation during the first five days of life. *Child Devel* 1968;39:35–52
82. Schulman CA. Heart rate response habituation in high-risk premature infants. *Psychophysiology* 1970;6:690–4
83. Schulman CA, Wade G. the use of heart rate in the audiological evaluation of non-verbal children; II. Clinical trials on an infant population. *Neuropediatrics* 1970;2:197–205

84. Schachter J, Williams TA, Khachaturian Z, *et al.* Heart rate responses to auditory clicks in neonates. *Psychophysiology* 1971;8:163–79

85. Gerber SE, Mulac A, Swain BJ. Auditory cardiovascular response of human neonates. In Mencher G (ed): *Early Identification of Hearing Loss.* Basel, Karger, 1976, pp 49–64

86. Himmelfarb MZ, Shanon E, Popelka G, *et al.* Acoustic reflex evaluation in neonates. In Gerber SE, Mencher GT (eds): *Early Diagnosis of Hearing Loss.* New York, Grune & Stratton, 1978, pp 109–119

87. McCandless GA, Allred PL. Tympanometry and emergence of the acoustic reflex in infants. In Harford ER, Bess FH, Bluestone CD, *et al.* (eds): *Impedance Screening for Middle Ear Disease in Children.* New York, Grune & Stratton, 1978, pp 56–67

88. Hecox K, Galambos R. Brainstem auditory evoked responses in human infants and adults. *Arch Otolaryngol* 1974;99:30–3

89. Galambos R, Hicks, G, Wilson M. The auditory brainstem response reliably predicts hearing loss in graduates of a tertiary intensive care nursery. *Ear Hear* 1984;5:254–60

90. Hyde M, Riko K, Corbin H, *et al.* A neonatal hearing screening research program using brainstem electric response audiometry. *J Otolaryngol* 1984;13:49–54

91. Kileny P. ALGO-I automated infant hearing screener: Preliminary results. *Semin Hear* 1987;8: 125–31

92. Jacobson JT, Javobson CA, Spahr RC. Automated and conventional ABR screening techniques in high-risk infants. *J Am Acad Audiol* 1990;1:187–95

93. Kemp DT. Stimulated acoustic emissions from the human auditory system. *J Acoust Soc Am* 1978;64:1386–91

94. Maxon A, White K, Behrens T, Vohr B. Referral rates and cost efficiency in a universal newborn hearing screening program using transient evoked otoacoustic emisssions. *J Am Acad Audiology* 1995;6:271–7

95. Thomson V. The Colorado newborn hearing screening program. Presentation at the American Public Health Association Annual Meeting, New York, NY, Nov. 1996

96. Grandori F, Lutman ME. Neonatal hearing screening programmes in Europe. Towards a consensus on good practice. *Audiology* (Guest Editorial), March 1996, pp 1–4

2

Preparing the Groundwork: Planning the Universal Newborn Hearing Screening Program

Lynn G. Spivak
Tina Jupiter

Introduction

Implementation of universal newborn hearing screening begins long before the first newborn in tested. Although screening for hearing loss may be a familiar and accepted procedure in the neonatal intensive care unit (NICU), this is not necessarily true for universal newborn screening that includes the well-baby nursery. Hospital personnel may not be as convinced of the need for screening all normal full-term babies, therefore, educating administrators and key individuals and departments regarding the importance of universal newborn screening will have to occur early in the planning process. By involving all key departments in the planning process, it is more likely that universal newborn screening will be positively received.

The carefully planned program will have the greatest liklihood of success. An essential element of any program is a solid and thorough preparation of the groundwork. This chapter will review essential elements of program preparation. The issues and recommendations discussed here represent the collective experience of over a dozen universal newborn hearing screening programs throughout the country. A survey of these programs revealed many common themes as well as situations that appeared to be unique to a given setting. Although not every situation, protocol, or problem discussed in this chapter will be experienced by every program, foreknowledge of the potential problems and solutions experienced by other programs will help future programs to avoid serious mistakes and oversights that will impede the implementation of a newborn hearing screening program. The goal of the chapter, therefore, is to prepare the reader to successfully handle the variety of issues that may be encountered during program planning.

The Community

It is useful to create interest and support for universal newborn hearing screening in the community as well as within the hospital. The needs and opinions of the community should not be overlooked during the planning stages. The program director must be familiar with the nature of the population that the hospital serves. Neighborhood leaders and organizations who are convinced that newborn hearing screening would be beneficial to the community can become powerful allies in the campaign to implement and organize a screening program.

Grass roots support for a newborn hearing screening program can be generated within the community through educational programs that focus on the value of early detection of hearing loss in infancy. The childbirth education class is an excellent forum in which to educate parents about communication development in childhood and the necessity for recognizing hearing impairment early in life. Parents who understand the rationale for early identification and the consequences of late detection will be more likely to support the program and comply with follow-up recommendations

The value of community awareness and marketing cannot be over emphasized. The marketing or public affairs department of the hospital can be a valuable resource for the screening program. Articles or announcements in local newspapers or local radio and television stations that focus on the hospital and the patients who benefit from newborn hearing screening programs help to heighten community awareness of the program, establish its value, and may even help to preserve the program if funding is threatened in the future. Participation in public events such as health fairs, and presentations to community and philanthropic groups will not only raise awareness of the program but may generate financial support as well.

The Proposal

The initial proposal for instituting a universal newborn hearing screening program may come from a variety of sources. Most typically, the program is requested by either pediatrics or audiology. In some hospitals nurses request, organize, and manage newborn hearing screening programs. Regardless of the source of the proposal, it is essential that an audiologist be involved in the planning, implementation, and supervision of the program. The audiologist, by virtue of his or her education, training, and experience with childhood hearing disorders and expertise in techniques for the diagnosis and management of hearing impairment in infants is the most appropriate professional to organize and supervise a newborn hearing screening program. Not every hospital has an audiologist on staff, however. In that case an audiologist from the community can be engaged by the hospital on a consulting basis. In some cases, it may be the community audiologist who makes the initial proposal to the hospital. Whether the audiologist is part of the hospital staff or an outside consultant, it is essential that, once the program is underway, he or she maintain a high profile in the nursery and among the pediatric staff to assure the hospital staff that the program is being carefully managed and to assert the audiologist's leadership role in the program. Attendance at hospital staff meetings at which important decisions regarding the program may be made is crucial.

It is impossible to have a successful screening program without multidisciplinary cooperation. The individual who takes on the mission of organizing newborn hearing screening must begin by generating a base of support within the hospital and the community. At the very least, the approval and support of administration, pediatrics, and nursing will be necessary. The program director must convince influential members of the hospital community that newborn hearing screening is important, cost-effective, and rapidly becoming standard of care. Key individuals who need to be brought on board as advocates for newborn hearing screening include the Chairpersons of Pediatrics, Obstetrics and Gynecology, and Otolaryngology, the Chief of Neonatology, and the Administrator of Nursing. Less obvious, perhaps, is the importance of involving the Director of Social Work in the early stages of planning. This should be done in anticipation of the important role social workers will play in infant tracking and follow-up.

In some hospitals, other departments may play important roles in the program. For example, the neurology department of one hospital became a key player in the implementation of a NICU screening program not only because the primary advocate for newborn hearing screening was a pediatric neurologist but also because the neurology department owned and controlled the use of the evoked potential equipment that was to be used in the screening program. In another hospital in which the neurology department routinely performed diagnostic auditory brainstem response (ABR) tests on selected NICU infants, the audiology department's proposal for newborn hearing screening was regarded as an invasion of their "turf." In this case, careful definition of procedures and delineation of the specific responsibilities of neurology and audiology were required before planning could proceed.

The program director should meet with individuals from key departments and be prepared to discuss specifics of program implementation, costs, and projected program outcomes. It is useful for the program director to offer to present information to collaborating departments during Grand Rounds or less formal in-service training sessions. The help and advice of key department heads or their designees should be solicited during the planning phases of the project. Support of powerful and influential medical chairpersons will prove invaluable when the project is eventually submitted to administration for approval.

The balance of the chapter will be devoted to a discussion of the key departments that must be involved in planning a universal newborn hearing screening program. Each department brings to the program a unique perspective, as well as particular issues, questions, and concerns. A major role of the program director during the program planning is to educate and inform the key players about universal newborn hearing screening. On the other hand, the cooperating departments can offer valuable information and advice to ensure the smooth integration of universal newborn hearing screening into the hospital routine. The successful director will not only convince the hospital staff of the value and feasibility of universal newborn hearing screening, but will also engage a multidisciplinary team of players who are fervently committed to newborn hearing screening.

Administration

The decision as to whether or not a newborn hearing screening program will be implemented ultimately rests with the hospital administration. Although strong professional and community support for newborn screening is important, without administration's approval the program will not go forward. Early in the planning stages, therefore, the project director must meet with the appropriate hospital administrators and prepare to introduce the concept of universal newborn hearing screening. Initial meetings with administration will be devoted to introducing the concept of universal newborn screening, explaining why such a program is needed, and exploring social benefits to the community and fiscal benefits to the hospital. The project director needs to know what is required to obtain approval for a new program, that is, what specific conditions must be met, what documentation is required, what professional endorsement within the hospital community should be secured, what human resource issues need to be addressed, etc. This information will guide the director in the preparation of a proposal that will address specific concerns and requirements of his or her administration and, thereby, increase the probability of success.

It will be necessary for the project director to be familiar with the stated mission of the hospital because administrative support for newborn hearing screening will be influenced by the priorities of the hospital. Armed with this knowledge, the project director can formulate a proposal that emphasizes the ways in which newborn hearing screening is consistent with and helps to fulfill the hospital's mission. For example, in a hospital in which charitable activity and service to the community is highly valued, the program director should stress the benefit to society of early identification of hearing loss. On the other hand, in an institution in which profitability and the bottom line are major concerns, the proposal should focus on financial benefits and cost-effectiveness of the program. The proposed project is more likely to capture administrative attention and approval if it is presented as an opportunity to enhance the mission of the hospital.

In the past, resources were available within institutions to develop programs that were judged to be worthwhile without regard to cost. In the current climate of cost containment, downsizing, re-engineering, and managed care, however, justification for any new program will have to address issues related to costs and how those costs will be covered. The program director should present a budget proposal to the administrator outlining costs of equipment, personnel, supplies (see White, Chapter 11 for a discussion of costs). A detailed business plan may be required by some hospital administrations. It is highly unlikely that any institution will be willing to invest in a program that cannot generate enough revenue to at least support itself. Thus, the program director will need to demonstrate how the program will be a financial asset as opposed to a liability to the hospital. Universal newborn hearing screening programs throughout the country have faced these issues. Not all solutions that have been proposed and implemented are applicable to all hospitals because critical factors such as reimbursement, legislative mandates, funding sources, etc. differ from state to state and from hospital to hospital. The program director will have to investigate ways in which his or her program can be supported. Direct revenue can be generated only if a fee can be charged for the screening. This may or may not be possible in a given institution. It is the responsibility of the program director to investigate the billing practices of the hospital and the potential for generating income from the hearing screening. The following questions and issues must be explored.

Can the Hospital Bill Patients for the Screening?

This question should be reviewed with the financial officer in charge of inpatient accounts. In some hospitals, procedures performed by salaried staff are included in the "bed charge" and cannot be billed as separated charges. The screening may be included in the overall charge determined by a Diagnostic Related Group (DRG), for example. In this case, newborn hearing screening simply becomes part of the overall charge for maternity.

Is the Charge for the Screening Reimbursable through Insurance?

Some universal newborn hearing screening programs report at least partial success in obtaining payment from insurance. In states like Rhode Island, where there is a legislative mandate for newborn hearing screening, insurance carriers may be required to reimburse for screening charges.[1]

Managed-care penetrance of the health-care industry has been steadily increasing and is destined to be the dominant form of third-party reimbursement for health-care costs. The impact of managed-care on the newborn hearing screening program must be considered. Terms of managed-care contracts should be reviewed carefully. Capitated plans in which the hospital receives a flat rate per covered life, for example, are not likely to cover screening as a separate or excluded charge. With plans that reimburse on a fee-for-service basis, however, there may be the opportunity for the hospital to include the cost of the hearing screening program when reimbursement rates for maternity are negotiated.

Can the Hospital Profit from Follow-up Services?

For institutions that provide outpatient hearing and speech services, the screening program will generate revenue from follow-up screenings, diagnostic evaluations, habilitation services, and hearing aid sales. Although these charges are not likely to cover the cost of the screening program, they may be used as examples of revenue sources that can help to offset screening costs.

What Nonmonetary Benefits of Newborn Screening will Interest an Administrator?

Although not contributing directly to revenue, there are other potential benefits of a newborn hearing screening program that administrators may consider as justification for the costs of the program. For example, a newborn hearing screening program can be used as a marketing tool. Directors of several newborn hearing screening programs reported that their administrations considered the programs to be valuable resources for positive publicity and good public relations. Additionally, some managed-care companies recognize the value of newborn hearing screening. The existence of a newborn hearing screening program has been found by some hospitals to provide a competitive edge over other hospitals in securing managed-care contracts.

Risk Management and Standard of Care

It can be argued that universal newborn hearing screening is standard of care in newborn nurseries. To establish standard of care, two requirements must be met. First, there must be the support and recommendation of major professional organizations for the procedure and, second, there must be the availability of technology to perform the procedure.[2] Universal newborn hearing screening meets both of these requirements and can, therefore, be justified as standard of care:

- Universal newborn hearing screening has been endorsed and recommended by many leading professional associations and committees including the American Academy of Audiology, the American Speech–Language–Hearing Association, the National Institutes of Health and the Joint Committee on Infant Hearing who endorsed universal detection of hearing loss in newborns.[3,4]
- The introduction of screening equipment that is relatively inexpensive and easy to operate by nonprofessional personnel makes universal newborn hearing screening practical and cost-effective thereby further supporting its adoption as standard of care.[5] As Ginsberg points out, the existence of technology alone does not mandate standard of care. "It does mean, however, that where the use of a device has been demonstrated to be effective in proscribed circumstances to avoid an untoward result and the technology becomes sufficiently simplified and available to be used regularly, the standard of care has evolved."[2]

When discussing costs of running a newborn screening program, administrators should also be made aware of the costs of not performing the screening. There is first and foremost the cost to the child whose diagnosis is delayed. There is, in addition, the higher cost to society for the education of a hearing-impaired child who has not developed sufficient speech and language skills to be educated in a mainstream setting.[1] Finally, there are the potential legal implications and associated costs of not identifying hearing loss in the newborn in spite of the availability of easy-to-use, affordable devices that have been used and adopted by a variety of medical disciplines.[2, 6] The failure to identify a disability in a newborn in spite of the availability of technology to detect the condition and the recommendation of respected professional organizations to perform the screening may constitute an emerging risk to hospitals that cannot be ignored.[7]

Informed Consent

Some hospitals may require the program to be reviewed by their Internal Review Board (IRB). The IRB may determine that it will be necessary to obtain informed consent from the newborn's mother or father before hearing screening can be performed. If informed consent is necessary, it should be secured early in the process, perhaps as part of the admissions protocol. The experience of hospitals that require informed consent has been that there is insufficient time within the short maternity stay for obtaining consent in addition to performing the screening.

If, on the other hand, the IRB accepts universal newborn hearing screening as standard of care, consent for the screening can be covered under the general consent for treatment that the mother signs prior to admission to the hospital. It is worth the time spent preparing a convincing argument in support of universal newborn hearing screening as standard of care for the IRB review. The experience of one major medical center underscores this point. The IRB of the hospital ruled that the proposed universal newborn hearing screening program was a *study* and not standard of care. As a result, parents were required to sign an informed consent form prior to the hearing screening. This practice proved to be time consuming and logistically unwieldy. Availability of staff did not always coincide with parents readiness to read, digest, and sign a lengthy consent form. Some mothers who might have otherwise readily consented to the hearing screening were intimidated by the consent form and either refused to sign or insisted on waiting until they could consult with their husbands. Another hospital that had similar requirements for obtaining informed consent reported that it took nurse practitioners 2 h each morning to secure all informed consents before screening could begin. These delays will obviously compromise the ability of the program to successfully screen all infants prior to discharge. One program reported that when they were permitted by their IRB to drop the requirement for informed consent, the refusal rate dropped from 12 to 0.5%. Whether or not informed consent is required, it is good practice to inform each mother that her baby will be screened prior to performing the screening. This gives the mother the opportunity to refuse the screening if she so chooses.

Pediatrics

It is through pediatrics that audiologists gain access to the newborn nurseries. Obviously the full support and cooperation of the pediatric administration, including the department chair and head of neonatology, is essential to development of a screening program. Without their blessing, there will be no screening program. The support of the full-time pediatric staff, house staff, and voluntary staff is also crucial. Having the full and enthusiastic support of the department leadership will be invaluable in winning the respect and support of the pediatric staff. It is sometimes at the invitation of pediatrics that screening programs are implemented. This is the ideal situation because there is no need to convince the department that the program is necessary. If, on the other hand, the impetus to begin a newborn hearing screening program comes from another source, that is, audiology or hospital administration, the first step toward establishing universal newborn hearing screening must be to convince pediatrics that the program is worthwhile.

While some pediatricians that we have encountered whole heartedly and unconditionally support universal newborn hearing screening, many others need to be educated about the purpose, feasibility, and potential benefit of the program to their patients (see Appendix A). The support of pediatricians is essential not only to the successful implementation and running of the newborn hearing screening program but also to the success of the follow-up program. Therefore, it is extremely important that the concerns of this important group of physicians be addressed early in the planning stages of the program.

Pediatricians express concerns about a wide range of issues ranging from cost-effectiveness to safety. Preknowledge of issues that are likely to be raised by pediatricians' will allow the program director to be prepared with answers and data that will help to neutralize pediatricians' objections. The following section reviews questions commonly asked by pediatricians concerning universal newborn hearing screening. Information intended to help formulate a response to these questions is included.

How Will the Test be Done?

The program director must be prepared to describe the test that is chosen for the program in detail. Pediatricians will want to know about how the infant will be handled, what preparation is needed, what is the background and training of the individual performing the test, and what risks there are to the safety and well-being of the infant. If at all possible, a hands-on demonstration of the screening technique should be planned.

Pediatricians also will be interested in published reports in the scientific and clinical literature that support the efficacy and safety of the screening test. The program director should be prepared to cite studies that evaluate screening methodologies as well as clinical studies that report outcomes of screening programs using the screening method chosen for the hospital's program. A list of suggested reference material is included in Appendix B of this chapter. Pediatricians will insist on justification for the method chosen based on hard data as well as technical, logistical, and pragmatic factors that are specific to the institution.

Programs surveyed around the country have suggested a variety of ways in which physician education can be accomplished. Presentation at Pediatric Grand Rounds has been used successfully by many programs to prepare pediatricians with the information they need to have regarding newborn hearing screening. Short lectures to small groups of physicians was also recommended. The lecture should include figures showing the incidence of hearing loss, relationship to other disorders, operating characteristics of the screening test being used, and importance of early intervention. Have available for distribution copies of relevant literature including published articles, program brochures, and samples of notification letters that will be sent to parents and physicians. Some program directors reported that a useful method for communicating information as well as generating good public relations was to visit the larger pediatric practices in their offices. A mailing targeted to all pediatricians in the hospital's catchment area is another effective method for announcing plans to begin a newborn hearing screening program. Having letters co-signed by the Chairperson of Pediatrics and/or the head of Neonatology will add credibility to the letter and increase the probability that it will capture the pediatrician's attention. If pediatricians are going to accept universal newborn hearing screening, it is vitally important that they be informed and involved from the beginning.

How Long Will the Test Take?

Experience of most facilities performing OAE and or AABR screening is that screening averages approximately 15 min per infant. Indeed, infants with normal, robust otoacoustic emissions (OAEs) may be screened in less than 5 min. It is important for pediatricians to understand, however, that the screening time could be significantly longer (30–45 min in some cases) for a fussy infant or an infant who fails his initial screen and needs to be rescreened.

There is no reason to expect delays in discharge or interference with nursery routines. It is the responsibility of the program director to establish schedules that will ensure that all infants are screened before discharge. The screening schedules must be integrated with the established nursery schedule. Pediatricians need to be assured that their patients will be available when they arrive in the nursery for examinations. On many occasions, screeners in our UNHSP at Long Island Jewish Medical Center (LIJ) have relinquished a newborn in mid-screen to accommodate the schedule of a busy pediatrician. Pediatricians must feel confident that the program director will be able to manage the program in a way that will not disrupt the smooth operation of the nursery and will be available in case difficulties should arise.

Is the Program Cost-Effective?

Program cost is an issue that concerns many pediatricians. Pediatricians will question the necessity of adding yet another screening test to the newborn care protocol. This will require justification based on benefits and costs. Benefits associated with early identification as well as risks associated with failure to identify hearing loss in infancy are covered elsewhere in this book. The program director must be prepared to discuss estimated costs of the program with physicians. Bases for estimating cost per infant screened and cost per infant identified are available in the literature[1,8,9] and are discussed in Chapter 11 of this book. The most extensive set of data related to screening costs comes from the RIHAP project. According to White,[7] the cost of screening in a large two-tier Screening Program (OAE followed by ABR for OAE fails) is approximately $25 per newborn. Based on a prevalence rate of 6 newborns per thousand, Johnson et al.[1] estimated the cost of identifying hearing loss to be $3,364 per infant. As Johnson et al.[1] point out, this is only a fraction of the cost of identifying far less prevalent diseases such as phenylketonuria (PKU), hypothyroidism, and sickle cell anemia for which every newborn is routinely screened.

What is the False-Positive Rate?

There is a sufficient number of reports in the professional literature that can be cited attesting to the ability of newborn hearing screening programs to achieve acceptably low fail and over-referral rates.[9] It is important to advise the pediatric staff that every program experiences a learning curve that may last several months until the program achieves its maximum efficiency.[9] Therefore, initial fail rates of a newly implemented program may be high. The experience of the New York State Newborn Hearing Screening Program demonstrates this point. During the first year of universal newborn hearing screening, the seven hospitals participating in the project reported an average fail rate of 4.4% with a range of 2.5 to 6.9%. Six months into the second year of the project, programs were reporting an average fail rate of 2.6% with a range of 1.8 to 5.5%. For each hospital, fail rates decreased with experience.

   One way to avoid unrealistic expectations on the part of the medical staff is to pilot the program on a small scale before full implementation. This will allow time for the screeners to hone their skills and for procedural difficulties to be worked out. If a pilot program per se is impractical, the program director can designate the first 2 to 3 months of the program as a time for program implementation, learning, and adjustment. Goals for fail rates, misses, and follow-up can be adjusted accordingly. For example, while the ultimate goal of the program may be to have an overall fail rate of less than 3% and a miss rate of no more than 1%, this will not be achievable until the program has accumulated significant experience and is functioning at full efficiency. The goal for the first month of the program, therefore, may be to have a fail rate in the range of 10 to 15% and a miss rate of no more than 25%. These goals can be adjusted down during the next few months until a predetermined target date (3–4 months post implementation, for example) has been reached.

Can I Do This in My Office?

Some pediatricians may be interested in the possibility of performing infant hearing screenings in their offices. Vohr, in Chapter 8, discusses this option for screening site. In-hospital screening is preferred over this approach primarily because it is more likely that all infants will receive the screen if they are screened in the hospital. In addition to costs associated with purchasing and maintaining equipment and training staff to competently perform the screen, pediatricians will be faced with logistical problems that may interfere with office-based screening such as unacceptable ambient noise levels and infants who may not be in an optimal state for testing when they arrive for routine physical examinations.

How Will Parents Be Notified?

A major concern among pediatricians is the manner in which parents will be notified of test results. Pediatricians are protective of new parents and do not want to falsely alarm them. Therefore, the method of parent notification needs to be decided in cooperation with the pediatric staff. Several screening programs have reported that the content of their notification letters was a major source of contention and several rewrites were required before all concerned parties agreed on the wording of the letter. This is an area in which compromise will be required; it is extremely important that pediatricians are comfortable with the information that is communicated to the parents of their patients.

Pediatricians may want to receive notification themselves about screening results for their patients. Pediatricians at some hospitals were anxious to be notified about passes as well as failures. One hospital handles this rather ominous chore by batching test results and mailing them to pediatrician practices in the area once a month. Pediatricians at other hospitals consider it a waste of time and paper to notify them about every infant who passes the screening. At Long Island Jewish Medical Center we routinely notify pediatricians only when their patients fail the screening. Notifying pediatricians about screening results is a good practice for three reasons: (1) Once a pediatrician is informed that his or her patient failed a screening test, he will often encourage parents to return for follow-up visits, (2) the letter serves as an opportunity for contact with pediatricians in the community as well as a reminder that the screening program is alive and well, and (3) communication with the pediatrician creates an opportunity to generate other referrals to the audiology clinic.

Nursing

The importance of nursing support for the program cannot be overemphasized. It is absolutely essential that nurses buy into the program. It is not enough for nurses to simply tolerate the program; their help and cooperation are essential to a successful program. Because the nursery-based newborn hearing screening program is likely to impact, either directly or indirectly, on the workload of nurses, nursing administration must be involved in the planning stages of the program and their full support must be secured. Programs have reported numerous obstacles encountered as a result of not having the support of nursing administration. The nurse managers of the well-baby nursery and NICU will play an important role in implementing screening. They will be responsible for assigning duties, designating work space, and helping to integrate the screening program into the operation of the nursery. It is necessary, therefore, that they fully understand not only why the program is important but also what is involved in screening newborns.

It is not unusual for nurses to be initially reluctant, skeptical, and suspicious of the program. Considering the crucial role nurses play in the success or failure of a newborn hearing screening program, it is vitally important that they be engaged and won over from the beginning. In-service training should be planned well in advance of program implementation. It has been the experience of many programs that once nurses fully understand and appreciate the purpose of screening and benefits of early intervention, they wholeheartedly support the program and become cooperative partners in the program. It is also fruitful to listen to nurses' opinions about your plans for implementing the screening program. Nurses have intimate knowledge of the physical layout and routines of the nurseries. They often have valuable suggestions, that is, modification of planned schedules or screening location, that can facilitate program implementation.

A survey of universal newborn hearing screening programs revealed that nurses tended to have more concerns than any other group of interested professionals. This section will deal with the most common concerns expressed by nurses.

Will My Work Load Be Increased?

The pressures imposed by managed care, hospital reengineering and downsizing have drastically effected work loads of all hospital employees, and nurses are no exception. They are expected to maintain high standards of care while, at the same time, take on more and more duties and responsibilities. Nurses are already overworked and understaffed. They are not likely to be receptive to a new program if it implies additional responsibilities and work for them. Screening programs differ with respect to nursing involvement. In some programs, nurses constitute the core of the program and may even perform the screening themselves. In other programs, a separate screening team performs all screening-related functions, relying on the nurse to cooperate in ancillary functions, such as diapering and feeding in preparation for the test, helping to locate a newborn, etc.

Nurse Screeners

Using nursing staff to perform screening has been a viable option for some programs. This approach has been adopted and appears to work well in small rural hospitals but has also been implemented in large urban hospitals as well. We have learned the most about how to plan a successful nurse-based screening program from programs that have encountered problems using nurses as screeners. Those problems will be reviewed here so that they may be avoided by future programs.

It should be cautioned that a nurse who is coerced against her will to add another job to her already busy schedule is not likely to perform satisfactorily. Therefore, it will be necessary to work out ways in which the right nurses are selected and that they be appropriately motivated. Ideally, the program director should have some input into the selection of candidates for the job of screener. The positive aspects of doing hearing screening should be stressed. For example, some nurses welcome the opportunity to learn a new skill and have a sense of being involved in an important project. In hospitals looking to reduce staff and promote multiskilling, participation in the screening program could enhance job security. One hospital offered tangible incentives such as paid expenses for professional conferences for nurses who agreed to participate in the program.

Specific routines must be established for carrying out the screening similar to routines that are established for other types of newborn screenings. Unless the nurse believes that the hearing screening is as important as other routine screenings and the consequences of missing screenings are just as severe, an unacceptable number of infants will be missed.

One program used nurse practitioners to carry out the screening. One of the advantages of using nurse practitioners was that these professionals were qualified to discuss results of the screening and counsel parents. The nurses were initially enthusiastic about the screening program and performed at a very high level. Unfortunately, they soon became bored and dissatisfied with their jobs. These highly trained professionals were clearly overqualified for the job of hearing screener (an argument also used against using audiologists as screeners!). The program now employs trained technicians.

In one large hospital, a team of 12 nurses was trained to perform the hearing screening. These nurses ran the gamut of skill levels, interest, and enthusiasm for the program. They also were selected from 3 different shifts to provide 24-h coverage and thereby ensure that no baby would miss the screening no matter what time of day or night he or she was discharged. The plan failed primarily because there were too many people with no provision for continuity. Nurses, who were busy with other duties, could not always complete screenings on all newborns in their care. The nurses just assumed that these infants would be screened by the next shift. No one person accepted responsibility for overseeing the program and ensuring continuity from shift to shift. This haphazard arrangement resulted in many missed screenings.

In large maternity units, it is more practical to have a dedicated screening staff. These technicians will be working side by side with nurses and will need their cooperation and assistance. The nursing staff must be assured that the screening program will not add to their workload and not interfere with the administration of their duties. The use of technician screeners will, however, create another set of questions and concerns.

Are Technicians Qualified to Handle Our Newborns?

Nurses have expressed legitimate concerns about nonmedical staff handling newborns. This concern should be shared by the project director. One solution is to enlist the help of nurses to train technicians in the proper handling of newborns and NICU infants. At Long Island Jewish Medical Center, for example, nurses run regular in-service training for screening technicians. Not only is this a benefit to the program, but it is an excellent opportunity to acknowledge the nurses' specialized skills and training and also involve them in an important way in the screening program.

Can Technicians Transport Newborns Within or Outside the Nursery?

This is an important issue for programs that plan to use designated sites either within or adjacent to the nursery to which the infant must be transported. Some hospitals have specific regulations prohibiting anyone except a nurse from removing an infant from the nursery or mother's room. The regulations concerning transportation of infants within the institution must be reviewed carefully. It is impractical in most busy maternity units to have a nurse on hand for the purpose of transporting infants back and forth from the test room. Therefore, if the hospital will not allow the technician to transport infants, the program will have to reconsider its plan to screen outside of the nursery or mother's room.

Transportation of infants in the NICU poses its own set of problems. Because infants will be screened shortly before they are ready to go home, they are likely to be medically stable enough to be transported to a designated quiet area within the NICU area. However, the recent trend to discharge smaller and sicker infants from the NICU may necessitate screening infants who are still connected to monitors, oxygen, I.V., and ng tubes (see Vohr, Chapter 8). These infants are most safely screened within the unit if a nurse is unavailable to accompany them to the screening site.

Who Will Notify Parents of Test Results?

This is an issue that needs to be discussed and negotiated as part of the planning process. The nurse has the most immediate and consistent contact with the mother during the postpartum period and may appear to be the most logical person to communicate screening results to the mother. In most universal newborn hearing screening programs, however, test results may not be immediately available. In this case, parents should be informed that screening results must be reviewed by the audiologist and they will be contacted if further follow-up is necessary. In some hospitals, pediatric and obstetrical staff may have strong feelings about when and by whom screening results are communicated to parents (see the Section on Obstretics and Gynecology in this Chapter). If results have been reviewed by the audiologist before the infant is discharged, the discharge planning conference may be a good time for the nurse to communicate screen results. One hospital reported that appointments for follow-up were scheduled before the mother and baby left the hospital. Some hospitals opt to inform parents only if infants fail the screening. Ultimately, it is the responsibility of the screening program to ensure that parents of all infants who fail or miss the screening are notified so that arrangements can be made for follow-up.

Obstetrics and Gynecology

Those with experience operating NICU-based hearing screening programs are used to working closely with neonatologists and pediatricians. As the operation expands into the well-baby nursery, another group of physicians is encountered. Obstetricians are not as likely to be as informed or sympathetic with the various issues and arguments surrounding newborn hearing screening as are pediatricians. Most of the programs that were surveyed reported that obstetricians offered no objections or concerns about newborn hearing screening. While some obstetricians enthusiastically support screening, the reactions of others ranged from indifference to outright opposition. It is important to understand the concerns of obstetricians, which may be very different from those of pediatricians.

Will My Patient be Unnecessarily Upset?

The obstetrician shares responsibility for the newborn with the pediatrician and is therefore legitimately concerned about any procedures involving newborns. He or she is, of course, primarily concerned with the well-being of his or her patient, the new mother. Like pediatricians, obstetricians are protective of their patients. One of the major concerns about newborn hearing screening that has been voiced by some obstetricians is that the new mother will be unduly alarmed if her infant fails the hearing screening. The first few days after birth is a time in which the mother should be allowed to bond with her newborn without the intrusion of "bad news." The audiologist, on the other hand, is anxious to inform the mother that her infant needs to return for a follow-up test to either rule out or confirm the presence of hearing loss within the first few months of life.

Clearly, this is an area that will require negotiation and compromise. A solution to this problem that has been adopted by some programs is to delay notification of parents until a week or two after discharge. In programs that use technicians for hearing screening, the screener is not qualified or permitted to convey screening results to parents. Thus, unless the supervising audiologist happens to be present, it is unlikely that parents will be given test results before discharge. In the LIJ program, parents of newborns who failed the screening are called 1 week after discharge to arrange for a follow-up appointment. Results are conveyed in nonthreatening language and possible reasons for the unsatisfactory results are explained including temporary blockage of the ear canal, temporary middle ear fluid, baby awake and fretful at test time, etc. The word "fail" is avoided; the need to repeat an unsatisfactory test is stressed. The phone call is followed by a letter to the parents and to the pediatrician (see Chapter 10 for a detailed description of methods for notification.) Although there will always be parents who will be unduly alarmed and upset at any suggestion that there could be something wrong with their baby no matter how carefully the information is conveyed, for the most part, parents accept the information calmly and schedule the follow-up appointment.[10]

In a recent survey of parents of infants who failed the in-hospital screening, it was found that the majority of parents did not experience any negative emotions or reactions as a result of being told that their infants needed a follow-up screening. On the contrary, parents reported feeling "informed, comforted, encouraged, and satisfied" about the screening process.[11]

Another point to emphasize is that only a small percentage of parents will need to be notified. The program director should be prepared with statistics from other successful universal newborn hearing screening to support the claim that, depending on the screening method used, fail rates in the normal newborn nursery can be under 2% (see Chapter 11).

Will I Be Held Responsible If My Patient's Baby is Found to Be Hearing Impaired?

The program director needs to be sensitive to the concerns of obstetricians about potential lawsuits. In our litigious society, doctors are besieged with malpractice claims that are often ungrounded, and skyrocketing malpractice insurance premiums. In some hospitals, it was reported that obstetricians were supportive of newborn hearing screening. They viewed the screening as one more way to help prove that the babies they delivered were normal and therefore considered its impact on malpractice claims to be positive.

On the other hand, obstetricians at one large medical center with a universal newborn hearing screening program feared that the program would make them vulnerable to lawsuits if hearing impairment was detected within days after birth. They reasoned that delaying detection of hearing impairment for a year or more would reduce the possibility of the impairment being connected with the delivery or prenatal care.

These concerns must be addressed directly. First, the obstetrician must be educated in the rationale for universal newborn hearing screening and early detection of hearing impairment. He or she must understand that delays in detection of hearing impairment are unacceptable. Second, the obstetrician will require information about the causes of congenital and acquired hearing loss in infants. Third, the program director should be prepared to present data to allay the fears of the obstetricians. How many successful lawsuits have been waged against obstetricians over this issue? As of this writing, we are aware of none.

As with other groups in the hospital, the best way to handle potential objections and misunderstandings is to engage the Department of Obstetrics in the planning stages of the program. If the hospital requires a committee or task force to discuss the program, a representative from obstetrics should be included. One of the hospitals surveyed involved the OB/GYN Department Heads in planning but made the mistake of not arranging for the information to be decimated through the ranks to the voluntary and house staffs. Although in this case, the department leadership was in strong support of the program, the concerns of the uninformed attending physicians were not adequately addressed before implementation.

The cooperation of as many people as possible who are involved in the delivery and care of the infant will ensure a more successful program. An informed, supportive obstetrical staff can be beneficial to the program in many ways:

- The obstetrician knows the maternal history and the prenatal history of the infant. He or she is in a position to alert the screening team to any known risk factors and may be instrumental in ensuring that an at risk baby is screened.
- The obstetrician can inform the parents that a hearing screening will be performed in the hospital. Literature about the hearing screening program as well as any other supporting literature can be made available to obstetricians to display or distribute in their offices. Thus, the parents will be prepared for the screening and not require lengthy explanations from the screener when it is time for their newborn to be tested.

Otolaryngology

Given their interest in medical treatment of hearing impairment and communicative disorders otolaryngologists should be a natural ally in the crusade to implement universal newborn hearing screening. Nevertheless, very few otolaryngologists have taken an active role in promoting universal newborn hearing screening.[12] It may be necessary to convince members of the ENT (Ear, Nose and Throat) department that their interest and support are needed for a successful program and that the program will be mutually beneficial.

Support of ENT is important to the screening program for several reasons. In many hospitals with audiology departments, audiology is part of or associated with the ENT department. The audiologist is the most appropriate professional to head up the screening program, therefore, audiology will have the major role in the planning and implementing of program. Depending on departmental organization and chain of command, the chairperson of ENT will most likely be part of the approval process and therefore must be sympathetic to the mission of the program. In addition, the chairperson of ENT enjoys greater influence and clout within the medical center than the head of the audiology who is usually not a medical doctor. Support of the chair will help gain hospital-wide acceptance. Bluestone[12] encourages otolaryngologists to become better informed about newborn screening so that they can advocate for new programs.

The screening program can also be beneficial to the otolaryngologist. Identified infants are potential patients for otolaryngologists. At the very least, these babies will require thorough otological evaluations prior to fitting with amplification and starting habilitation. Furthermore, screening programs are capable of identifying babies with chronic middle ear disease.[13] These infants will require ongoing medical care and some may even become candidates for surgery. A close association with a cooperative otolaryngology department will facilitate management of hearing impaired infants identified by the program.

Medical Records

Screening results should become a part of the newborn's permanent medical record. The program director needs to meet with the Director of Medical Records to determine how, when, where, and by whom screening information will be recorded. Several hospitals reported using a three-part form, one of which was sent to medical records. Some hospitals use a pre-inked stamp and enter screening results directly into the progress note section of the newborn's chart. Many nurseries are adopting a care map system to track patient care (See Chapter 9). At LIJ, in addition to stamping the infant's chart, a notation that the screening was performed is entered on the care map. Inclusion of the hearing screening as part of the care map is another validation of the importance of the program and provides an excellent means of monitoring the effectiveness of the program.

Follow-Up

A screening program is only as good as the follow-up program. The greatest weakness of any screening program is often the inability to adequately follow infants who have failed the hearing screen. The protocol for follow-up must be established as part of the planning process. Simmons[14] has recommended that for any child that fails a hearing screening, a retest should occur with 2 weeks of discharge. Most hospitals surveyed recall infants within 3 months of the initial screen. Hospitals located in small towns report greater success in recalling infants for follow-up than hospital in large cities. Hospitals that do not offer outpatient audiological services must make arrangements with audiologists in the community who are willing to perform follow-up screening and diagnostic evaluations and report back results to the hospital program. Reporting mechanisms and data management protocols should all be in place before the program screens the first newborn (see Chapter 9).

Special Considerations for Inner City Hospitals

There are specific problems associated with implementing a screening program in an inner city hospital that need to be addressed in the planning stages of the program. The lack of compliance with follow up testing is an area that is especially troublesome. There are several reasons why follow-up in inner cities is difficult

- Many infants are discharged to foster care and are lost to the system.
- Parents sometimes give false addresses or phone numbers when admitted to the hospital making it difficult or impossible to find them after discharge.
- Some mothers may be living in temporary shelters prior to their admission and are placed in different housing after the birth of the child.

Given the considerable challenges of following infants in inner city neighborhoods, it is imperative that effective follow-up strategies and protocols be in place before the screening program begins. There are a number of strategies can be used to contact families (see Chapter 10), however, not all of the traditional follow-up methods are effective in poor, urban environments. The least effective method is a follow-up letter. Families may move without a forwarding address or report an incorrect address and be unreachable by mail. Similarly, phone calls may be ineffective. In addition to being mobile, many inner city families do not have telephones and may rely on neighbors or relatives to take phone messages for them.

One of the most successful methods of following urban infants is to schedule the screening follow-up appointment at the same time as the well-baby or NICU follow-up appointment. A large percentage of inner city families receive their routine medical care in hospital out-patient clinics. Combining follow-up hearing screening with regular pediatric appointments, therefore, is an excellent way to follow otherwise difficult-to-find infants. Another successful strategy is to register all infants who fail their screening with the state's infant high-risk tracking program. In our experience, this provides another effective mechanism for locating hard-to-find infants. The hospital social worker can also be enormously helpful in tracking infants who are frequently lost when they enter foster care. By alerting the foster care agency that an infant requires follow-up testing, the social worker can help to ensure compliance with the follow-up program.

In some hospitals, infants may have prolonged stays in the nursery because their families are unwilling or unable to care for them. These are the "boarder babies," who are waiting to be put in foster care. Many states have addressed this problem so that the number of boarder babies has been decreasing. However, it is likely that infants will remain in a nursery for at least several days. In those cases infants can be retested before they are placed in foster homes. The strategy of performing repeat screenings and even diagnostic evaluations before discharge can be incorporated into any hearing screening program in which there is a large probability that follow-up will be difficult. Strategies for successful follow-up of inner city infants will require the collaborative efforts of administration, audiology, pediatrics, and social work, as well as local child find programs.

After Implementation

The educational and advocacy responsibilities of the program director do not end when the program is finally approved and implemented. Ongoing staff education is of paramount importance for the continued success of the program. The majority of hospitals surveyed stressed the importance of keeping key hospital staff updated and apprised of the program's progress. Periodic reports, updates, and refresher in-service training sessions help to perpetuate interest and enthusiasm for the program.

References

1. Johnson JL, Mauk KM, Taekawa RP, Sia CK, Blackwell PM. Implementing a statewide system of services for infants and toddlers with hearing disabilities. Semin Hear 1993;14:105–19
2. Ginsberg WH. When does a guideline become a standard? The new American Society of Anesthesiologists guidelines give us a clue. Ann Emerg Med 1993;22:1891–6
3. American Speech–Language–Hearing Association Joint Committee on Infant Hearing. 1994 Position Statement. ASHA 1994;36:38–41
4. National Institutes of Health. Early identification of hearing impairment in infants and young children. NIH Consensus Statement 1993;11:1–24
5. Marlowe JA. Legal and risk management issues in newborn hearing screening. Semin Hear 1996;17:153–64
6. Meister S. Emerging risk: Failure to detect hearing disability in newborns. QRC Advisor 1993; 10:1–4
7. White KR, Behrens TR. The Rhode Island hearing assessment project: implications for universal newborn hearing screening. Semin Hear 1993;14:1–119
8. Turner RG. Factors that determine the cost and performance of early identification protocols. J Am Acad Audiol 1992;3:233–41
9. Maxon AB, White KR, Behrens TR, Vohr BR. Referral rates and cost efficiency in a universal newborn screening program using transient evoked otoacoustic emissions. J Am Acad Audiol 1995;6: 271–7
10. White KR. Universal newborn hearing screening using transient evoked otoacoustic emissions: Past, present, and future. Semin Hear 1996;17:171–83
11. Abdala de Uzcategui C, Yoshinaga-Itano, C. Parent's reactions to newborn hearing screening. Audiol Today 1997;9:24–7
12. Bluestone CD. Universal newborn screening for hearing loss: Ideal vs. reality and the role of otolaryngologists. Otolaryngol Head Neck Surg. 1996;115:89–93
13. Maxon AB, White KR, Vohr BR, Behrens TR. Feasibility of identifying risk for conductive hearing loss in a newborn universal hearing screening program. Semin Hear 1993;14:73–87.11
14. Simmons FB. Diagnosis and rehabilitation of deaf newborns, part II. ASHA 1980;22:475

APPENDIX A

To evaluate pediatricians reactions to the Universal Newborn Hearing Screening Program at Long Island Jewish Medical Center, a brief questionnaire was sent to 600 pediatricians in the Queens–Long Island area of New York. All of the physicians surveyed were attending physicians associated with the Long Island Jewish Medical Center and many had patients who had participated in the Hearing Screening Program at the hospital. Surveys were returned by 114 physicians (19%). The results are summarized below.

- Over 70% of the physicians supported universal newborn hearing screening and thought that screening for hearing loss was just as important as screening for metabolic disorders such as PKU, hypothyroidism, and sickle cell anemia.
- The major concern about the program expressed by pediatricians was the potential to cause unnecessary parental anxiety because of a high false-positive rate.
- Almost all the physicians (over 85%) indicated that they considered the major benefit of a newborn hearing screening program to be the identification of hearing impairment in infancy providing the opportunity for early intervention.
- Preference for test type was equally split between OAE and ABR. Most of the physicians who choose OAE indicated that they did so because they thought it was fast and safe while most of those who chose ABR did so because they thought it was accurate.
- Over 70% of the pediatricians wanted to know the results of the screen regardless of whether the infants passed of failed the hearing screen.
- When asked if they would encourage their patients to return for follow-up testing, 96% answered affirmatively.

Overall, pediatricians who responded to this survey approved of hearing screening and supported the program. They seemed to understand the value of early intervention and were willing to cooperate with our efforts to identify hearing-impaired infants.

APPENDIX B
SELECTED ANNOTATED REFERENCES

Buttross SL, Gearhart JG, Peck, JE Early identification and management of hearing impairment. Am Fam Physician, 1995;51:1437–46, 1451–2

(The family physician is in an excellent position to identify hearing impairment at an early stage during well-child visits. Children at high risk for hearing loss should be referred for auditory function tests, including OAE testing. The advantages and limitations of each test should be understood by the family physician.)

Downs MP. Universal newborn hearing screening—The Colorado story. Int J Pediatr Otorhinolaryngol 1995;32:257–9

(In 1992, the Colorado State Public Health Department inaugurated a state-wide program of universal newborn hearing screening. A preliminary report covers the screening of 14,191 infants. Research from the University of Colorado confirms that children receiving intervention by 3 months perform significantly higher at 40 months than those identified later.)

Galambos R, Wilson MJ, Silva PD. Identifying hearing loss in the intensive-care nursery: A 20-year summary. J Am Acad Audiol, 1994;5:149

(The outcome of a study on hearing loss in graduates of one third-level and two second-level intensive-care nurseries is reported. Initial hearing-threshold estimates were obtained by ABR analyses at the time of discharge from the hospital. The goals were to identify, test, and fit hearing aids on those who needed them. Approximately half of the fittings occurred within 1 year of the hospital test that initially diagnosed the loss.)

Goldberg B. Universal hearing screening of newborns. An idea whose time has come. ASHA 1993;35:63–4

(One out of every 1000 children in the United States is born deaf, with an estimated 6 out of 1000 diagnosed as having significant sensorineural hearing loss. Less than 50% of these children are identified until almost 3 years old. This article discusses the recent NIDCD grant funding research leading to the development of model systems for neonatal hearing screening.)

Maxon AB, White KR, Behrens TR, and Vohr BR. Referral rates and cost efficiency in a universal newborn hearing screening program using transient evoked otoacoustic emissions. J Am Acad Audiol 1995;6:271–7

(Although the value of identifying hearing loss before 1 year of age is widely recognized, the feasibility of universal newborn hearing screening using TEOAE is sometimes questioned because it is presumed that the technique has a high false-positive rate and is not cost-efficient. This paper presents new data for 4253 infants from an operational universal newborn hearing screening program using a TEOAE procedure that answers those arguments.)

Morlet T, Collet L, Duclaus R, Lapillonne A, Salle B, Putet G, Morgon A. Spontaneous and evoked otoacoustic emissions in pre-term and full-term neonates: Is there a clinical application? Int J Pediatr Otorhinolaryngol 1995;33:207–11

(Evoked OAEs and spontaneous OAEs recorded in 93 preterm and full-term neonates revealed that this technique is potentially useful for auditory screening in neonatology units.)

National Institute of Health. *Consensus statement: Early identification of hearing impairment in infants and young children* (NIH Consensus Statement, 11). Bethesda, MD, U.S. Government Printing Office, 1993

Norton SJ. Application of transient evoked otoacoustic emissions to pediatric populations. Ear Hear 1993;14:64–73

(TEOAEs, which are sensitive to mild to moderate degrees of cochlear hearing loss up to about 40–50 dB HL, can be measured rapidly and noninvasively in infants and children. Potential applications in pediatric audiology include screening for hearing impairment in neonates, separating peripheral hearing loss and central auditory dysfunction, and monitoring cochlear status in children receiving ototoxic drugs.)

Norton SJ, Widen JE. Evoked otoacoustic emissions in normal hearing infants and children: emerging data and issues. Ear Hear 1990;11:121–7

(Evoked OAEs are a promising tool for evaluating cochlear status in children. Preliminary data from normal hearing subjects ranging from birth to 29.9 years are discussed. Issues related to further application of evoked OAEs to pediatric populations are discussed.)

Picton TW, Durieux-Smith, A, Moran LM. Recording auditory brainstem responses from infants. Int J Pediatr Otorhinolaryngol 1994;28:93–110

(ABRs can be reliably recorded from infants in the first few months of life, and are useful in screening for hearing impairment. At present, ABRs are mainly used for screening infants who have been treated in neonatal intensive care units. Because the majority of infants with hearing impairment are not seen in these units, it might be worthwhile to use ABRs in a more widespread screening program.)

Stewart DL, Pearlman A. Newborn hearing screening. J Kentucky Med Assoc 1994;92:444–9

(This study reported 2 years' experience at Kosair Children's Hospital where 1987 infants admitted to well-baby, intermediate, or intensive-care nurseries were screened using the ALGO-1 screener, a modified ABR. The positive predictive value of the test was 96%. Therefore, it was concluded that the use of the modified ABR in the newborn is a timely, cost-efficient method of screening for hearing loss and should be used for mass screening of all newborns.)

White KR, Behrens TR (eds.). The Rhode Island hearing assessment project; implications for universal newborn hearing screening. Semin Hear 1993;14: 1–119

(The Rhode Island Hearing Assessment Project (RIHAP) was initiated in 1990 to evaluate the feasibility, validity and cost-efficiency of using TEOAEs to screen infants for hearing loss. As of this date, over 12,000 infants have been screened by RIHAP. The procedures and current results are summarized, and implications for policy and practice related to neonatal hearing screening are discussed.)

White KR, Culpepper B, Maxon AB, Vohr BR, Mauk GW. Transient evoked otoacoustic emission-based screening in typical nurseries: A response to Jacobson and Jacobson. Int J Pediatr Otorhinolaryngol 1995;33:17–21

(Jacobson and Jacobson recently questioned whether TEOAE-based newborn hearing screening could be implemented in a typical nursery setting. This article presents data based on dozens of currently operational TEOAE-based programs, which demonstrate that the concerns raised by Jacobson and Jacobson are not representative of what is being experienced by operational newborn hearing screening programs.)

White KR, Vohr BR, Maxon AB, Behrens TR, McPherson MG, Mauk GW. Screening all newborns for hearing loss using transient evoked otoacoustic emissions. Int J Pediatr Otorhinolaryngol 1994;29:203–17

(This study reported on 1850 infants from the well-baby nursery and neonatal intensive-care unit who were screened with TEOAE using a two-stage process. The results suggest that TEOAE is a promising technique for screening newborns for hearing loss and should be evaluated further as a tool for universal newborn hearing screening.)

3

Models for Universal Newborn Hearing Screening Programs

MARK S. ORLANDO
BETH A. PRIEVE

Introduction

The design of a universal newborn hearing screening program will depend on many factors unique to each hospital. Therefore, an enormous organizational effort is needed to implement and run a successful Universal Newborn Hearing Screening Program (UNHSP). A concerted effort in a preimplementation phase will hopefully foresee problem areas and provide time to develop strategies and procedures that can solve such problems. One important consideration that will circumvent problems is choosing a screening protocol that best suits your hospital.

Previous programs have used a variety of nonphysiological test procedures such as: public awareness campaigns, high-risk registries/indicators, high-risk hearing screening by maternal interview, high-risk registries tied to the infant birth certificate, behavioral observation audiometry performed in audiological facilities, hospital crib-o-grams or by home health visitors/nurses. Although it appears that a number of these programs have been successful in certain geographical areas or communities, all have certain limitations that put into question the feasibility and success when used as a UNHSP.[1] More importantly, the 1994 report of the Joint Committee on Infant Hearing (JCIH) recommends that physiological measures be used for screening.

Currently, the auditory brainstem response (ABR) and evoked otoacoustic emissions (EOAE) are the only practical and objective methods meeting the JCIH[2] guidelines. Each tool has its own unique advantages and disadvantages. Neither is a behavioral test of hearing, but each is a good predictor of auditory function and is able to identify hearing loss. Both tests require normal peripheral auditory function, such as patent ear canals and normal middle ear and cochlear function. The ABR also requires normal auditory neurological function.

There are a variety of hearing screening models from which to choose. An existing model may be appropriate, however, designing your own UNHSP is often necessary. The design of a UNHSP will depend on factors unique to each setting such as: screening tools, program philosophy, severity and configuration of hearing loss, prior experience, personnel, typical length-of-stay for mothers and their infants, space, referral rates, and funding. The goal of this chapter is to provide a discussion of these factors and how they may influence your program.

Auditory Brainstem Response Screening

The ABR is a physiological measure of the auditory system to stimuli presented to the ear. Three or four electrodes are pasted to the scalp to record EEG activity that is altered by auditory stimuli. For screening purposes, short-duration "clicks" are presented to each ear via earphones. Because the alterations in EEG activity due to the stimuli are small, the response is differentially amplified and averaged, thus reducing random EEG activity and enhancing the changes due to the response of the auditory system to the click stimuli. The ABR assesses the integrity of the auditory system, mechanical and neural, through the level of the inferior colliculus of the brainstem. Although the ABR evoked by click stimuli lacks frequency specificity and is not a behavioral test of hearing, the ABR correlates well with hearing sensitivity in the important mid-to-upper speech frequencies from 2000–4000 Hz.

The intensity of the clicks can be changed by the examiner, and the lowest intensity of the click that evokes an ABR correlates with hearing threshold. Hearing screening with ABR has been shown to be reliable and has high sensitivity and specificity.[3–10]

ABR hearing screening can be administered in either an automated or nonautomated delivery system. The nonautomated procedure requires careful consideration of stimulus, patient, and recording parameters. In the nonautomated procedure, trained audiologists are needed to test and subjectively analyze waveforms to determine replicability of a response. Because highly trained/educated professionals are needed to administer and interpret the test, the nonautomated procedure can be expensive.

In an automated delivery system, a pass-refer outcome is determined by either comparing the infant's ABR waveform to a template,[4] using a binomial-probability waveform analysis[11] or a statistical cross-correlation analysis that compares noise and signal electroencephalogram (EEG).[12] The stimulus and recording parameters have been predetermined and do not require a highly educated/trained audiologist for the administration and the interpretation of results. Therefore, the automated procedure is less expensive than a conventional nonautomated ABR.[13] The automated equipment is often portable and battery powered, which will reduce environmental electrical artifact. Although automated ABR hearing screening equipment has been shown to be reliable and has a high sensitivity and specificity when screening small samples,[4–10] the clinical feasibility as a tool for a large UNHSP has not been published.[7]

As with any physiological test that is correlated with behavioral hearing, there are instances in which the relationship does not hold. A few case studies have shown abnormal ABR responses but normal behavioral responses to auditory stimuli.[14–18] In these cases, an auditory neural pathology likely compromises the ABR responses but does not affect the behavioral responses to sound. Hyperbilirubinemia and auditory neuropathy are likely two conditions that can compromise the ABR.[14–18] Those infants may be inappropriately diagnosed with hearing loss and fit with amplification prior to obtaining any behavioral responses to sound. Therefore, appropriate behavioral follow-up by qualified audiologists is essential when using ABR hearing screening and diagnostic evaluation protocols to assess auditory sensitivity in predicting a hearing impairment.

Evoked Otoacoustic Emissions Screening

Evoked otoacoustic emissions (EOAEs) are sounds that are generated in the cochlea in response to stimuli presented to the ear. They travel through the middle ear and into the ear canal, where they can be measured with a miniature microphone. It is thought that the EOAE has no physiological purpose in and of itself, but reflects the cochlear transduction process (e.g., ref. 19). Although it is uncertain exactly how EOAEs are generated, there is good evidence that outer hair cells are involved.[20] Because most hearing loss involves loss of outer hair cells, the lack of an EOAE is a good predictor of hearing loss.[21–23] Evoked otoacoustic emission measurements are fast, noninvasive, require no electrode preparation or placement, and can be easily elicited from well babies and infants in the neonatal intensive care unit (NICU).[19,24–41]

Evoked otoacoustic emission is a general term used to describe the broad category of OAEs evoked by sound. The two types of EOAEs that are used in UNHSPs are transient evoked otoacoustic emissions (TEOAEs) and distortion product otoacoustic emissions (DPOAEs). TEOAEs are frequency-specific responses evoked by brief acoustic stimuli such as clicks or tone bursts. They generally appear up to 20 msec after stimuli are delivered to the ear. DPOAEs are generated in response to two continuous pure-tones, referred to as "primaries" and occur at frequencies that are mathematically related to the frequency of the primaries.[22,42,43]

Transient Evoked Otoacoustic Emissions Screening

The most widely used EOAE technique in UNHSPs is the TEOAE.[44] TEOAEs can be elicited in nearly all individuals with hearing sensitivity better than 25–35 dBHL.[21,45] Unlike ABR, TEOAEs appear to be an "all-or-none" response; that is, a TEOAE will most likely be elicited in any frequency region in which an infant has normal hearing. Thus, TEOAE level can identify persons with hearing loss, but cannot predict behavioral hearing sensitivity.[46]

TEOAEs were first used in a UNHSP in the United States beginning in February 1990, with the development of the Rhode Island Hearing Assessment Project (RIHAP).[47] The primary purpose of the RIHAP was to determine the validity and cost-effectiveness of TEOAEs for universal newborn hearing screening. White et al.[32] reported that after one TEOAE test, the referral rate for the outpatient rescreen was 26.9%. Of the 81% of infants that returned for outpatient rescreening at 4–6 weeks of age, 82% passed the outpatient rescreen. The high percentage of false-positive findings from inpatient TEOAEs screening was but one reason that Bess and Paradise[48] argued against universal newborn hearing screening. Maxon et al.,[49] however, reported the RIHAP inpatient screen refer rate with transient EOAEs was reduced to only 7% at discharge. Maxon et al.[49] concluded that screener experience, reduction of internal and external noise, and improvement of the conditions of the external ear canal could account for the reduction in the referral rate from 26.9 to 7%. Infants were screened just prior to discharge with most infants being screened between 24–72 h of life when they were fed and ready for sleep. For those infants who failed screening shortly after birth, a second screen was conducted at discharge. External noise was reduced by using a probe tip providing the tightest fit and the quickscreen option on the Otodynamic Analyzer ILO88™ (Hatfield, Herts, United Kingdom), which reduces low-frequency ambient and patient noise. In addition, screeners used a probe refit technique by inserting the probe, removing and cleaning the probe, and refitting the cleaned probe for screening (See Vohr, Chapter 8).

Distortion Product Otoacoustic Emissions Screening

No published data exist regarding the effectiveness of the DPOAE procedure to detect hearing loss when used in a UNHSP. However, the DPOAE has been shown to be able to evaluate newborns and infants at risk for hearing loss.[29,50,51] DPOAEs are also good detectors of hearing loss in adults[52] and in a mixed population of children and adults.[53] Although claims have been made that DPOAEs can predict hearing sensitivity, this area has not been rigorously studied.

Combined Evoked Otoacoustic Emission and Auditory Brainstem Response Screening

Although there are no published guidelines at the present time that are based on empirical data, the National Institutes of Health (NIH) convened a consensus of professionals in 1993 to discuss early identification of hearing loss and its habilitation. The consensus panel recommended universal newborn hearing of all NICU and regular-nursery infants within the first 3 months of life. They further stated, screening hearing of infants ideally should occur prior to hospital discharge using a two-stage inpatient screening procedure, TEOAEs followed by ABR screening for infants who failed the TEOAE screen. The NIH consensus statement[54] recommended the two-stage inpatient screening procedure because the panel was concerned with the potential numbers of overreferrals if using only TEOAE for screening.

Dalzell et al.[55] have implemented a variation of the NIH recommendation by using a "three-stage inpatient screen." The authors reported results from a UNHSP that uses a three-stage inpatient screen procedure (TEOAEs, repeat TEOAEs for infants failing the initial screen, and the administration of an ABR for those failing the initial and repeat TEOAE screens) with 3194 healthy newborns prior to discharge. The referral rate (infants that did not pass hearing screening bilaterally) based on administration of one TEOAE screen was 22.8%.

After repeated TEOAE screen(s), the referral rate was reduced to 5.5%. The referral rate for an outpatient screen was further reduced to 2.7% by the administration of the ABR. Nearly all (92%) of the initial TEOAEs failures had a repeat TEOAE screen prior to discharge, while 78% of the repeat TEOAE failures had an inpatient ABR screening. Dalzell et al.[55] concluded that a UNHSP using TEOAE screening and rescreening followed by an ABR screening for those infants that fail the TEOAE screen can achieve very low (less than 3%) refer rates at discharge.

Factors Influencing Protocol Decision

Philosophy of the Program

There are many factors that may influence the UNHSP protocol. The first and most important decision is the underlying philosophy of the Universal Newborn Hearing Screening Program. It is imperative that the director and all involved decide what type, severity, and configuration of hearing loss they want to identify. If the goal is to identify only bilateral hearing loss, the screeners would need to test and "pass" only one ear, which could significantly reduce test time and ultimately overall cost of the program. Some programs take this approach, as it is controversial to habilitate unilateral hearing loss. However, children with unilateral hearing loss are 10 times more likely to repeat a grade than children with normal hearing in both ears.[56] Listening strategies for unilateral hearing can be initiated at a young age. In addition, medical intervention for otitis media during childhood and protection from noise exposure would likely be more aggressive if it is known that the child has only one ear upon which to rely.

Examples of how philosophy affects decisions are as follows. If the UNHSP wants to identify bilateral, severe or profound hearing losses, the program should screen one ear with ABR using a click level of approximately 60 dB nHL. The number of referrals for further testing will be very low; however, the program will miss all infants with a unilateral hearing loss and those infants with a bilateral mild or moderate hearing loss. If the UNHSP intends to identify infants with a bilateral mild hearing loss, even if the underlying etiology is conductive, EOAE screening of both ears might be the procedure of choice.

Severity of Hearing loss

The second important factor to consider is the severity of hearing loss the UNHSP intends to identify. Although the TEOAE level[46] does not correlate well with behavioral threshold, TEOAEs can identify even a mild hearing loss. Therefore, TEOAEs are an excellent choice if the UNHSP intends to detect a mild, moderate, severe, or profound hearing loss.

Depending on the click level chosen for screening, ABR can identify different severities of hearing loss. For example, if the goal of the UNHSP is to identify a severe or profound hearing loss, a click level of 60 dB nHL can be used. If the goal of the UNHSP is to identify a mild hearing loss, a lower click intensity should be used. The click intensity for automated ABR screeners is often set at 35 dB nHL. The 35 dB nHL level, however, would likely pass infants that are minimally hearing impaired.

Habilitation of a mild hearing loss may be controversial because the majority of mild hearing losses in early childhood are likely to be conductive. Because conductive hearing loss is often transient in nature, many may feel they do not want to screen for conductive loss. On the other hand, these data lead some directors of UNHSPs to advocate for screening for even mild hearing loss, hoping they can identify infants who have early otitis media and, thereby, preventing possible speech and language delay.

Configuration of Hearing Loss

The choice of screening tool will have little effect on the detection of different configurations of hearing loss. The ABR evoked by click stimuli correlates best with behavioral thresholds in the 2000 to 4000 Hz range, while TEOAEs and DPOAEs can provide information about cochlear function in the 500–1000 Hz region. Both screening tools, however, have high false alarm rates for identification of low-frequency hearing loss.[53,57,58] Therefore, the detection of hearing loss in the 500–1000 Hz range by ABR and TEOAE are equally poor. Therefore, the only practical choice may be to identify hearing loss in the mid-to-high frequencies. Although this is a compromise, it is justifiable based on the fact that most permanent sensorineural hearing loss involves the higher frequencies.

Prior Experience

In some cases, prior experience with a particular tool may influence your protocol decision. If you have a person who is an expert at infant ABR, perhaps this is the best method for your program. Also, if the hospital already has equipment, the screening program may be limited to what is on hand. Fortunately, ABR and EOAE are able to identify hearing loss, so either tool is appropriate.

Personnel

The model and type of screening selected will be dictated, to a large extent, by the type of personnel who will be performing the screening. Successful programs have used audiologists, nurse/nurse practitioners, technicians, or volunteers to screen infants (See Orlando and Sokol, Chapter 4). Athough technicians and other nonaudiologist personnel can screen infants using EOAEs or automated ABR, if the UNHSP intends to screen infants with a nonautomated ABR procedure, it is imperative that the screener not only be an audiologist but an audiologist with extensive experience in assessing infant auditory sensitivity with the ABR.

Length-of-Stay

External forces, such as insurance reimbursement, has significantly reduced the length of stay of all infants and their mothers. Only recently have State and Federal legislative bodies begun to formerly debate length of stay mandates. Numerous bills were introduced into the 104th National Congress to require providers and health plans to follow the recommendations for inpatient care for mothers and their infants issued by the American Academy of Pediatric (AAP) and The American College of Obstetricians and Gynecologists (ACOG). Although all bills that were introduced required similar lengths of stay, bills did vary with respect to allowable exceptions, target population, and means of enforcement. Under a conference agreement passed by the House of Representatives and the Senate and signed into law by President William Clinton on September 26, 1996, health insurance plans will be required to follow AAP and ACOG recommendations for a 48-h length of stay for mothers and their infants following normal vaginal deliveries and a 96-h length of stay following caesarean sections beginning on January 1, 1998. The law, however, does not provide for minimum lengths of stay for health plans that do not provide health-care coverage for hospitalization following childbirth.

If your hospital has a short length of stay for mothers and infants, it is possible that the referral rate for an outpatient test may be higher. The higher referral rate for very young infants is likely a result of the flaccid and debris-filled ear canals causing a very mild conductive hearing loss. Further, short lengths of stay may preclude a multistage inpatient model because so little time exists to test infants more than once.

Length of stay is not as much of an issue in the NICU. The length of stay for infants in the NICU is often weeks or even months. The NICU infant, however, provides for a greater number of scheduling concerns. NICU infants require many more medical/surgical procedures. Often NICU infants are attached to potentially noisy monitors and may be more difficult to screen if they are unable to be moved to a quieter location. Unexpected discharges to a hospital nursery closer to home or transfers within a hospital may also make it difficult to schedule the NICU infant for screening. Moreover, infant readiness to screen for hearing is difficult to judge, especially without the assistance of nursing and/or physician staff. Therefore, screener schedules in the NICU will likely be dictated by physician exams, other medical procedures, feeding schedules, and early discharges (See Smillie, Chapter 7).

Screening Environment

The UNHSP will likely need to negotiate for space with hospital administration and/or the Department of Obstetrics and Gynecology and/or Pediatrics. Ideally, space should be assigned to the UNHSP and used solely for hearing screening. Space used solely by the UNHSP will prevent scheduling conflicts and reduce noise during screening. The screening space can also serve as an outpatient re-screen room, depending on the specific protocols of the UNHSP.

Space should be close to the nursery or nurseries, quiet, and available during the majority of the screening day. The room should be designed to store supplies and equipment and ideally contain general office equipment, such as: a desk, desk chair, phone, and other equipment that the UNHSP deems appropriate. The room should also have a rocking chair, and shades or window coverings, especially for outpatient rescreens, if mothers wish to nurse their infants to soothe them for screening. Although almost all hearing screening procedures do not require infants to sleep, reducing the ambient environmental noise as much as possible will decrease the time needed for data collection, especially if using EOAE screening. Window curtains, acoustic dividers, damping ceiling exhaust fans and placing an infant in a modified isolette may be required to reduce the ambient environmental noise. Johnson et al.[47] reported that the ambient environmental noise was reduced by about 10–15 dBA with room modifications and further reduced by 10 dB using a modified isolette with a closed lid.

Most institutions will have little, if any, space available for a UNHSP. Thus, hearing screening will often be performed in less than ideal noise conditions. Infants will most likely be screened in a well-baby nursery or the mother's room. Therefore, ask parents to turn off the television or radio and ask other family members and friends to be quiet, that is, no talking, or preferably, to leave the room while the infant is screened. If the mother's room is still noisy, an alternative site, such as an infant holding room, can often be used. Encourage parents to follow you for screening, however, check hospital procedures and precautions before transporting any infant.

The UNHSP procedure of choice may vary from the NICU to the well-baby nursery. Screening in the NICU has potential problems for both ABR and EOAE testing. Although some NICU infants are able to be moved to a quieter room for screening, such as a breast feeding/pumping room, most infants will be connected to monitors and will need constant nurse supervision. With these NICU infants, hearing screening may occur at the patient's cribside. NICUs are often acoustically noisy environments making hearing screening difficult. Excess noise can often be decreased or eliminated in the screening environments for well babies, such as the mother's room, holding room, or a dedicated screening room, where the acoustically noisy NICU is unlikely to be modified. Neonatal intensive-care infants are most often in isolettes, which when closed, can reduce ambient room noise. Each isolette, however, contains heating elements with fans to heat and circulate air, and motorized mattresses to change infant pressure points. Infants are often oxygenated via nasal canulae producing high-level noise, which may preclude a valid hearing screen.

Each UNHSP will need to work closely with the NICU staff to find optimal screening conditions for NICU infants. Ideally, the UNHSP will screen NICU infants just prior to discharge, when the infant is healthy, connected to as few monitors as possible, capable of being sustained on room air, and can be moved to a quieter environment. Realistically, the UNHSP will likely move from infant to infant and screen in the noisy NICU environment.

Some programs have found that the NICU is too noisy for measuring OAEs. The likelihood of evoking a measurable OAE is highly affected by the level of the ambient noise. Therefore, the ABR, either automated or nonautomated, may be needed to reduce the number of NICU referrals. Although a UNHSP based solely on an automated ABR may be found to be cost prohibitive, a two- or three-stage inpatient screening procedure where NICU infants are first screened with EOAEs followed by a repeat EOAE and/or automated ABR may be cost-effective.

Referral Rates

There is considerable concern regarding referral rates for UNHSPs. The goal of a UNHSP is to identify all newborns with hearing loss while minimizing the number of normal hearing newborns who are referred for follow-up. Obviously, there is a delicate balance between identification of hearing loss (sensitivity) and over-referrals (specificity). This balance is influenced by an number of factors including the incidence of hearing loss in the population, the tool chosen for screening, the expertise of the screeners, the environment, and most importantly, the criteria chosen for "passing" the test. The only way to determine which method has the lowest referral rate while identifying the targeted hearing loss is to screen every infant with each tool using equivalent "pass" criteria and then to recall all infants for follow-up. As of this writing, such data are not available.

There are two referral rates over which to be concerned. The first referral rate is how many infants are referred for the outpatient screen. The outpatient referral rate needs to be kept as low as possible because of the costs and inconvenience associated with unnecessarily recalling infants for follow-up. The second referral rate over which to be concerned is the number of infants who will need to undergo diagnostic testing. Because diagnostic testing is costly, the number referred for dignositic testing should be kept low and approximate the actual incidence of hearing loss in the population. Thus, if you are testing for a bilateral, severe sensorineural hearing loss, the referral rate for dignositic testing should be around 0.1%.[59] If you are screening for mild, unilateral hearing loss, which includes infants with conductive hearing loss, the referral rate could be as high as 2.6% to 3.2%.[32,60] To reduce the referral of normal-hearing newborns for diagnostic testing, many UNHSP use an outpatient rescreening for infants who failed their inpatient screening. Only those infants that do not pass the outpatient rescreening are referred for diagnostic audiological evaluation.

There are few published referral rates for UNHSPs. Most of those published used TEOAEs as the screening tool. As cited earlier, referral rates for outpatient rescreening from the first cohort of infants from the RIHAP program were somewhat high at 26.9 %.[32] Recently, White[44] reported considerably lower outpatient referral rates (5–12%) from 7 TEOAE UNHSPs throughout the United States. Roughly 80% of the infants rescreened as outpatients meet the passing criteria, resulting in less than 1% of the newborns from TEOAE UNHSPs being referred for diagnostic audiological evaluation. This percentage is consistent with what would be expected for reported incidence of congenital hearing loss.[44]

It is important to note, however, that even though few infants are referred for diagnostic audiological evaluations, many infants are rescreened on an outpatient basis. If 80% of the infants referred for the outpatient rescreen are believed to have normal cochlear function and auditory sensitivity, almost all are over-referred. Trying to follow even 10% of the infants that are referred for outpatient rescreening can account for hundreds of infants. Often the time spent on the telephone scheduling infants, rescheduling infants, and tracking down parents of infants who did not show for a scheduled appointment can be exorbitant. Therefore, as few outpatient referrals as possible are needed for a successful UNHSP.

Models of UNHSPs

Successful UNHSP have been in existence in the United States since the early 1990s. A successful program, regardless of hearing screening method, should ensure a valid screen and rescreen, if necessary, of all infants prior to hospital discharge. The following describes three different models that have been successfully implemented in UNHS programs.

Auditory Brainstem Response Program

Figure 3–1 describes a UNHSP based on automated ABR (AABR) using the Algo II Newborn Hearing Screener. The hospital in this example averages 4500 births annually, including 375 NICU infants. The typical length of stay for well babies is 48 h. The screening protocol is identical for NICU and well babies. Newborn hearing screening is a standing order for all infants admitted to the nursry. In the past year, only one infant has been missed prior to discharge and that infant was successfully recalled for outpatient screening. Refusals are not typical and occur only once or twice a year. Initially, well babies are screened at 2–6 h of age using a simultaneous 35-dB nHL screening option available on the Algo II (see Kurman and Spivak, Chapter 5). Unilateral as well as bilateral "refer" results are immediately rescreened. The UNHSP is directed by an audiologist who supervises three nursing assistants and one clerical assistant who have been trained to operate the Algo. The clerical assistant additionally handles secretarial responsibilities associated with the program. Personnel time allotted to the UNHSP by these four individuals amounts to 1.75 FTEs (Full Time Equivalents). The referral rate at time of discharge for this program was 1.7% with only 76 infants requiring any follow-up services as outpatients. Infants in need of an outpatient screen are recalled at age 2–3 weeks. A two-level, nonautomated ABR screen and tympanometry are completed by the audiologist to obtain preliminary findings regarding degree and type of hearing loss prior to completing a full diagnostic ABR. Ongoing contact is maintained with the primary-care physician to encourage prompt follow-up and appropriate family support. Although this program is universal, the risk indicators cited in the 1994 Position Statement of the Joint Committee on Infant Hearing are used to monitor for delayed and progressive hearing loss. Infants with risk indicators who pass any stage of the screening process are recalled for follow-up evaluation at 6 months of age as a routine service of this program.

Transient Otoacoustic Emissions Program

The second model is one based entirely on TEOAEs. Although this model uses TEOAEs, the flow chart presented in Figure 3–2 would be applicable to programs using a DPOAE screening procedure as well. The infants in well-baby, step-down, and NICU nurseries undergo the same protocol. Infants are screened as close as possible to discharge. More than one administration of the screen may take place before discharge if the infant does not pass. Inpatient and outpatient EOAE rescreenings are an effective means of reducing the number of infants referred for diagnostic audiological evaluations. Infants failing the inpatient

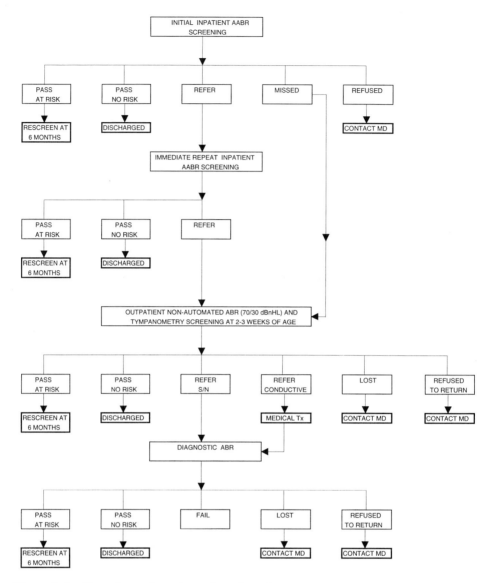

Figure 3–1.   Flow chart of a universal newborn hearing screening program using an automated auditory brainstem response (ABR) screening procedure.

TEOAE screen return in 4 weeks for an outpatient rescreen. Those failing the TEOAE outpatient rescreen are referred for diagnostic ABR and to early intervention. This model is used in a hospital where the number of annual births is approximately 4000, and of those, 900 are NICU births. Typical length of stay in the well baby nursery is 40 h, although some mothers choose to leave in 24 h.

An audiologist and part-time technician perform the inpatient well-baby screens. Neonatal nurse practitioners screen the infants in the step-down and

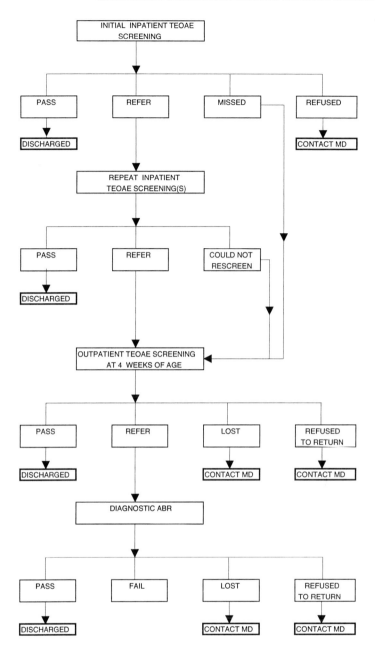

Figure 3–2. Flow chart of a universal newborn hearing screening program using transient evoked otoacoustic emission (TEOAE) screening procedure.

NICU nurseries and perform well-baby screening on some weekends. The directors of the program are a neonatologist and an audiologist. A clerk is hired for 1/3 time to help with the database and infant tracking. The referral rate for outpatient re-screens during the first 9 months of the program was 7% and the referral rate for diagnostic ABR was 1.5%. In the second year of the program, referral rates for outpatient rescreens dropped to 5%.

Combined TOAE and ABR Program

The third model is from a hospital that has approximately 4000 births per year (900 of which are NICU infants) with a typical 48-h length of stay. Although this procedure seems complicated, the procedure provides an opportunity for greater flexibility while attempting to minimize the number of inpatient ABR screenings and reduce the number of outpatient referrals (Fig. 3–3). The director of the program is an audiologist. Other personnel include an audiologist coordinator, audiologist screeners, paid technician screeners, a part-time secretary, and database manager. Although the procedures are similar in the Birthing Center and in the NICU, well babies in the Birthing Center are screened by paid technicians and NICU infants are screened by audiologists. Audiologists had been screening all at-risk infants in the NICU for almost 12 years prior to initiating universal newborn hearing screening. Audiologists have continued to screen in the NICU because they were familiar with NICU procedures, were known by NICU physicians and staff, and collaborated with NICU faculty on a variety of patient-care and research activities. In addition, TEOAE's are often difficult to obtain in the acoustically noisy NICU environment. Neonatal ICU infants are unable to be moved to a quieter location for screening. The loud NICU environment, early transfers to a NICU closer to parents home, and the need to perform ABR hearing and auditory function tests resulted in the audiologist as the preferable screener in the NICU.

Well babies and NICU babies are initially screened with TEOAEs followed by a TEOAE rescreen for those infants that failed the initial TEOAE screen. Rescreening the initial TEOAE failures significantly reduces the number of infants referred for an inpatient ABR. Infants failing the TEOAE rescreen are then screened with a nonautomated ABR by audiologists prior to discharge. Infants that are referred for outpatient TEOAE screening are scheduled to return at 3–4 weeks of age. Those failing the outpatient rescreen are then scheduled to return at approximately 3 months of age for a diagnostic ABR test. When hearing loss is diagnosed, early intervention is contacted, as parents permit, and habilitation and enrollment in programming initiated often well before 6 months of age. The referral rate for outpatient rescreens during the first 9 months of the program was 3.8% and the rate of those referred for diagnostic ABR was 0.9%. In the second year of the program, the outpatient referral rate was reduced to 3.1%.

Conclusions

Few will argue the importance of a UNHSP in detecting all infants with hearing impairments. Even the most successful high-risk indicator programs detect only

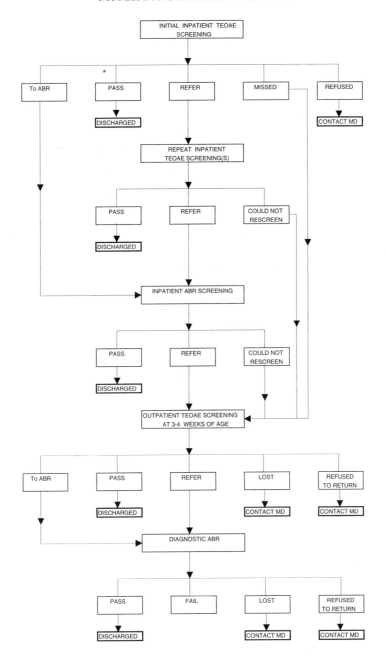

Figure 3–3.   Flow chart of a universal newborn hearing screening program using a combined transient evoked otoacoustic emission (TEOAE) and auditory brainstem response (ABR) screening procedure.

50–60% of all infants with hearing loss.[61–63] The goal of any UNHSP, regardless of the screening method or procedure, is to perform a valid hearing screening on all infants prior to hospital discharge. Ultimately hearing screening of all infants should decrease the age at which intervention is initiated.

It is clear that there is no "one" model for UNHSPs. Each program must carefully consider what type and severity of hearing loss it wishes to identify. Then, based on available screening tools, program philosophy, prior experience, personnel, typical maternity length of stay, space, referral rates, funding, etc., an appropriate protocol must be developed. Although many the issues that determine the nature of the hearing screening program do not change over time, others may change significantly. One area that continually changes is technology. Expect the technology for automated ABR and EOAE to change dramatically in the next few years. Technological advances may influence which tool hospitals choose for screening. Those wanting to implement a screening program must keep abreast of the emerging research on UNHSPs. The research should be critically evaluated with respect to the feasibility of incorporating new findings in each UNHSP.

Acknowledgments

Some of the screening models were projects funded by a grant from the New York State Department of Health. Beth Prieve was also supported by grant #R29 DC0208 from the National Institute for Deafness and other Communication Disorders.

References

1. Mauk GW, Behrens TR. Historical, political and technological context associated with early identification of hearing loss. Semin Hear 1993;14:1–17
2. Joint Committee on Infant Hearing. 1994 position statement. ASHA 1994;36:38–41
3. Hecox K, Galambos R. Brain stem audiotory evoked responses in human infants and adults. Arch of Otolaryngol 1974;99:30–3
4. Peters JG. An automated infant screener using advanced evoked response technology. Hear J 1986;39:25–30
5. Kileny PR. Algo-1 automated infant hearing screener: prelimanary results. Semin Hear 1987;8:125–31
6. Kileny PR. New insight on infant ABR hearing screening. Scand Audiol 1988;30(Suppl):81–8
7. Hall JW, Kileny PR, Ruth RA, et al. Newborn auditory screening with Algo-1 vs. conventional auditory brainstem response. ASHA 1987;29:120–4
8. Jacobson JT, Jacobson CL, Spahr RC. Automated and conventional ABR screening techniques in high-risk infants. J Am Acad Audiol 1990;1:187–95
9. Stewart DL, Bibb KW, Pearlman A. Automated newborn hearing testing with the ALGO-1 screener. Clin Pediatr 1993;32:308–11
10. Herrmann BS, Thonrton AR, Joseph JM. Automated infant hearing screening using the ABR: Development and validation. Am J of Audiol 1995;4:6–14
11. Marsh RR. Concurrent right and left ear auditory brain stem response recording. Ear Hear 1993;14:169–74
12. Ozdamar O, Delgado RE, Eilers RE, et al. Automated electrophysiologic hearing testing using a threshold-seeking algorithm. J Am Acad Audiol 1994;5:77–88
13. Weber BA. Screening of hie-risk infants using auditory brainstem response audiometry. In Bess FH (ed): *Hearing Impairment in Children*, Parkton, MD, York Press, 1988, pp 112–132
14. Worthington D, Peters JF. Quantifiable hearing and no ABR: Paradox or error? Ear Hear 1980;1:281–5

15. Kraus N, Ozdamar O, Stein L, et al. Absent auditory brain stem response: Peripheral hearing loss or brain stem dysfunction? Laryngoscope 1984;94:400–6
16. Berlin CI, Hood LJ, Cecola RP, et al. Does type I afferent neuron dysfunciton reveal itself through lack of efferent suppression? Hear Res 1993;65:40–50
17. Sininger YS, Hood LJ, Starr A, et al. Hearing loss due to auditory neuropathy. Aud Today 1995;7:10–13
18. Stein L, Tremblay K, Pasternak J, et al. Brainstem abnormalities in neonates with normal otoacoustic emissions. Semin Hear 1996;17:197–213
19. Kemp DT, Ryan S. The use of transient evoked otoacoustic emissions in neonatal hearing screening. Semin Hear 1993;14:30–45
20. Lim DJ. Cochlear micromechanics in understanding otoacoustic emission. Scand Audiol 1986; 25(Suppl):17–23
21. Kemp DT. Stimulated acoustic eimissions from within the human auditory system. J Acoust Soc Am 1978;64:13–1391
22. Lonsbury-Martin BL, Martin GK. The clinical utility of distortion product otoacoustic emissions. Ear Hear 1990;11:144–50
23. Prieve BA. Otoacoustic emissions in infants and children: Basic characteristics and clinical applications. Semin Hear 1992;13:37–52
24. Johnsen NJ, Bagi P, Elberling C. Evoked acoustic emissions from the human ear III. Findings in neonates. Scand Audiol 1983;12:17–24
25. Martin GK, Whitehead ML, Lonsbury-Martin BL. Potential of evoked otoacoustic emissions for infant hearing screening. Semin Hear 1990;11:1–203
26. Lafreniere D, Jung MD, Smurzynski J, et al. Distortion-product and click-evoked otoacoustic emissions in healthy newborns. Arch Otolaryngol Head Neck Surg 1991;117:1382–9
27. Norton SJ: Application of transient evoked otoacoustic emissions to pediatric populations. Ear Hear 1993;14:64–73
28. Norton SJ. Emerging role of evoked otoacoustic emissions in neonatal hearing screening. Am J Otology 1994;15:S4-12
29. Smurzynski J. Distortion-product and click-evoked otoacoustic emissions of preterm and full-term infants. Ear Hear 1993;14:258–74
30. Smurzynski J. Longitudinal measurements of distortion-product and click-evoked otoacoustic emissions of preterm infants: Preliminary results. Ear Hear 1994;15:210–23
31. Kok MR, van Zanten GA, Brocaar MP, et al. Click-evoked otoacoustic emissions in 1036 ears of healthy newborns. Audiology 1993;32:213–24
32. White KR, Vohr BR, Behrens TR. Universal newborn hearing screening using transient evoked otoacoustic emissions: Results of the Rhode Island Hearing Assesment Project. Semin Hear 1993; 14:18–29
33. White KR, Vohr BR, Maxon AB, et al. Screening all newborns for hearing loss using transient evoked otoacoustic emissions. Int J Pediatr Otorhinolaryngol 1994;29:203–17
34. Brown DP, Taxman SI. Five years of neonatal hearing screening: A summary. Infant–Toddler Intervention 1993;3:135–53
35. Goldberg B. Universal hearing screening of newborns. ASHA 1993;35:63–4
36. Brass D, Kemp DT. The objective assessment of transient evoked otoacoustic emissions in neonates. Ear Hear 1994;15:371–7
37. Bergman BM, Gorga MP, Neely ST, et al. Preliminary descriptions of transient-evoked and distortion-product otoacoustic emissions from graduates of an intensive care nursery. J Am Acad Audiol 1995;6:150–62
38. Marco J, Morant A, Caballero J, et al. Distortion product otoacoustic emissions in healthy newborns: Normative data. Acta Otolaryngol 1995;115:187–9
39. Popelka GR, Karzon RK, Arjmand EM. Growth of the $2f_1$-f_2 distortion product otoacoustic emission for low-level stimuli in human neonates. Ear Hear 1995;16:159–65
40. van Zanten GA, Kok MR, Brocaar MP, et al. The click-evoked oto-acoustic emission in preterm-born infants in the post conceptional age range between 30 and 68 weeks. Int J Pediatr Otorhinolaryngol 1995;32;S187-97
41. Salamy A, Eldredge L, Sweetow R. Transient evoked otoacoustic emissions: Feasibility in the nursery. Ear Hear 1996;17:42–8
42. Kemp DT, Chum R. Properties of the generator mechanism of stimulated emissions. Hear Res 1980;2:213–32
43. Harris F, Probst R. Reporting click-evoked and distortion product emission results with respect to the audiogram. Hear Res 1991;12:399–405
44. White KR. Universal newborn hearing screening using transient evoked otoacoustic emissions: Past, present and future. Semin Hear 1996;17:171–83

45. Stevens JC. Click-evoked oto-acoustic emissions in normal and impaired adult ears. Br J of Audiol 1988;22:45–9
46. Stover L, Norton S. The effects of aging on otoacoustic emissions. J Acoust Soc Am 1993;94: 2670–2681
47. Johnson M, Maxon AB, White KR, Vohr BR. Operating a hospital-based universal newborn hearing screening program using transient evoked otoacoustic emissions. Semin Hear 1993;14:46–56
48. Bess FH, Paradise JL. Universal screening for infant hearing impairment: Not simple, not risk-free, not necessarily beneficial, and not presently justified. Pediatrics 1994;98:330–4
49. Maxon AB, White KR, Behrens TR, Vohr BR. Referral rates and cost efficiency in a universal newborn hearing screening program using transient evoked otoacoustic emissions. J Am Acad of Audiol 1995;6:271–7
50. Jacobson JT, Salata J, Strasnick B. A comparison of automated ABR and distortion product OAEs in high-risk infants. Paper presented at the American Auditory Society, Dallas, TX, 1995
51. Hall JW, Baer JE, Chase PA, et al. Transient and distortion product otoacoustic emissions in infant hearing screening. Poster presented at the 6th Annual American Academy of Audiology Convention, Richmond, VA, 1994
52. Stover L, Gorga MP, Neely, ST. Towards optimizing the clinical utility of distortion product otoacoustic emission measurements. J Acoust Soc Am 1996;100: 956–67
53. Gorga MP, Stover L, Neely ST. The use of cumulative distributions to determine critical values and levels of confidence for clinical distortion product otoacoustic emission measurements. J Acoust Soc Am 1996;100:968–77
54. National Institutes of Health. Early identification of hearing impairment in infants and young children. NIH Consensus Statement 1993;11:1–25
55. Dalzell LE, Orlando MS, Seeger C, et al. 3-stage newborn hearing screening reduces failures at discharge. Poster presented at the American Academy of Audiology National Convention, Salt Lake City, UT, 1996
56. Bess FH, Tharpe AM. Case history data on unilaterally hearing-impaired children. Ear Hear 1986;7:14–19
57. Gorga MP, Neely ST, Bergman BM, et al. Otoacoustic emissions from normal-hearing and hearing-impaired subjects: Distortion product responses. J Acoust Soc Am 1993;93:2050–60
58. Prieve BA, Gorga MP, Schmidt A, et al. Analysis of transient-evoked otoacoustic emissions in normal-hearing and hearing-impaired ears. J Acoust Soc Am 1993;93:3308–19
59. National Institutes on Deafness and Other Communicative Disorders. A *Report of the Task Force on the National Strategic Research Plan*. Bethesda, MD, Author, 1989
60. Hull FM, Mielke PW, Willeford JA, et al. National Speech and Hearing Survey (Final report, Porject No. 50978). U.S. Department of Health, Education and Welfare. 1976 (ERIC Document Reproduction Service No. ED 129 045)
61. Elssmann SF, Matkin ND, Sabo MP: Early identification of congenital sensorineural hearing impairment. Hear J 1987;40:13–17
62. Epstein S, Reilly JS. Sensorineural hearing loss. Pediatr Clin North Am 1989;36:1501–20
63. Mauk GW, White KR, Mortensen LB, et al. The effectiveness of screening programs based on high-risk characteristics in early identification of hearing impairment. Ear Hear 1991;12:312–19

4

Personnel and Supervisory Options for Universal Newborn Hearing Screening

Mark S. Orlando
Heidi Sokol

Introduction

The success of any Universal Newborn Hearing Screening Program (UNHSP) will depend on its personnel. The need for highly trained, educated personnel to administer and interpret auditory brainstem response (ABR) testing had limited the feasibility of implementing universal newborn hearing screening in the past.[1] The development of automated Auditory Brainstem Response and Otoacoustic Emissions (OAEs) instrumentation, which can be operated by technicians, however, makes universal newborn hearing screening practical and cost-effective. In addition, the publication of guidelines within audiology and related professions advocating universal newborn hearing screening has promoted its acceptability among health-care professionals, hospital administrators, and the community.[1,2] This chapter will focus its discussion on the personnel and the supervisory responsibilities needed to implement a successful UNHSP.

Personnel

Personnel and staffing options vary widely and personnel choices should be made based on practical issues specific to each hospital. There are a number of primary and support personnel needed in a UNHSP. Primary personnel include a director, a screening coordinator, and screeners. Support personnel may include a database manager and a secretary. Additional peripheral support personnel also may be needed, although the peripheral support personnel are unlikely to be financially supported by the UNHSP.

Director

The director is the primary point of contact among the UNHSP, the community and hospital physicians, as well as hospital administration. The director may be instrumental in allocating or obtaining space for screening, ensuring adequate support, and assuring that the hearing screening protocols are consistent with Federal, State, and hospital regulations. The director should be involved in the development of all procedures used in the UNHSP and be thoroughly knowledgeable about the operation of the program. He or she should be responsible for disseminating information about the program to the community.

It is likely that the director will be someone from either Neonatology or Audiology. There are advantages and disadvantages of having directors from either profession. Audiologists are highly educated professionals who are trained to diagnose and treat hearing impairment and do so on a daily basis. The audiologist will understand the full spectrum of audiological screening methods and procedures while the neonatologist may be knowledgeable only about the specific procedure used by his universal newborn hearing screening program. The audiologist is better able to understand and/or recommend appropriate follow-up diagnostic audiological evaluations, better able to assist parents through the often complicated process of fitting amplification, and is probably more familiar with community support services for infants and children with hearing impairments than the neonatologist.

The neonatologist, however, is likely to be more familiar with hospital procedures and protocols, especially those procedures and protocols that deal with newborn infants. The neonatologist may have a better rapport with not only hospital physicians and professional staff, but also primary-care physicians within the community. The importance of the rapport between the neonatologist and hospital physicians within the Departments of Pediatrics and Obstetrics and Gynecology and primary-care physicians within the community should not be underestimated, especially when trying to negotiate for space and ensuring follow-up on all infants that are referred for outpatient screens and diagnostic evaluations. In addition, because many hospital administrative personnel are physicians, the neonatologist may be better able to gain administrative support, especially during the development and implementation of a UNHSP.

Audiology Coordinator

Although the professional background of the Director of the UNHSP may vary, the Coordinator of the program should be a certified audiologist with extensive experience with the screening method used in the program and with pediatric audiological assessment and habilitation. The coordinator is the one individual who can assume the responsibilities of all universal newborn hearing screening personnel, is responsible for training and supervision of the screening staff, and often serves as the primary contact between the UNHSP and the community.

The Audiology Coordinator should be responsible for the day-to-day operations of the UNHSP and must possess good organizational skills. Responsibilities of the coordinator include:

- establishing and evaluating screening protocols and procedures;
- training and supervision of screening staff;
- education of the community and providers of follow-up services;
- maintenance of quality assurance;
- setting screener schedules;
- checking consistency of the results from week to week;
- interpretation of screening results;
- dissemination of results to primary-care physicians in a timely manner; and
- monitoring and evaluation of follow-up diagnostic audiological procedures.

Supervisory responsibilities of the audiology coordinator are reviewed in detail later in this chapter.

Qualifications for the practice of audiology are strictly defined by the Certification Board of ASHA and, in most states, by licensure laws. Regulations regarding the practice of audiology impose limitations on the audiologist's ability to delegate testing responsibilities and provide supervision to technicians, volunteers, and other support personnel. Exceptions to these regulations are sometimes made, however, applications should be made to the state licensure board prior to implementing a UNHSP.[1]

The size of the program will dictate which responsibilities the audiology coordinator will assume and which will be delegated to other Universal Newborn Hearing Screening staff. For example, a large program may require a full-time screening coordinator to run the day-to-day operations, such as assuring that all infants are screened, developing screeners' schedules, as well as training and supervising the screeners. A smaller program, on the other hand, may require only a part-time audiologist to consult and interpret screen results, leaving the day-to-day operations to other hospital staff.

Screening Personnel

The importance of screening personnel in a UNHSP should not be underestimated. Screeners are responsible for screening infants, maintaining equipment, and may even be required to perform other clerical duties, such as photocopying results and assisting the coordinator in sending notification of final results to primary-care physicians. In addition to being able to perform the screening procedure, screeners should be familiar with the nursery's system for newborn identification and protection, have the necessary skills to recognize the signs of an infant in distress, and take appropriate preliminary steps to promptly obtain medical assistance. Screening staff should know emergency procedures for obtaining assistance and may even be required to complete specialized emergency medical training, such as CPR.

At least two screeners are needed for any program to provide screening coverage 7 days a week and to cover for screener vacations and sick time. Although two screeners are highly desirable, having a large staff of screeners may not be beneficial. Programs that split up screening responsibilities among many screeners (such as volunteers or nurses from different shifts) may provide for an atmosphere in which no one person takes responsibility for making sure that all infants are screened.

The specific educational or work background of the screener is unlikely to predict screener success. Individuals with a wide variety of backgrounds have developed into excellent screening personnel. Successful programs are using audiologists, nurses or nurse practitioners, technicians, volunteers, and even graduate students in preprofessional programs as screeners. The following will discuss the advantages and disadvantages of each type of screener.

Audiologists

The Rhode Island Hearing Assessment Program reported that although audiologists were successful screeners, they were overqualified for the job and, as a result had the highest turnover rate and reported that they felt constrained by the rigid screening protocols.[3] Audiologists, furthermore, are among the highest paid categories of screeners, which could dramatically increase the cost of the UNHSP. On the other hand, the advantages of having audiologists as screeners are that they will require the least amount of training, are the most qualified personnel to discuss the screening procedures with parents and answer questions, and are qualified to interpret results and communicate them immediately to parents.

NURSES AND/OR NURSE PRACTITIONERS

Nurses and nurse practitioners constitute another group of highly educated professionals who can be trained to screen hearing. As is the case with audiologists, however, nursing salaries will tend to drive up the costs of the program. An obvious advantage of using nurses for screeners is that nurses are well acquainted with the newborn nursery and the neonatal intensive care unit (NICU) and would be comfortable handling and performing screening procedures on newborn infants. Nurses or nurse practitioners, however, are unlikely to be hired solely to perform the duties of a hearing screener. Therefore, unlike a dedicated screening technician, nurses and nurse practitioners will be required to perform additional functions. When the nursery census is low, nursing staff will likely be able to fit hearing screenings into their daily routines. However, when the census is high or shortages in staff occur due to sickness or vacation, hearing screening could easily become the least important of the nurse's responsibilities and, therefore, may be postponed or even eliminated (see Spivak and Jupiter, Chapter 2, for a further discussion of nursing issues).

VOLUNTEERS

The volunteer is the least costly type of screener but may also be the least conscientious screening personnel. Unless volunteers are extremely dedicated, hearing screening may become a low priority on any given day. This would significantly reduce the effectiveness of any UNHSP. Although screening procedures are not complex and can be learned by volunteers, the number of hours that a volunteer is willing to work may be insufficient for him or her to achieve mastery of the screening procedures. Johnson et al.[3] reported that a screener needs to work a minimum of 20 h per week to develop and maintain optimum skills. Furthermore, the turnover rate of volunteers may preclude the development of a well-trained and consistent staff.

A graduate student from preprofessional programs, such as audiology, speech pathology, medicine and education, is a viable alternative to the traditional hospital volunteer. Student volunteers have the added incentive of gaining valuable experience in an area related to their course of study and may even be able to earn academic or practicum credit for their work. Thus, the commitment, quality of work, and consistency of these volunteers may match that of salaried staff (Fig. 4–1).

State and/or hospital regulations and union contracts may dictate which, if any patient-care activities can be performed by volunteers. Exceptions to State and hospital regulations and union contracts may be possible, but these will have to be thoroughly investigated prior to enlisting volunteer screeners. For example, graduate students in training for professional careers are often able to perform patient-care activities as long as they are enrolled in an accredited university program, have professional liability insurance, and are closely supervised by certified, and/or licensed professional staff. The hospital and University should enter into a formal affiliation agreement and sign a contract that clearly delineates responsibilities and liabilities of both parties. In summary, the decision to use volunteers as screeners should not be made lightly. If the UNHSP is considering using volunteers, it should check with hospital administration, la-

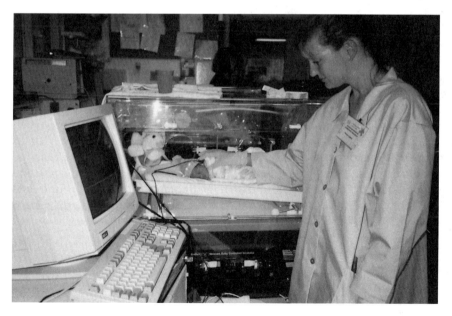

Figure 4–1.   A screener performs an OAE screen on a premature infant in an isolette in the NICU of Schneider Children's Hospital.

bor relations, and the Legal Affairs Department regarding limitations of the use of volunteers in the hospital.

PAID TECHNICIANS

Paid technicians, dedicated to the screening program, represent a relatively inexpensive type of screening personnel. The screener who is employed by the hospital is contractually committed to the program and his or her attendance, punctuality, and job performance must conform to hospital guidelines. He or she will have a vested interest in performing well to remain employed. For all screeners, expertise and screening performance improves with practice. Paid screeners, who are likely to work longer hours and more consistently than volunteers or other nondedicated staff, perform the greatest number of screening tests, develop the most expertise and, therefore, obtain the greatest number of valid results. Johnson et al.[3] reported that paid technicians were the most successful screeners. Successful screeners, regardless of educational background, were those who were competent and comfortable with newborns, conscientious about their work, computer literate, and able to be flexible within the screening protocol.[3]

Support Personnel

Two categories of support personnel may be required for the program: a secretary and a database manager. Secretarial personnel may be required to schedule outpatient screenings and/or diagnostic audiological evaluations, answer the telephone, photocopy results, register infants, and perform many other day-to-day clerical operational responsibilities.

Computer literacy of support personnel is essential. This is particularly important in large UNHSP, which must follow an enormous number of infants. The job of recording results, sending reports, keeping track of statistics, and tracking infants becomes close to impossible without computerized systems. Although the National Center for Hearing Identification and Management has developed a user-friendly database management system for newborn hearing screening programs, a database manager may still be required, especially for large programs that generate enormous amounts of data or if a noncommercial database and tracking system is used. It is the responsibility of the database manager to check data integrity on a daily or weekly basis, develop procedures to send reports to physicians and parents, and arrange data in a format that is understandable to the screeners, coordinator, and director (see Moore, Chapter 9, for a thorough discussion of data management).

Supervisory Responsibilities

Professional oversight of the newborn hearing screening program is the job of the coordinating audiologist. In most programs, the screening staff is recruited, selected, and trained by the audiology coordinator. As was mentioned earlier, the coordinator is also responsible for setting screener schedules, directly supervising screeners, and reviewing test results.

Recruiting Screeners

The coordinator needs to have an appreciation of the traits and qualities that a successful screener must possess to assemble a high-caliber screening staff. The screeners are the first individuals that the hospital staff associates with the screening activities. Screeners, therefore, are an important part of the program's public image and their professionalism, work ethic, appearance, and demeanor should reflect positively on the program. Screeners should have cheerful, pleasant personalities and look upon their work as a fulfilling endeavor. A competent screener should possess the ability to:

- learn the skills needed to perform OAE and ABR screenings;
- follow proper screening protocols;
- safely handle babies in the NICU and well-baby nursery (WBN);
- interact with parents in an appropriate manner;
- establish and maintain a good working relationship with hospital staff;
- troubleshoot equipment;
- maintain accurate records;
- work in a physically demanding job; and
- maintain a calm and patient demeanor in an often hurried and frenetic atmosphere.

As was mentioned earlier, the specific experience and educational background of the screener is often unimportant. It is important, however, that the screener understands the goals of the program and his or her role in accomplishing those goals.

Screener Training

Proper training of screeners is crucial to the smooth and efficient operation of a UNHSP. Although time is typically a rare and valuable commodity in any screening program, the time invested in training will improve accuracy, efficiency, and productivity of the screening staff. Training should be given to all new screeners and should consist of didactic as well as practical, hands-on training. The help of a neonatal nurse or nurse educator should be enlisted to teach new screeners techniques for baby handling, proper disinfection, and operation of monitors and other patient-care equipment (Fig. 4–2). An outline of the Long Island Jewish Medical Center's (LIJ) screener training course can be found in Appendix A.

TEST INTERPRETATION

The audiologist coordinator is responsible for review and final scoring of the screening results. Nevertheless, it will be necessary for screeners to be thoroughly instructed in pass–fail criteria adopted by the program and be able to make a preliminary determination about the outcome of the screen. Only in this way, will the screener be equipped to make an immediate decision on the validity of the screen as to whether or not an infant should be rescreened. In hospitals where results are to be given to parents immediately following the screen, audi-

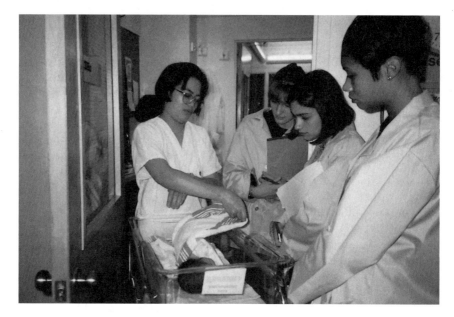

Figure 4–2.   A nurse demonstrates proper swaddling techniques to a group of audiology graduate students who work as screeners in the LIJ UNHSP.

ologist screeners are the only screeners qualified to screen, interpret findings, and disseminate results.

WHEN A NEWBORN FAILS A HEARING SCREENING

It is important for the coordinator to stress to screeners that if a newborn fails an initial screen they must continue to screen the infant until it is proven that all steps were taken to rule out any factor that could have resulted in a false-positive finding. Screeners should be told to be aggressive and thorough in trying to keep the false-positive rate as low as possible without sacrificing test sensitivity. A high false-positive rate will negatively affect the efficiency of the program, and lessen the credibility of the results.

Avoiding a false-positive finding should be a priority of any UNHSP. False-positive OAE findings are likely caused by a poorly fitted probe, vernix in the ear canal, a partially collapsed ear canal, or excessive ambient or infant noise. False-positive ABR findings are caused by poor electrode impedance; improperly placed transducer; collapsed ear canal; and excessive ambient, infant, or electrical noise. If a newborn fails the screening, the coordinator should emphasize the importance of the troubleshooting techniques outlined in Tables 4–1 and 4–2. If, after several attempts, the infant continues to fail the screening, the infant should be rescreened later in the day or the next day.

INTERACTING WITH PARENTS

The nonprofessional screeners should not be permitted to communicate results to parents, give advice, or make recommendations. Their responsibilities are

Table 4–1. Techniques for Minimizing False-Positive Findings with OAE Screening

1. Reposition the probe in the ear canal.
2. Inspect the probe tip for debris and clean with a fine needle or a hearing aid cleaning loop and retest. (The "serviceable" probe for the ILO88 allows for the occluded tubing to be quickly replaced.)
3. Massage the ear canal with a gentle circular motion anterior to the tragus and by gently tugging on the pinna. This manipulation may dislodge debris in the ear canal and may dilate a partially closed canal.
4. Use a larger probe tip, if possible. A larger probe tip may further open the ear canal.
5. Ambient noise can often be reduced by moving to a quieter area of the nursery or by placing the infant in an closed isolette.

limited to: greeting the mothers of the infants, explaining what the screening involves, safe handling of the infants, performing the screen, returning the baby to the mother or to the nursery, and completing required paperwork.

Parents, in most hospitals, are encouraged to question anyone taking their newborn out of their presence for any period of time and to ask questions about any procedure being performed. Screeners should, therefore, anticipate questions and keep parents, as well as nursing staff, well informed. It may be important, therefore, to have scripts written for nonprofessional screening personnel. Each script should have possible scenarios that are likely to occur and wording of acceptable responses that screening personnel can follow. For example, screeners should introduce themselves by using their complete names and title. They should inform mothers and/or parents that they are there to screen their infant's hearing. Additional information can be added such as, when the project was started, how long the procedure will take, and general procedures. Screening personnel can give the mother and/or the parents a brochure that explains the importance of hearing screening. This will allow parents the opportunity to read about hearing screening while the infant is being screened.

When the screening is complete, nonprofessional screening personnel should inform parents that an audiologist will interpret the results. If a rescreen is

Table 4–2. Techniques for Minimizing False-Positive Findings with ABR Screening

1. Check electrode impedance. If electrode impedances are high (generally, above 5 K ohms), remove electrodes, reprepare skin, and reapply electrodes. Teaching good skin preparation and electrode application techniques will prevent this problem.
2. Ambient noise can often be reduced by moving to a quieter area of the nursery. If this is not possible, the infant may be isolated from room noise by using noise attenuating circumaural earphones (i.e., earphones used with the Algo™ Natus Medical, Inc., San Carlos, CA.) or by placing the infant in an isolette.
3. Excessive electrical artifact may necessitate that the screening operation move to an electrically quieter area, away from nursery equipment. Some techniques for reducing electrical artifacts include braiding electrode wires, moving the infant away from the computer monitor, and making sure that transducer cables and electrode leads are separated.

needed, parents should be told that it will be completed before their infant is discharged. Screening personnel also should inform the parents about how the program handles reporting screening results to the infant's primary-care physician.

Screening personnel will often need a different script to cover the situation in which an infant fails the screening and repeat screening is required. Parents should be informed that an additional screen may be attempted before the infant is discharged. If difficulties in scheduling preclude another screen, the parents will be contacted by a member of the screening staff and arrangements will be made for them to return for an outpatient hearing screening. If parents ask about results, screening personnel can reiterate to parents that the results need to be interpreted by an audiologist. If parents are insistent upon receiving the results, screening personnel can assure parents that an audiologist will contact them with the results as soon as possible.

The screener should always maintain a friendly, professional demeanor with parents. He or she should always try to accommodate parent's wishes and allow parents to observe the screening.

Although the screening protocol should be designed to make the hearing screening a positive experience, sometimes the screener does not feel comfortable handling a parent's concern or criticism. If parents have any concerns or criticisms, the parents should be given an opportunity to discuss their concerns with the coordinator immediately. These situations are rare, and may be successfully defused by the coordinator, avoiding complaints to the nursing staff, physicians, or administration. If the coordinator cannot resolve the problem to the parent's satisfaction, the coordinator should speak with the mother's nurse privately and follow hospital protocol regarding complaints.

In summary, screeners should be cognizant of how they relate to the parents. They should be informed during their early training that the universal hearing screening program is usually well accepted. But screeners should remember that mothers are often tired, may not feel well, and are concerned about any procedure being performed on their infant. If screeners approach parents appropriately, the parents will likely find the hearing screening beneficial.

INTERACTING WITH PHYSICIANS AND OTHER PROFESSIONALS

If a physician or other hospital personnel asks for results, screening personnel are told to explain to the physician that they are nonprofessional screening personnel and that the test results need to be interpreted by an audiologist. The screener should defer all inquiries about results, test procedures, and protocols to the coordinating audiologist.

SECURITY

In some hospitals newborns reside in the mother's room, while in other hospitals infants stay in the nursery and are brought to the mother for feeding. The coordinator should stress to the screeners that when they remove a baby from the nursery to perform the test in another room, the parents, as well as the nursing staff must be informed. All screening programs should avoid a situation in which the mother or nurse is unable to locate an infant. The protocols of the nursery governing transporting infants, notification of the location of the baby, and verification of the infant's and mother's identity must be rigorously observed.

CONFIDENTIALITY

Screening personnel must be informed and reminded about the patient's rights to confidentiality and privacy. Discussions regarding a patient's findings should never occur in hallways, elevators, and other public areas.[1,4] Medical records are an important component in any risk management program.[1] All entries made by nonprofessional and professional personnel must be accurate, relevant, and appropriate because a patient's medical chart is difficult to alter. In fact, when changes must be made, they may need to be completed in chronological order leaving the original entry intact. All hospitals will have specific policies and procedures for completing the medical record and for changing errors. These policies must be thoroughly reviewed with the screeners. Entries in the mother's and/or infant's medical chart should be timely and complete and made only by authorized personnel. Personal comments from family members and other medical professionals as they relate to an infant should never be included.

Screener Schedules

The newborn hearing screening schedules should be arranged to maximize the likelihood of screening all infants; missing an infant should be a rare event. Given a sufficient length of stay (48 h), a good time to schedule newborns for screening is the day before discharge. If the baby fails the initial screening, there is another opportunity to rescreen the baby the morning of discharge. The short length of stay in most hospital maternity units requires 7-day-a-week coverage to ensure that all newborns, including those born and discharged on weekends and holidays are screened. The scheduling of screeners will vary depending upon the specific routines and schedules of the nursery as well as the personnel involved in the screening program.

PAID SCREENERS

Paid screeners (audiologists or paid technicians) should have schedules that are designed to meet the needs of the screening program and are consistent from week to week. The coordinator needs to monitor the screener's accrued vacation and/or personal time. Adequate notice must be given before vacation time can be granted to allow sufficient time to arrange coverage. A mechanism for emergency coverage in case the screener is unexpectantly absent due to illness or an emergency must be in place. Emergency coverage may be provided by supervisory staff, overtime assignments, or on-call per diem screeners.

NURSES

If hearing screenings are to be administered by the nursing staff, the coordinator will have to work with the nursing supervisor to set screener schedules. Time for screening can be integrated into the nurse's daily routine as long as there is a mechanism to ensure that the screening is performed before discharge. Making the hearing screening part of the infant's Care Map is one way to ensure that each baby receives a screening prior to discharge.

VOLUNTEERS

Volunteers must commit to working during times required by the program and work a consistent schedule. A volunteer who cannot make this kind of commitment can be used in other aspects of the program such as data entry, clerical work, etc. where more flexible scheduling can be accommodated.

STUDENT SCREENERS

Student screeners' schedules may vary depending upon the arrangement between the university and the screening program. Students may work in the program through a work-study agreement, internship, traineeship, etc. For the universal screening program to maintain a full complement of screeners, they should be available to work year-round, including holidays and intersession breaks during which the schools are closed.

Scheduling Screening in the WBN

Newborns in the WBN are a challenging population to screen. Although they must be sleeping or resting quietly to perform the screening, babies in the WBN are often engaged in other activities such as feeding, being bathed, having their diapers changed, undergoing medical examination and lab tests, and, of course, being admired by family and friends. Finding the right time for screening will require creativity and adaptability. If possible, it may be advantageous to visit each new mother the day prior to the screening, inform her about the test, and give her any pamphlets or written material describing the program. In this way, the mother has time to discuss the screening with her husband, nurse, or pediatrician before the baby is screened.

   The best time of day to screen will depend upon the nursery schedule. For example, in some nurseries the early morning hours between 6:00 and 9:00 A.M. may be the best time to begin screening because most of the infants will be in the nursery. Screening babies in one location is less time consuming than having to locate infants in their mothers' rooms. On the other hand, early morning hours are often a popular time for physicians to perform rounds, making screening difficult. Mothers may be unwilling to have their newborns screened while visiting with family and friends. In addition, infants may tend to be more irritable, due to overstimulation by visitors. A careful study of the nursery routines will be required before implementing screening schedules.

Scheduling Screening in the NICU

The high volume of infants in WBN poses the greatest challenge to universal newborn hearing screening programs, nevertheless, the regularity and predictability of the WBN schedule makes setting schedules to accomplish universal screening relatively easy. The situation is much more complex in the NICU. Because the date and time of discharge of any given baby may be uncertain, programs tend to miss more infants in NICU than WBN. Thus, creative scheduling to minimize missed babies must be instituted. Some babies may be extremely premature, require life-saving intervention, and may be in the NICU for many months. Other babies may be in the NICU for only a short stay for observation or short-term phototherapy. The charge nurse, or case manager specialist should be given the responsibility to inform the screening team of the imminent discharge of any baby in her care. In large hospitals the nurse educator or nursing coordinator may be enlisted to compose a daily discharge list for the screeners.

Large screening programs may decide to use different staff to cover the NICU and WBN. In many screening programs, however, the same personnel who screen in the WBN will also screen in the NICU. There is a tendency to focus on WBN because of the large numbers of infants as compared to the NICU. Screening staff must be reminded to make an equal effort to screen all infants regardless of location.

Tracking infants that are transferred between units can be difficult. Tracking infants is easier if the same individual(s) screens in all units. It will be necessary to institute a reliable communication system to identify which babies are in need of screening. One approach is for the UNHSP to designate which infants require screening by placing a small sticker on the bassinet name tag. These identifying stickers may contain the telephone number of the screening program and instructions to the nursery staff to call prior to the infant's discharge. Alternatively, a sticker may indicate that the screening has been completed. In this case, infants without stickers are targeted for screening. Stickers will work well if they are used solely by the UNHSP staff. Overuse of stickers will decrease their novelty and, in turn, their effectiveness.

When NICU babies are nearing discharge, they are more likely to be in an open crib, not attached to intravenous lines and monitors, and, therefore, may be much easier to test if they can be transported to a quiet screening environment. Often NICU infants are unable to be relocated to a quiet environment for screening. Screening in a open isolette in the NICU may be impossible due to the excessive ambient environmental noise. Screening NICU infants in a closed isolette may be prudent to reduce excessive environmental noise.

NICU babies may be screened at any time of day or night, however, it is advisable to avoid times with high levels or activity such as rounds or feeding times. It also may be important for the screening staff to be consistent about the time of day or night that they will be screening in the NICU. A consistent screening schedule will allow nursing staff the opportunity to prepare for screening by making sure the infants are fed, diapers changed, and that infants are likely to be asleep.

Evaluating Screeners

ONGOING INFORMAL EVALUATIONS

Evaluating all screening personnel (audiologist, nurses, volunteers, and paid technicians) is an ongoing process. The coordinator can accomplish this by periodically working along side the screeners. During this time, the coordinator can observe screening techniques, re-instruct and provide praise and constructive criticism. The coordinator should observe each screener's routine to ensure the use of proper disinfection techniques. Feedback from the screeners should be encouraged and they should be made to feel comfortable discussing issues as they arise. For example, a screener may be having some difficulty interacting with a nursery staff member. Discussing problems with the coordinator as they occur and working toward a resolution can prevent a potentially damaging situation.

FORMAL EVALUATIONS

In addition to the ongoing informal evaluations, the coordinator should formally evaluate screeners on a regular basis. Formal evaluations are likely required by the hospital and may be linked to raises and promotions. The formal evaluation should include observations, written evaluation, and meeting with each screener. Sample evaluation forms are included in Appendix B of this chapter. It is suggested that the coordinator perform formal evaluations on salaried screeners and volunteers. Job performance of staff nurses and staff audiologists will, most likely, be rated by their department administrators, but their screening performance should be judged by the program supervisor.

The first formal evaluations should be given near the end of any probationary period for salaried screeners or after 3 months of service for volunteers. Subsequent formal evaluations for all screeners should be given at least on a yearly basis. The formal evaluation can be divided into the following four areas:

1. *Preparation*: The coordinator should meet with the screener to discuss the evaluation procedure and to set a date for observation. In this way, the screener will know in advance the skills on which he or she will be rated.
2. *Observation*: The coordinator should observe the screener test several infants. The screener's technique, as well as his or her compliance with safety and disinfection policies and accuracy of recordkeeping, should be assessed.
3. *Result Analysis*: The number of passing scores, failing scores, and missed screenings for each screener is recorded to assess efficiency and productivity.
4. *Formal Meeting*: The coordinator and the screener discuss the observation and the screener receives a written evaluation. Areas that need improvement and goals for the next evaluation period should be included.

Conclusion

There are a variety of staffing options from which to choose. Although most successful UNHSPs are headed by a director from either audiology or neonatology and an audiology coordinator, backgrounds of screening personnel vary widely. Each hospital must carefully consider which type of screening personnel is needed within the context of the specific program.

Screening staff will most likely be supervised by the coordinating audiologist. The coordinating audiologist should be responsible to recruit, train, set screener schedules, and informally and formally evaluate screeners on a regular basis. The size of the program, screening protocol used, as well as specific human resources requirements and hospital regulations will all impact on the nature of the screening staff. Therefore, each UNHSP must carefully evaluate its own strengths and weaknesses with respect to the screening environment, hospital regulations, screening protocols, etc and hire staff that they feel can result in a successful UNHSP.

References

1. Marlowe JA. Legal and risk management issues in newborn hearing screening. Semin Hear 1996;17:153–64
2. Meister, S. Emerging risk: Failure to detect hearing disability in newborns. QRC Advisor 1993;10:1–4
3. Johnson M, Maxon AB, White KR, Vohr, BR. Operating a hospital-based universal newborn hearing screening program using transient evoked otoacoustic emissions. Semin Hear 1993;14: 46–56
4. Balsamo RR, and Brown MD. Risk management. In Sanbar SS, Gibofsky A, Firestone MH, LeBlang TR (eds): Legal Medicine. St Louis, Mosby, 1995, 237–261

APPENDIX A
SCREENER TRAINING CURRICULUM

I. Lecture
  A. Universal Newborn Hearing Screenings
   -brief history
   -rationale for newborn screening
   -risk factors for hearing loss
   -prevalence of congenital hearing loss
   -benefits of early detection of hearing loss
  B. Overview of Anatomy and Physiology of the Ear
  C. OAE and ABR screening
   -what they measure
   -limitations
   -OAE vs. ABR: pros and cons
  D. When a Newborn Fails a Hearing Screening
   -importance of minimizing false-positive
   -reasons for failure
   -procedures for reducing fail rate
  E. Newborn Hearing Screening Protocol
   -OAE
   -ABR
   -Outpatient rescreen

II. In-Service by Nurses

The coordinator is not an expert on the care and management of newborns. For this reason, the help of nurse educators from the WBN and the NICU is enlisted to teach the new screeners proper infant handling techniques, nursery protocols, and procedures for an emergency.

The following topics are covered:
  A. Responsibilities of various nursing staff
  B. Proper handling of newborns
  C. Disinfection techniques
  D. Nursery regulations regarding proper attire
  E. Security protocols
  F. What to do in an emergency
  G. Judging an infant's readiness for testing
  H. Recognizing warning signs of distress
  I. Common medical conditions of infants in the NICU
  J. NICU equipment
   - procedures for disconnecting and reconnecting monitors, i.v. and central lines, ng tubes, oxygen, isolettes, etc.

A discussion of the above topics can be found in Rowan, Chapter 6 and Smillie, Chapter 7.

III. "Hands-On" Clinical Training

Techniques for performing the OAE and ABR screen are demonstrated and practiced.

A. OAE
  1) Operation of test equipment
     -calibration
     -test selection and procedures
     -care and routine maintenance
  2) Entering patient information
  3) Valid test parameters (stimulus intensity and spectrum)
  4) Obtaining a good probe fit
  5) Pass criteria
  6) Troubleshooting
  7) Practice recording OAE
Criteria for Mastery:
  A. Twenty-five valid tests completed on adult subjects
  B. Twenty-five valid tests completed on newborns
B. Automated ABR
  1) Operation of test equipment
  2) Entering patient information
  3) Proper technique for application of electrodes
  4) Proper earphone placement
  5) Troubleshooting
Criteria for Mastery:
  A. Ten valid tests completed on adults
  B. Ten valid tests completed on newborns

On-site training will be required for screeners to achieve mastery of the screening techniques with newborns. New screeners typically have difficulty obtaining an adequate probe fit, experience frustration in learning to use the equipment efficiently, have problems quieting crying or active newborns, and are especially hesitant about handling babies in the NICU. The best way for the coordinator to assist the screeners during this initial learning period is to work with them in the nursery until they demonstrate mastery of the techniques and are comfortable with the nursery environments and routines.

APPENDIX B

1. Instructions and evaluation form for newborn hearing screeners. Reprinted with permission from Karl White, the National Center for Hearing Assessment and Management.
2. Screener evaluation form used in the Long Island Jewish Medical Center Universal Newborn Hearing Program.

Instructions

This form was designed to assist supervisors in providing feedback to screeners on their screening techniques. In addition to pointing out where improvement is needed, the supervisor should also be sure to note and reinforce proficiencies. Although there are many variables that influence the way that a screening session occurs, and although not all screening sessions will follow the outlined sequence exactly, the feedback form provides a checklist of critical activities and decision points.

The screening supervisor should begin the feedback session with the equipment turned off so that each screener has the opportunity to move through all of the screening steps. A left and a right ear screening session should be observed. The screening steps are listed sequentially; however, credit should be given if the screener performs the steps in a different, but equally appropriate order (i.e., swaddles the infant before turning the computer on, rather than after, etc). A "P" (pass), and "I" (improvement needed), or an "INO" (item not observed during the screening sequence) should be recorded for each item listed. If the screener performs a step incorrectly, or continues with the screening session without making the proper adjustments, "I" should be recorded in the corresponding blank. If no conditions arise where it would be appropriate for a screener to carry out specific steps, however, "INO" should be recorded.

Under **Screening**, the supervisor will frequently need to use the left- and right-hand columns to document a screening session. In other cases, only the column on the left side will be marked with a "P" or an "I" and the items corresponding with the column on the right will not be observed (INO). For example, if the infant is quiet during the left ear screening session, the probe is positioned correctly, and the screening proceeds successfully without interruption, each blank in the column on the left (for the left ear) would be marked with a "P" and it would not be possible to observe the "troubleshooting" activities corresponding with the right-hand column ("INO" would be recorded for each item). However, if during the screening session on the right ear the stimulus waveform were not present, and the screener removed the probe from the infant's ear to check for debris, the supervisor would mark a "P" in the column on the right (under right ear) for the item "✓ probe tip for debris." If removing debris solved the problem, the waveform could be observed, and the proper stimulus spectrum shape were noted, the supervisor would return the left-hand column to mark "P" for each of those items. In some screening sessions, the screener will thus "cycle" through a sequence of steps more than once.

Screener's Feedback Form (Level I—Beginner)

The purpose of this form is to assist supervisors in reinforcing good screening practices and in providing feedback where improvement is needed. Items are marked according to the following key: *P = Pass, I = Improvement needed, INO = Item Not Observed because the screener did not have to perform the task.*

1. Preparation

Equipment ___ Turns on computer (CPU & Monitor)	**Software** ___ Accesses HI*SCREEN
___ Turns on ILO88 analyzer	___ Enters infant demographic info.
___ Connects probe to analyzer	___ Selects infant name for
Subject ___ Follows hospital sanitation procedures	screening
___ Swaddles infant correctly	

2. Screening

(*Left*)	(*Right*)	**Software**			(*Left*)	(*Right*)
___	___	Confirms infant to be screened				
___	___	Confirms ear to be screened				
(*Left*)	(*Right*)	**Subject**				
___	___	Positions infant correctly				
___	___	Manipulates pinna & tragus, examines ear canal size & angle				
___	___	Obtains good probe fit				
___	___	Positions cord correctly				
(*Left*)	(*Right*)	**Checkfit**			(*Left*)	(*Right*)
___	___	Stimulus waveform present				
		➥ If not, ✓ that ILO88 analyzer is "on"			___	___
		✓ probe tip for debris			___	___
___	___	Proper stimulus spectrum shape				
		➥ If not, manipulates ear			___	___
		refits probe (✓ tip for debris)			___	___
		repositions cord			___	___
___	___	Stimulus intensity 78–83 dB				
		➥ If not, presses "∧" twice			___	___
___	___	Noise level at or below green/yellow bar				
		➥ If not, calms infant			___	___
		refits probe (✓ tip for debris)			___	___
		reduces environmental noise			___	___
___	___	Begins screening				
(*Left*)	(*Right*)	**Screening data collection**			(*Left*)	(*Right*)
___	___	At 40 quiet samples, response present				
		➥ If not, & noise reject level >48 dB & noise floor does **not** taper off, escapes & returns to **Step 2—Subject**			___	___
		➥ If not, & noise reject level <=48 dB & noise floor tapers off, escapes & returns to **Step 2—Subject** (trying a larger probe tip).			___	___
___	___	Band reproducibility levels meet or exceed program "pass" criteria				
___	___	Number of quiet samples meet or exceed program "pass" criteria				
___	___	Terminates screening				
___	___	Saves data file				

3. Wrap up

___ Removes infant's name from screening list
___ Records screening activity according to program protocol
___ Communicates screening activities to parents according to program protocol
___ Exits HI*SCREEN and turns off screening equipment

Long Island Jewish Medical Center—Universal Newborn Hearing Screening Program

Screener Evaluation Form

Screener's Name _____ Evaluation Period _____

Date of Conference _____ Screener's Signature _____

Supervisor's Signature _____

Rating Scale:

4 = outstanding performance
3 = above average
2 = average performance
1 = below average / unacceptable

Basic Skills

Rating

1. Attendance and punctuality. _____

2. Performs clerical and recordkeeping duties in an accurate and organized fashion. _____

3. Administers otoacoustic emissions screening accurately. _____

4. Administers ABR screenings accurately. _____

5. Handles newborns properly and according to protocol. _____

6. Respects patient confidentiality. _____

7. Establishes and maintains effective relationship with nursing staff and other hospital personnel. _____

8. Interacts appropriately with parents and presents information in a clear and accurate manner. _____

9. Is realistic about the number of babies to be tested and works at an appropriate pace. _____

Supervisor's Comments

_____
_____
_____
_____
_____
_____

5

Instrumentation for Newborn Hearing Screening

Barbara Kurman
Lynn G. Spivak

Introduction

The proliferation of newborn hearing screening programs throughout the country has resulted in the development and marketing of numerous instruments designed to perform quick, efficient, and cost-effective screening. One of the most important decisions the director of a newborn hearing screening program must make is the selection of screening equipment. Purchase of instrumentation represents not only a significant one-time capital investment, but also a commitment to ongoing associated expenses including maintenance, replacement parts, and supplies. Limited capital budgets will provide few if any opportunities to rectify a bad decision, leaving the screening program to deal with equipment that is inappropriate for its needs. Selection of equipment must be based on a thorough investigation of systems that are commercially available, and careful consideration of the specific needs of the program. The purpose of this chapter is to provide the reader with information needed to select instrumentation that will be compatible with the goals and objectives as well as the unique conditions and logistics of the screening environment.

Before a specific instrument can be selected, the choice of screening method must be made. The reader is referred to Chapter 3 for a thorough discussion of different screening models. The following will review the various program options, highlight important issues that should be considered in instrument selection, and finally present a detailed catalog of equipment that is currently available for newborn screening.

ABR, OAE, or Both?

The auditory brainstem response (ABR) has long been considered the "gold standard" of newborn screening, however, it was thought by many to be impractical and too costly for use as a mass newborn screening test. The introduction of the ALGO I™ (Natus Medical Inc., San Carlos, CA) automated ABR screener, however, paved the way for the use of ABR in a universal screening program.[1] This instrument with its simplified operation, rapid data acquisition, and automated scoring made it possible for reliable and accurate ABR hearing screening to be performed by trained, nonprofessional personnel.[2–4] Subsequently, other ABR screeners with the capability of performing automated routines have been developed. The ability to use technicians, nurses, and in some cases, trained volunteers to perform the hearing screening represented a significant reduction in the cost and time required to screen newborns and has brought the use of ABR for universal hearing screening within the realm of feasibility.

The most recent technological advance in the field of auditory diagnosis, otoacoustic emissions (OAEs), has emerged as a viable alternative to ABR for newborn screening. First described by David Kemp[5], the OAE test has been shown to be a reliable and cost-effective method for screening hearing in newborns.[6–9] Because recording OAEs is generally faster and less expensive than recording ABRs, and the results of OAE testing compare favorably to ABR testing, some authors have recommended that OAE be used as the primary screening method for newborn hearing screening.[6,9,10]

While at first glance, OAEs may appear to be the ideal choice for universal newborn hearing screening programs, there is a major drawback. OAE-based hearing screening programs tend to produce higher fail rates than ABR-based programs.[9,11] This is especially true in well-baby nurseries (WBN), where because of short length of maternity stay, infants may be tested within hours of birth. Blockage of the external auditory meatus (EAM) with debris and retention of fluid in the middle ear are among the common conditions that may prevent a newborn from passing the OAE screen (see Vohr, Chapter 8). For this reason, the National Institutes of Health (NIH) in its 1993 consensus statement endorsed a two-stage screening protocol combining OAE and ABR.[12] By rescreening OAE failures with ABR, the fail rate for the program can be reduced significantly. The experience of the Long Island Jewish Medical Center (LIJ) program, for example, has been that approximately 7% of all newborns fail the initial OAE screen, but immediate rescreening with ABR reduces this failure rate to under 3%.

Issues Related to Choice of Equipment

The choice of screening device will be driven by a number of issues . The program director will need to know the answers to the following questions before an informed decision can be made.

What Kind of Information is Expected from the Screening?

Programs will differ in terms of what information they expect from newborn hearing screening. It is important therefore to be clear about the expected outcomes of the newborn hearing screening and make certain that the chosen equipment is capable of providing the required data. For example, some programs using ABR as the screening method accept the presence of Wave V at a predetermined intensity level as criterion for a pass, while others may also include the latency of wave V in the criteria. In the latter case, obviously, the selected instrument must have the capability of supplying latency information.

For What Type of Hearing Loss am I Screening?

The type and degree of hearing loss that the program expects to detect is also a factor in test choice. For example, there is some evidence that OAE screening may be more sensitive than ABR for detecting mild conductive hearing loss.[8,13] On the other hand, if information beyond a simple "pass" or "fail" is desired, an ABR screener with the capability of screening at multiple levels and/or seeking threshold would be a more appropriate choice.

Who Will Be Doing the Screening?

If audiologists will be performing the screening, the choice of screening equipment is essentially limitless. Standard, manual diagnostic equipment requiring operator test interpretation is appropriate for the audiologist to use. If nonprofessional screeners are to be employed, however, the equipment choices are limited to those that perform simplified, automated screening protocols and, ideally, are self-scoring. The audiologist's role in a program employing technician screeners is supervision, training, and review of test data for quality assurance. It will be necessary for the equipment to store, print out, or display test data collected by technicians in a convenient form for later review by the audiologist. It should be kept in mind that equipment requiring manual scoring will require more of the audiologist's time than equipment that provides automated scoring.

Will the Equipment Be Dedicated to the Screening Program?

Budgetary constraints may require that the equipment chosen for the screening program function in more than one capacity. For example, the equipment might be used as a screening device in the newborn nursery in the morning and as a diagnostic system in the outpatient audiology department in the afternoon. Instruments such as the ALGO II™ (Natus Medical Inc., San Carlos, CA), or GSI 55 (Grason-Stadler, Inc., Milford, NH) have limited or no diagnostic capabilities and, therefore, would be inappropriate choices for such an application. The need to have diagnostic capabilities, of course, must be weighed against the need to have professional operators performing the screen. There are some instruments that have features that make them potentially capable of fulfilling both needs.

Where Will the Screening Take Place?

Screening may take place in the nursery proper, in a quiet room separated from the main nursery area, or in the mother's room. The equipment must be compatible with the screening environment. In this regard, the program director should consider the following issues:

- *Ambient noise*: High noise levels often encountered in the NICU or a fully occupied well-baby unit may prevent effective use some systems. OAE testing may be difficult or impossible in high-noise situations unless provisions are made to isolate the infant from the noise. ABR screening levels may be dictated by ambient noise levels. Systems that provide for noise attenuation, such as the circumaural earphones used with the ALGO II,™ may be suitable for noisy conditions.
- *Electrical interference*: In addition to ambient noise, interference from electrical noise must also be considered. ABR testing is particularly susceptible to electrical interference from nursery equipment. This is an important consideration in the neonatal intensive care unit (NICU) where infants are often tested while connected to monitors and life-support systems that may produce electrical artifact. ABR testing may be more successful using battery powered equipment. Alternatively, an OAE-based system could be chosen. OAE testing is unaffected by electrical noise.
- *Portability*: The program director needs to consider the size and portability of the equipment. These may not be major issues for programs in which infants are transported from the nursery or mother's room to the screening site. Nevertheless, one should consider the possible, occasional need to move the screening operation to another area, as well as the need move equipment for storage in a secured place.
- *Power source*: For programs in which the equipment must be transported to the mother's room or to an infant's isolette, the source of power must also be considered. Battery-powered equipment will avoid the necessity of having to power down and reboot equipment between tests and, as mentioned above, will isolate the equipment from possible interference from line current.

Should the ABR and OAE Systems Be Combined in One Computer?

Some programs find it convenient and cost effective to have more than one screening system, for example ILO88 (Otodynamics, LTD., UK) and Smart Screener™ (Intelligent Hearing Systems, Miami, FL), installed in a single PC. This concept was taken a step further by Sonamed Corporation (Brookline, MA) which produces an integrated ABR and OAE screening instrument. Although combined systems save space and the cost of a computer, they sacrifice flexibility. Large hospitals with high-volume nurseries may have more than one screener assigned to a shift. The major disadvantage of combined systems is that only one person can use the system at any given time. If the OAE and ABR systems are housed in separate computers, however, one screener could be performing ABR rescreens while another screener performs the OAE screen. One system can also take over for another in case of a breakdown.

What is the Cost of the Equipment?

While the initial cost of the equipment is an important consideration, one must also consider the ongoing costs of supplies, replacement parts, repairs, and maintenance. Some devices require the use of expensive disposable supplies that significantly increase the cost of the test. The program director should calculate the projected cost of supplies and materials required by the each device to make accurate cost comparisons. See Appendix A for information about equipment and supply costs.

Computers

All hearing screening devices are computer based. Some manufactures package their systems in dedicated computers while others sell the hardware and software that can then be installed into any computer meeting the minimum requirements for power, speed, and memory. While some systems require full-size PCS, others can be installed in smaller lunch box or laptop computers. As mentioned above, the size, portability, and power supply requirements of the host computer must be considered. All manufactures are careful to state the minimum computer requirements for their own test equipment. Once the minimum requirements are met, additional features of the host computer are limited only by the program budget. The cost of the hardware dedicated to the various test instruments are fairly similar. Thus, many of the equipment decisions will not be dominated by the system or test mode per se, but by the expense of the host computer and peripherals.

Screening Devices

Before embarking on a detailed description of test equipment that is suitable for newborn hearing screening, a few caveats must be made:

- First, it will be assumed that the screening program to be developed will follow the recommendations of the NIH[12] and the Joint Committee on Infant Hearing (JCIH)[14] and make use of either ABR or OAE technology, or a combination of both.
- Second, the discussion will be limited to products available for sale and clinical use in the United States (i.e., systems that have Food and Drug Administration [FDA] approval). Equipment availability is different in other parts of the world.
- Third, it is not the intention of this chapter to endorse or recommend any particular system. The product review was intended to describe the features of each system in an objective fashion to provide the information that the program director will need to make the most appropriate choice for his or her particular situation.
- Finally, development of computer processing hardware as well as test hardware and software are ongoing and rapidly changing. No sooner is one system introduced on the market then it is revised and improved. Although instrumentation described here is current as of the publication date of this text, a certain amount of information outdating is, unfortunately, unavoidable. Therefore, the reader is advised to consult with the manufacturer or distributer of the equipment in which he or she is interested before committing to a purchase.

At the end of this chapter, a manufacturer's reference guide is provided to further assist the reader in planning and acquisition of equipment.

Otoacoustic Emissions Equipment

OAE testing equipment can be divided into two main classifications based on the type of emissions that they record: transient otoacoustic emissions (TOAE) and distortion product otoacoustic emissions (DPOAE). To date, there is only one OAE device with FDA approval that is able to perform both TOAE and DPOAE tests. It is possible, however, to house tests from different manufacturers in a single host computer.

Transient Otoacoustic Emissions

David Kemp, who is credited with discovering OAEs, is the principal owner of the U.S. patent on the TOAE system. His product, known as the ILO88 is manufactured by Otodynamics, Ltd. (England, UK), which markets and sells its product in the United States through its distributor network. The ILO88 may be purchased in the United States through special instrument distributors (SIDS) authorized to sell the system. Not only was the ILO88 the first OAE system to receive FDA approval, it was also the device chosen by the well-publicized Rhode Island Hearing Assessment Project. For those reasons, the ILO88 enjoys the largest representation in the literature concerned with OAEs and newborn screening. The TOAE system is available in three configurations: the ILO88 board kit, the ILO88 Echoport, and the ILO88i.

BOARD KIT

In this configuration, the ILO88 consists of an external preamplifier and a board and software that are installed in a host computer. This version of the ILO88 requires a full-sized expansion slot in the host computer. The special instrument distributor often recommends a specific host computer. In some cases, the distributer provides the computer and installs the board and software as part of the purchase. The ILO88 board kit can be upgraded to include the chip and processing capabilities of DPOAE. A new version of the ILO88, known as the ILO88i, is now available to be internally mounted through an Industry Standard Architecture (ISA) bus card.

ECHOPORT

The Echoport consists of the computer board housed in an external box, with a built-in preamplifier and receptacle for the probe. The software is identical to that used in the standard ILO88. Unlike the board kit version, however, the Echoport cannot be upgraded to perform the DPOAE test. Because the Echoport is external to the computer, a small laptop or notebook computer can be used as the host computer. The Echoport can be powered by either line current or batteries. Coupled with a laptop computer, the entire screening system can be battery operated. In this way, the system is completely electrically isolated, a feature that may please the hospital's Biomedical Department. A battery-powered system is advantageous especially if line current, or electrical noise presents a problem. This configuration also offers the greatest amount of portability.

ILO88I

This latest version of the ILO88 features all the same software capability as the ILO88 but with the ease of internal mounting of the hardware directly through the ISA bus card. This space is usually located at the site of the floppy disk in most computers. With this type of configuration, it is usually not necessary to open the external housing of the computer and expose the internal boards and chips. This type of configuration, however, required a larger portable PC or a desktop PC.

PROBE

There are two types of probes currently available for the ILO88. The most commonly used probe is the NS type probe or "nonserviceable" probe. As the name implies, this probe cannot be serviced or cleaned and great care is necessary to avoid clogging it with wax or vernix. Each probe is said to have a "use" life of 500 tests. Thus, in the planning of a newborn screening program, the annual birth census should be considered in estimating the number of probes that will have to be purchased. The newest probe available is the "serviceable" probe. This probe can be taken apart at its head, allowing a replaceable coupler to be inserted within the probe housing. These couplers should be purchased in quantity, and replaced approximately weekly. In addition, replacement heads and lids are recommended for periodic change to increase the probe life. Kemp reports that with frequent replacement of the coupler, the probe life can be doubled, to perhaps 1000 tests.

Both ILO88 systems are shipped with multiple probes: usually two newborn probes and two adult probes. However, any combination of sizes can be requested. It is recommended that at least one adult probe be purchased. In this way, the adults who will be performing the test can learn the proper test technique by testing each other. The adult probe can also be used to perform biological calibration checks if necessary. The instrument package also includes a glass calibration cavity. It is recommended that the calibration cavity be used on a daily basis to test probe function. ILO88 probes require disposable probe tips that come in four sizes for newborn testing.

DEVICE FEATURES

A complete description of the ILO88 is beyond the scope of this text. The interested reader is referred to Kemp, Ryan, and Bray[15] and Kemp and Ryan[16] for a comprehensive description of the system and its application to newborn screening. The following discussion will be limited to a brief overview of the most commonly used, default test parameters.

After the patient's identifying information is entered, the initial screen, known as "check fit" is displayed. At this point, the examiner has the opportunity to assess the adequacy of the probe fit by monitoring the level and spectrum of the stimulus in the ear canal. The test is easy to administer once the probe fit has been achieved. During the test, the screen displays an enormous amount of information, allowing the examiner to continuously monitor test conditions as well as the accumulating OAE data. Although the ILO88 display appears overly busy and confusing at first, with a little practice the examiner easily learns to navigate around the screen. The TOAE test is very fast. In a normal-hearing, quiet baby, the test could take as little as 15–30 sec per ear. In a baby with no measurable TOAE response, the test time averages about 4 min. At the end of the test, the examiner can assess the quality of the data on the computer screen and, if desired, compare the test results with stored normative data. The test results can be stored on the computer's hard drive or disk. A hard copy printout is also an option. The decision of a "pass" or "fail" is determined by the user's own criteria. Automated scoring of the ILO88 test is being developed.

One consistently negative comment that is made regarding the ILO product is the poor documentation accompanying the product. The company reports, however, that this situation will be rectified.

Distortion Product Otoacoustic Emission Systems

Unlike TOAE technology, there is no single patent holder on the technology for distortion product OAE measurement. Thus, there are seven FDA approved and commercially available products on the market. This section will review each of them. It is important to note that almost all of the instruments noted below are sold through the SID arrangement. Due to contractual arrangements with the manufacturers and territorial considerations, not all products are available through the same SIDs. However, any manufacturer will accept an order directly, and then make the necessary arrangements for installation and in-service through its authorized representative (SID).

ILO 88 DPI

This newly FDA-approved device is the only system to jointly house TEOAE and DPOAE within the same hardware. The hardware itself is mounted as described in the section describing the ILO 88i. However, with this new addition in the OAE arena, Otodynamics has captured the coveted combination of TEOAE *and* DPOAE test capabilities in one hardware system. Until January, 1997 Otodynamics offered a DPOAE (ILO 92) product for sale as a "research tool." However, it did not have FDA approval and, therefore, could not be used in the mass screening market. Certain features of the original Otodynamics DPOAE product received FDA approval: specifically and most importantly, the ability to perform the DP test and obtain a "DP gram." The new, FDA-approved DPOAE system is known as the ILO 88DPi. With the introduction of this device, TEOAE and DPOAE tests became available from the same manufacturer. However, due to the nature of the software contraints, the two tests must be run separately. It is currently necessary to switch from the TEOAE test mode and enter the DPOAE test mode from the main menu. The manufacturer reports that changes in the software will ultimately make this a more seamless operation.

The DP screen looks different from the TEOAE screen. The DP gram presents the user with a clear measure of the actual DP emission, the noise floor, and the ability to "zoom" in on particular data points for closer analysis. This test, which is a DOS-based program, can be automatically run from factory default parameters. Stimulus levels, noise floor parameters, F1 and F2 ratio options, and many other features can be changed by the user. A typical DP test on a normal newborn may take approximately 1–1 1/2 min. Like the TOAE system, the DP system uses disposable probe tips, and the probe itself is "serviceable" in the same manner described earlier in the TEOAE section. The manufacturer does not indicate what constitutes a "pass or fail," which is user or site determined. The system is shipped with 1 newborn, 1 adult TEOAE probe, 1 newborn and 1 adult DP probe, and 1 general purpose TEOAE probe. Additional research applications are available through the manufacturer, but may require additional software purchases or approval by the hospital's Investigational Review Board.

GRASON STADLER GSI 60

This unit may be purchased as a board kit, factory installed within a computer, or as a new portable version, with a laptop computer. The GSI 60 operates on a Windows platform and is compatible with Windows 95™ (Microsoft Corporation, Seattle, WA). The probe design is based on the probe used in the GSI 33 Middle Ear Analyzer and utilizes the same, nondisposable probe tips. However, disposable probe tips for this have recently become available, and will be described later in this chapter. The GSI 60 probe is easy to clean, and a cleaning wire is provided. A probe fit test is available, which can save test time by ensuring a good probe fit before the test begins.

The software allows the user to store a great deal of demographic data. All test parameters are under examiner control including criteria for acceptable noise floor. The examiner can create customized test protocols that can be saved, recalled, and implemented at will. Grasen-Stadler (Grason-Stadler, Inc., A Welch Allyn Co., Milford, NH) claims that the GSI 60 is the only device capable of performing a "simultaneous" test, that is, a two tone pairs separated by at least one octave are presented simultaneously. This method of stimulus presentation drastically reduces test time. The average test time for a normal hearing newborn, utilizing the screen protocol shipped from the factory is approximately 1 to 2 min. With the "simultaneous" test protocol, this test time can be a low as 30 sec to 1 min.

The screen displays the DP responses marked with audiometric symbols and colors, that is, red "O's" for the right ear and blue "x's" for the left ear. There are display options under the control of the examiner. For example, all data from either one ear or both ears can be superimposed and the data can be plotted as a function of F2 or the as a function of the geometric mean.

This is the only system available with factory-installed normative data, which was developed in the laboratories of Frank Musiek at Dartmouth Medical Center, and Brenda Lonsbury-Martin at Miami Medical Center. Although the availability of normative data may assist the tester in determining pass–fail criteria, there is no effort made by the manufacturer to dictate the pass–fail criteria or suggest how the normative data should be used.

Other features of the GSI 60 include a full interrelational database that allows the examiner to sort data by a number of parameters including referral physician, age, date of test, type of test, etc. The optional printout provides the examiner with information about the actual distortion product in decibels for each stimulus pair, the level and frequency of the distortion product recorded, and the noise floor. Although the screening function of the GSI 60 is the focus of this discussion, it should be pointed out that the GSI 60 can also function as a sophisticated research tool and full diagnostic DPOAE system.

As a portable system, the new configuration allows the GSI 60 board to be encased in its own housing and operate on battery or AC current. Thus, the design is similar to that of the ILO 88 Echoport. The battery is rechargeable within 8 hr, and because it is externally connected, it can be run off a notebook or laptop computer. The sofware is identical in all versions; portable or housed within the computer. The portable version does not require the use of a docking station, because the board is external to the computer. This version also does not require an isolation transformer. Because this can also be battery run, biomedical departments are not as concerned with electrical or safety issues (Fig. 5–1).

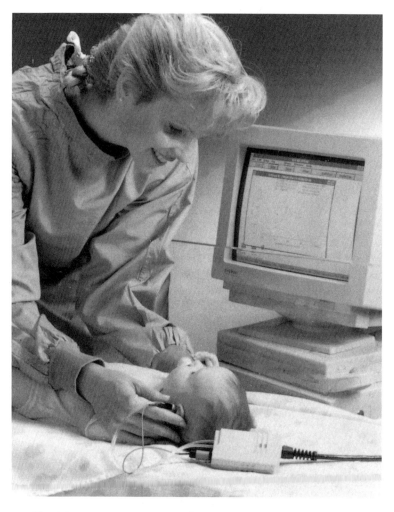

Figure 5–1.   The GSI 60 DPOAE system. (Photo courtesy of Grasen Stadler, Inc.)

MIMOSA ACOUSTICS CUBE DIS™ DISTORTION PRODUCT OAE SYSTEM

The development of the original software for this product, was a collaborative effort by AT&T Bell Laboratories (Murray Hill, NJ), Etymotic Research (Elk Grove Village, IL), and others. The marketing rights to this product were acquired by Mimosa Acoustics (Mountainside, NJ), which subsequently revised the software, hardware, and design several times. The unit operates in a laptop environment with a docking station to house the processing board. The company reports that it is working on a plan to limit the need for a docking station and processing board, and is moving toward a plan to miniaturize this portion (Fig. 5–2).

The probe and preamplifier were designed and manufactured by Etymotic Research (Elk Grove Village, IL). A single probe size is used for all ages. The probe tips are all disposable and come in an assortment of sizes. The probe, which is serialized to the preamplifier, must be replaced along with the preamplifier if either breaks down. The preamplifier is powered by two 9-volt batteries. This feature helps to reduce the noise floor and limit the possibility of ground loop interference.

The Cube Dis™ software program was originally written in DOS, but knowledge of DOS is not necessary to operate the system. A Windows™ (Microsoft Corp., Seattle, WA) compatible version is also available that looks exactly like the DOS version. Access to Lotus™ (Lotus Development Corp., Cambridge, MA) is available through a down-load routine to an ASCII file. Single keyboard

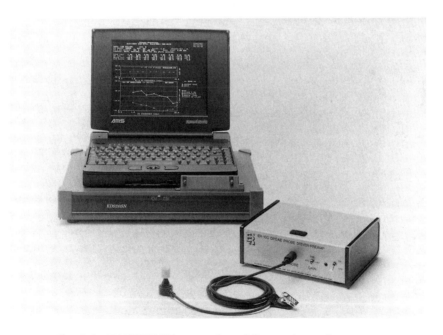

Figure 5–2. The Cube Dis™ DPOE system from Mimosa Acoustics.

strokes enable all the test functions. Although not extensive, the demographic data storage portion of the system is adequate and the menu is easy to follow.

One of the unique features of this product is the required probe calibration within the actual test ear before the test begins. The probe calibration is an assessment of the energy transfer function of the probe signal through the ear canal. The system automatically assesses the calibration and informs the examiner whether or not it is acceptable. Unacceptable calibrations can be redone with the aid of "help prompts" that allow the examiner to troubleshoot the situation. The computer makes adjustments for the results of the calibration run and alters the output of the probe to compensate for this transfer function information.

Test parameters may be selected individually for each test or stored for repeated use. The unit tests from the high to low frequency region. This is the only system capable of testing up to 11 kHz. The examiner can easily rerun a curve, and superimpose the results immediately. The ease and speed of this unit makes it practical to rerun tests in those cases that appear borderline. Typically, with 2 points per octave and a 5-octave range, the test takes about 2 min to perform.

The screen display is in color, making the noise floor easily discernable below the stimulus pair. The transfer function obtained during the calibration procedure is plotted at the bottom of the screen although this information does not directly assist the examiner in assessing the DP data. The original calibration data can be recalled. The stimulus levels, frequencies, DP levels, and noise floor are all displayed on the screen and on the hard copy. The data is automatically saved to the hard drive. The manufacturer makes no effort to determine pass–fail criteria; interpretation of test data is entirely in the hands of the examiner. The system is shipped from the manufacturer with the original Cube-Dis™ test software as well as the Cube-Dis R™, which includes an artifact rejection algorithm. The product is available from Mimosa Acoustics (Mountainside, NJ) and its authorized local representative.

MADSEN CELESTA 503 COCHLEAR EMISSIONS ANALYZER

This unit is the only "Kemp approved" DP system on the market. Otodynamics Ltd. (England, UK) licensed the technology to Madsen (Minnetonka, MN) for sale in the United States, Canada, and Europe. The Celesta can be interfaced with any IBM-compatible PC via the serial COM port. There are no boards to install, therefore, similar to the Otodynamics' (England, UK) Echoport, this instrument can be used with a laptop computer.

The system uses the probe design of the Madsen 901 (Minnetonka, MN) impedance bridge. It also uses the same nondisposable tips and shoulder harness that are supplied with the Madsen 901 (Minnetonka, MN). The probe is available in one size designed for use by all ages. This probe assembly can be separated and cleaned much like the impedance probe is cleaned.

The software is written in DOS and some knowledge of DOS is helpful. The examiner can customize the test signal bandwidths as well as change probe tone levels. The screen display contains extensive information but is quite easy to read. On-screen options, as well as presentation of data in graphic and tabular form make the interpretation of the data fairly easy. The Celesta can also display test results as a "normalized DP gram." Like the Cube-Dis,™ the demographic information field is somewhat limited. Data is stored by patient name, date, or patient number.

The Celesta does not specify pass–fail criteria requiring that decision to be made by the examiner. However, normative data collected from the National University Hospital of Copenhagen is incorporated into the system and can be displayed on the screen and on the hard copy. It should be noted, however, that these data were not obtained from neonates and, therefore, may not be applicable for newborn screening purposes.

The average test time can be as little as 1 min. The documentation for the Celesta is fairly complete and the instrumentation is easy to learn. This product is available through Madsen (Minnetonka, MN) and its authorized local representative or SID.

VIRTUAL MODEL 330 OTOACOUSTIC EMISSION SYSTEM

This distortion product system is the only system designed for MacIntosh™ (Apple Computer, Cupertino, CA) as well as DOS/PC-based computers. This product was the first DP system to obtain FDA approval and become commercially available. Virtual Corporation (Portland, OR) ceased operations and their technology has been purchased by Maico Hearing Instruments (Minneapolis, MN). A description of the Virtual 330 is included in this chapter for completeness and because the reader may come across Virtual instruments in his or her facility or in the literature. The hardware for both the MacIntosh™ and PC systems consists of a probe assembly and an interface box. The MacIntosh™ version can be housed with other Virtual products within the same computer making it a complete audiological laboratory. The PC version requires the installation of an internal board. The probe design is based on the Virtual Model 310 impedance design. The probe is difficult to clean and probe tubes are difficult to change. There are reports, however, that plans to change the probe design would rectify this problem.

The operation of the MacIntosh™ and PC versions are somewhat different with the PC version requiring more keystrokes than the MacIntosh™ version to run the test and store the data. Both versions allow the examiner to customize the screen and select test parameters. The examiner can select recording bandwidth, stimulus levels, number of data points per octave to test, and also adjust the noise floor rejection levels. The test data are presented extremely clearly on the screen and in the optional hard copy print out. DPs can be plotted as a function of F2 or the geometric mean and a plot of the physiological noise floor can be included with the data. The system also provides for the recording of extensive demographic information. The documentation for the Virtual DP system is fairly complete.

The Virtual does not provide a calibration routine nor is the examiner given any information regarding the probe fit. Thus, test validity is difficult to assess until the test run is completed. Neither statistical analysis of the test data nor normative data are provided. Like other systems, the Virtual does not determine the pass–fail criteria for the examiner. The basic test time is approximately 1 to 2 min.

The product had been available through Virtual Corporation and its local representative or SID. However, since Maico (Minneapolis, MN) has purchased the rights to the Virtual technology, it is unclear whether support exists for Virtual products. Consult your local special instrument distributor for further information.

BIO-LOGIC SCOUT™ AND RANGER™ OAE SYSTEMS

Bio-logic (Bio-logic Systems Corp., Mundelein, IL) was the first manufacturer to combine OAE and ABR devices in a single unit. Although Bio-logic's OAE and ABR systems (Bio-logic Systems Corp., Mundelein, IL) reside within the same computer, the software is not interrelational and the database is not shared. The OAE and ABR products are, therefore, treated by the computer and by the user as two separate instruments. For this reason the following discussion will be limited to the OAE portion of the system, the Scout™, Ranger™, and Sport™. The Bio-logic ABR system (Bio-logic Systems Corp., Mundelein, IL) will be described in the section devoted to ABR devices.

Of the three OAE systems produced by Bio-logic (Bio-logic Systems Corp., Mundelein, IL), the Scout is the more complete. The Sport™ is the portable version of the Scout™. Many features, however, are shared by all. systems. The software programs for the Ranger™, Scout™, and Sport™ are DOS based, and all systems can be operated on a notebook or desktop type of computer. The preamplifier is battery operated with externally attached 9-volt batteries so there is no concern regarding line current and ground loop artifacts. Both systems use the Etymotic Research Design ER 10C probe with many sizes of disposable tips.

The systems are easy to use. Both the Scout and Ranger use a "check -fit" for initial assessment of probe fit. The waveform and the signal spectrum are displayed to provide feedback about the quality of the probe placement in the ear canal and help the examiner to determine the integrity of probe placement. Both systems sweep the tonal pairs from high to low frequency over a range of 10 kHz to 100 Hz. Both systems monitor the level of the two probe tones—L1 and L2. The measurement parameters are user defined and preprogrammed protocols are available. Either system can be purchased with an optional printer that comes with documentation from the manufacturer.

The Scout™ and the portable Sport, ™ offer several advanced features that are not available in the Ranger™. The Scout™ gives the user the ability to define measurement based stopping rules by setting the maximum averaging time, overall noise level, and signal-to-noise ratio criteria. The purpose of these"stopping rules" is to minimize the test time while at the same time maximize the DP response. An automatic Test Replication Option is available in the Scout™ but not the Ranger™. On-line adjustment of the artifact rejection level is also available, which helps to maximize the DP response over the noise floor. Finally, the Scout™ offers many user-defined protocols while the Ranger™ is limited to just one. The approximate test time for both systems is 1–2 min.

Neither the Ranger™ nor the Scout™ determines the pass–fail criteria for the examiner. The data must be evaluated by the audiologist before a determination is made. The automated features of the Scout,™ including preprogrammed stopping rules and automated test replication, however, may be useful for screening

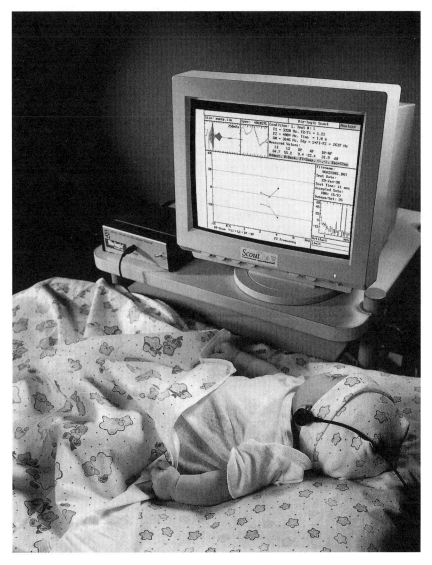

Figure 5–3. The Bio-Logic Scout™ DPOAE system. (Photo courtesy of Bio-logic Systems, Inc.)

programs that use nonprofessional screeners. The Sport™, their newest addition, features a hand-held unit that connects to the computer. It utilizes a rechargeable battery, which therefore eliminates the need for AC coupling or power cords. Again, this feature helps to reduce electrical interference and the need for isolation transformers. The Ranger,™ Scout,™ and Sport™ can be obtained through Bio-logic Systems Group (Mundelein, IL) and its authorized local representative or SID (Fig. 5–3).

THE CLARITY[R] SYSTEM FROM SONAMED CORPORATION

This is the only true, interrelational OAE/ABR screening product on the market. Both the OAE and ABR portions of this product share the same database so that demographic information need only be entered once for each newborn. The examiner can easily switch from OAE to ABR testing without leaving the program. It has a single user interface. Unlike other systems, the Clarity[R] system runs entirely in a Windows environment. The Clarity[R] may reside in a desktop- or notebook-type computer, but utilizes external bioamplifiers and preamplifiers for the ABR portion of the system. The company prefers to sell its Clarity[R] with its own mobile cart, which houses all the supplies as well as the monitor, printer and computer.

The OAE portion of the Clarity[R] is a DPOAE instrument. The system provides an insert earphone fit test to determine proper placement prior to running the OAE. The stimuli range is from 30 Hz to 12 kHz. The Clarity[R] product literature describes the system's ability to present multiple, simultaneous tone pairs, a feature that was first introduced by Grason Stadler (Milford, NH).

The examiner has several options for changing test parameters and data display, however, these choices are more limited than those available on other OAE systems on the market. The examiner can define the number of responses per octave and opt to perform either an intensity series or a frequency series. Responses from the right and left ears or multiple responses from the same ear can be overlaid. The portion of the program allowing changes in test parameters is protected by a security feature that permits access only to authorized individuals.

A fully automated response detection mode is incorporated into the OAE portion. According to the manufacturer, the examiner does not have to determine the pass–fail status of the OAE test. This is a unique feature of the Clarity[R] and simplifies decision making for nonprofessional screeners. The approximate test time is 1 min.

The system generates a complete report including OAE and ABR data, which is stored as a single patient file. The documentation from the manufacturer is somewhat limited. This is a relatively new product, and thus does not enjoy a wide user base. The Clarity may only be obtained directly from the SonaMed Corporation (Brookline, MA) and thus there is currently no local support (Table 5–1).

Auditory Evoked Potentials

Automated ABR Systems

THE SONAMED CLARITY[R]

The ABR portion of the SonaMed Clarity[R] (SonaMed Corp., Brookline, MA) can function as either a manual or an automated screener. The clinician selects the test protocols from a screen. Selections include an insert phone fit identification test, electrode impedance test, automated response detection, and response display. There is an automated protocol that selects the stimulus, ear, repetition

Table 5–1. Summary of OAE Systems Indicating Key Features of Each Device

	OAE Systems											
	TOAE	DPOAE	DOS	Windows	Laptop	Check Fit	Auto Protocols	Auto Stop Rules	Change Parameter	Norms	Simultan Mode	Data-base
ILO 88	•		•			•		•	•	•		
ILO 88 Echo Port	•		•			•		•	•	•		
ILO 88i	•	•	•		•	•		•	•			
ILO Dpi	•	•	•			•		•	•	•		
GSI-60		•	•	•		•	•	•	•	•	•	•
Celesta 503		•			•				•			
Virtual 330		•			•				•			
Scout™		•			•	•	•		•			
Ranger™		•	•		•	•	•	•	•			
Sport™		•	•		•	•		•	•			
Cube Dis™		•	•	•	•	•			•			•
Clarity^R		•		•	•	•	•		•		•	•

rates, time domain, maskers, and acquisition parameters. The clinician has the ability to override the automatic response detection mode and utilize a manual mode. A complete diagnostic ABR can be performed in the manual mode, making this system suitable for screening programs that must share equipment with the audiology or neurology department.

This unit is the only one on the market that can provide seamless ABR and OAE testing within the same system and within the same software and database. The database information is used for all patient information and report generation. The unit may currently be purchased directly from the SonaMed Corporation (Brookline, MA).

SMART-SCREEN™ FROM INTELLIGENT HEARING SYSTEMS

The ABR-based infant hearing screener is designed for use by a nonprofessional screener under the supervision of an audiologist. The system is DOS based, however, a new Windows 95 program will soon be released. The system may be installed in a full-size or lunch box PC. The examiner has a choice of transducers, including insert or supra-aural earphones, and bone vibrator. Either reusable silver-silver chloride electrodes or pregelled disposable electrodes can be used with the Smart Screener. The electrode impedance tester is built into the bioamplifier, which is battery powered. The touch screen option simplifies operation of the computer. The system is very flexible in that all stimulus and recording parameters can be adjusted and preset by the audiologist. The test parameter section can be accessed only by authorized individuals having the proper password.

The Smart Screener™ performs two full tests at each intensity level. When a predetermined signal-to-noise ratio is achieved, the averaging stops. The probability of a response is determined by a cross-correlation, statistical analysis and is reported as "probable response" or "no response."

The examiner can choose from a number of preprogrammed, automated, screening protocols or he can design his own. An automated threshold seeking option uses "chained stimuli," allowing the system to acquire responses from a range of intensity levels virtually simultaneously in 10- or 20-dB steps. The data is displayed on the screen, and can be printed out and stored in the patient record. There is a companion clinical ABR device, the SMART EP, ™ which will be discussed in the section devoted to full-scale diagnostic devices. The Smart Screen™ is available through Intelligent Hearing Systems (Miami, FL) and its authorized local representative or SID.

NATUS ALGO II

Originally marketed by Algotech, the ALGO™ was the first automated ABR screener to be marketed. The technology was bought by Nicolet and then by Natus Medical, Inc., which developed the most recent version known as the ALGO II. ™ Although the ALGO™ has undergone extensive research and development over the past 10–12 years, the response recognition algorithm, based on windowed template matching, has been in use since the 1980s (Fig. 5–4).

The ALGO II™ is extremely easy to use and is arguably the most foolproof screener on the market. The ALGO II™ has many features that make this instrument an excellent choice for nonprofessional screeners who must work with

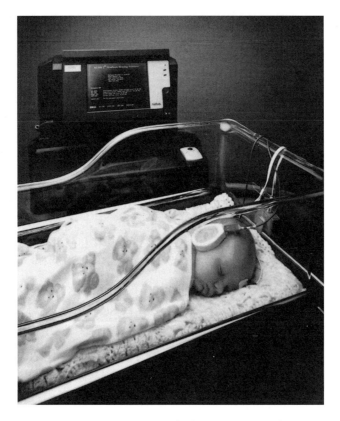

Figure 5–4. A newborn being screened with the Algo II.™ (Photo courtesy of Natus Medical, Inc.)

minimal supervision from the audiologist. The system monitors adequacy of test environment and will not run unless preset criteria for electrode impedance, level of myogenic activity, and ambient noise are met. Color-coded stimulus delivery tubes are inserted into clear plastic, circumaural cushions that allow the operator to view the covered ear and monitor the position of the earphone. Disposable electrodes are pregelled and application requires little or no skin preparation. The simplified three-electrode montage, forehead to nape with a common electrode on the cheek or shoulder, permits the operator to test both ears without switching electrode position in the preamplifier. The screen is simple and easy to read, supplying only essential information regarding electrode impedance, noise levels, ear being tested, and test outcome.

Several different automated protocols are available. The original protocol performs a screening test at one stimulus level, 35 dB. The ALGO II™ can test the right and left ears either sequentially or simultaneously or test each ear individually. There is also an automated two-stimulus level protocol that sequentially tests at 70 and 40 dB. Unlike the single-level protocol, this test mode allows the examiner to view the waveforms at the end of the test. In all modes, testing automatically terminates when the probability of a response, or likelihood ratio, reaches a preset criterion. If the criterion is not met, averaging will continue to a maximum of 15,000 responses. The system then scores the test as either a "pass" or "refer." Depending on infant state, ambient noise levels and robustness of the response, the ALGO II™ takes from 7–20 min to perform a screen.

The ALGO II™ uses proprietary supplies, that is, all disposable supplies including pregelled electrodes and circumaural earphone cushions must be purchased from Natus. Because supplies are not reusable and only can be obtained from Natus, the cost of an ALGO™ screen is higher (slightly less than $10 per test) than a screen performed by other ABR systems.

The ALGO II™ is a DOS-based system, and is internally protected at many levels. Natus (Natus Medical, Inc., San Carlos, CA) sells its system as a complete package: software, hardware, computer, printer, and cart. The company advertises that an OAE system can be housed within the Natus lunch box (Natus Medical, Inc., San Carlos, CA) style computer. Unlike the Clarity™, however, the OAE and ABR instruments operate as separate systems and information cannot be shared in a database.

Natus (Natus Medical, Inc., San Carlos, CA) prides itself on providing a "turnkey" operation to its customers. The company provides excellent documentation, a training videotape, and marketing materials. The ALGO™ is the most popular product in the automated ABR newborn screening domain. It should be noted, however, that this instrument was designed solely for screening purposes and has very limited diagnostic capabilities. The ALGO II™ is available directly from Natus Medical, Inc. (San Carlos, CA). All support and service must also be obtained through Natus.

Non-Automated ABR Screeners

GRASON STADLER GSI 55 ABR SCREENER

This unit is the only battery-operated ABR screener on the market. It is portable, weighing only 7 lbs, and easy to operate. The unit comes with a built-in electrode impedance check, monaural insert earphones with assorted size tips, a built-in printer, and travel case. The GSI 55 (Grason-Stadler, Inc., A Welch Allyn Co., Milford, NH) utilizes either standard nondisposable electrodes, or disposable electrodes, which are accommodated by a quick disconnect cable. Up to two waveforms at a time can be stored on the screen, marked, and printed. Because the GSI 55 (Grason-Stadler, Inc., A Welch Allyn Co., Milford, NH) runs entirely on batteries, there is reduced possibility for electrical interference from nursery equipment or line current. The test time with this unit may vary from 5 to 20 min, depending upon ambient noise levels and infant state. The manufacturer provides acceptable documentation.

Although the GSI 55 (Grason-Stadler, Inc., A Welch Allyn Co., Milford, NH) is a popular screener, due to its low price and portability there are, however, some important limitations. This one channel instrument has limited flexibility with respect to selection of stimulus and recording parameters and has no storage capability. The unit must be operated manually because there are no automated test protocols. Even more importantly, determination of pass or fail requires a professional who is trained in interpretation of ABR waveforms. These factors limit the usefulness of this system for programs employing nonprofessional screeners. The GSI 55 may be obtained through Grason-Stadler (Grason-Stadler, Inc., A Welch Allyn Co., Milford, NH) or its authorized local representative.

Clinical ABR Systems with Automated Protocols

This section will discuss clinical ABR instruments that have the capability of performing automated ABR routines and, therefore, can be considered for use in a screening program. The host computers of each clinical ABR system can house an OAE unit, thereby creating a complete screening system able to perform the recommended NIH protocol as well as follow-up diagnostic evaluations. It is important to note that *none* of the clinical ABR systems have automated response recognition capabilities and do not score tests as "pass or fail." An audiologist or other qualified professional will need to review and interpret each screening.

SMART EP™—AUDITORY EVOKED POTENTIAL SYSTEM

The Smart EP™ is the companion clinical ABR system to the Smart Screen, ™ which was reviewed above. The two systems are fully compatible and share the same hardware. The ideal test protocol recommended by the manufacturer is for screening to be performed with the Smart-Screen, then, if necessary, the Smart-EP™ software can be easily accessed for additional diagnostic data. The Smart EP™ can function as a screener itself. The device can be programed to perform automated test routines, however, unlike the Smart Screen™, the Smart EP™ will not automatically score the test as a "pass" or "fail." Standard reusable electrodes or pre-gelled disposables can be used. The examiner has the option of using a variety of transducers, including insert earphones, bone vibrator, and standard headphones. It is possible to use the Smart EP computer to host an OAE system. Thus, one could create a complete ABR/OAE screening and diagnostic package. The Smart EP™ may be obtained from Intelligent Hearing Systems (Miami, FL), or its authorized local representative or SID.

NICOLET COMPASS AUDITORY EVOKED POTENTIAL SYSTEM

This DOS-based instrument functions as a complete clinical ABR system. The Compass may be purchased in a desktop configuration, or as a notebook with a docking station, called the Portabook. All types of stimulus transducers are available for the Compass, including insert earphones, bone vibrator, and standard headphones. Either reuseable electrodes or disposable pregelled electrodes can be used.

The Compass provides the audiologist with enormous flexibility for creating test protocols that can be operated easily by trained, nonprofessional screeners. The examiner can initiate an automatic sequencing of tests based on user-defined protocols for either screening or threshold search with a single keystroke. The software provides function key options that help reduce interactive time with the equipment leaving more time for actual testing and reducing the potential for errors. Data retrieval is also accomplished quickly with a single keystroke.

Most OAE systems can be loaded and run through the Compass as the host computer thus making this a complete OAE/ABR screening and clinical package. The Compass is available for purchase through Nicolet Biomedical (Madison, WI) and through its authorized local representative or SID.

THE NICOLET SPIRIT™/BRAVO™

The dual platform OS2 (International Business Machines Corporation, Armonk, NY)/Windows™-based Nicolet Spirit (Nicolet Biomedical Inc., Madison, WI) is a full clinical evoked potential instrument. The Spirit™ and/or Bravo™ may be purchased as a desktop system or in a notebook docking station configuration. All types of stimulus transducers are available as are electrode options. Although is was not designed as a screening instrument per se, the Spirit™ has the proprietary "Maximum Length Sequence" (MLS) test, which uses high repetition rates in its test protocols. With repetition rates as high as 1600 clicks/sec, a test could be conducted in less than 5 min. The MLS, therefore has been regarded by some to be a viable tool for hearing screening.[17] Like traditional ABR, the responses obtained from the MLS test must be interpreted and scored by a qualified professional.

An additional feature of the Spirit™ (Nicolet Biomedical Inc., Madison, WI) that makes it suitable for a screening program, is the availability of preprogrammed protocols. The manufacturer supplies several protocols, however, the examiner can create his or her own. With the multiple software options available for the Spirit, ™ the unit can be configured as a versatile clinical unit in addition to its use as a screener.

A basic word-processing capability is standard in the system and an optional report writing software package is available for greater flexibility and creativity. Most OAE systems can be loaded and run on the Spirit, ™ making it a complete ABR/OAE screening/clinical package. The Nicolet Spirit™ and/or Bravo™

Table 5–2.   Summary of ABR Systems Indicating Key Features of Each Device

			ABR Systems				
	DOS	*Windows*	*Battery Powered /Option*	*Laptop*	*Auto Score*	*Auto Protocols*	*Change Parameters*
ALGO II™	•				•	•	
Smart Scr.™	•			•	•	•	•
Clarity^R		•					•
GSI-55			•				•
Smart EP™	•	•		•		•	•
Compass/ Portabook	•			•		•	•
Spirit/ Bravo™		•		•			•
Traveller^R	•						•

may be obtained from Nicolet Biomedical (Madison, WI), and its local authorized representative or SID.

BIO-LOGIC TRAVELER EXPRESS[R] AND NAVIGATOR E[R]

According to the manufacturer specifications, the portable Bio-logic Traveler Express[R] is essentially the same as the desk top Bio-logic Navigator E[R] (Biologic Systems Corp., Mundelein, IL). This DOS-based system comes with either one or two channels and is preconfigured from the factory to include both screening and diagnostic test protocols. Thus, the Traveler[R] could function as the ABR system for the hearing screening program as well as the diagnostic clinical program. The Traveler[R] can utilize either reusable or disposable electrodes. A single keystroke command can initiate an automated test protocol that can perform the test and store the data. ABR data can be downloaded to another computer for analysis and report generation or performed on the host Traveler.[R] Although the test sequences can be run automatically, as with other clinical units, the data must be interpreted and scored by a professional. As mentioned above, the Bio-logic Traveler[R] can be combined with the Bio-logic Scout™ or Ranger™ OAE system (see description in OAE equipment section) or other OAE systems to provide a complete package for a screening and clinical protocol. The Bio-logic Traveler is available through Bio-logic Systems Group (Mundelein, IL), or its authorized regional representative (Table 5–2).

Associated Products

Grason Associates, Inc., (Berlin, MA) recently released a line of "single-use" eartips. These tips, which are available in 12 sizes, can be used for OAE systems, acoustic immittance instruments, and audiometric insert earphones. While equipment manufacturers neither endorse or rebut these claims, Grason Associates (Berlin, MA) claims to have developed its products to fill the void left by

Table 5–2.   (*Continued*)

ABR Systems						
User Defined Protocols	*Combine w/ OAE*	*Disposable Electrodes*	*Data-base*	*Full Diagnostics*	*Latency Information*	*Threshold Search*
	•	•				
•	•	•	•			•
•	•	•	•	•	•	
•		•			•	
•	•	•	•	•	•	•
•	•	•	•	•	•	•
•	•	•	•	•	•	•
•	•	•	•	•	•	•

those manufacturers whose tips are nondisposable. Single use, or disposable tips obviate the need for sterilization and may be a practical solution to infection control problems. These tips are available from the manufacturer, or the local SID in your area.

EarCare Products (Glen Cove, NY) manufactures disposable earphone covers, which are acoustically transparant and made of elasticized polypropylene fabric. These "bonnets" fit over all standard earphone cushions, which normally come in contact with the patient's ear. Here too, disposable cushion covers may help to address any question about the need sterilize or disinfect stimulus transducers.

References

1. Thorton AR, Obenour J. Auditory response detection method and apparatus. U.S. Patents #4,275,744, 1981. Reviewed in J Acoust Soc Am 1981;70:1814
2. Kileny PR. New insights on infant ABR hearing screening. Scand Audiol 1988;30(Suppl):81–88
3. Jacobson JT, Jacobson CA, Spahr RC. Automated and conventional ABR screening techniques in high risk infants. J Am Acad Audiol 1990;1:187–105
4. Marlowe J. Screening all newborns for hearing impairment in a community hospital. Am J Audiol 1993;2:22–5
5. Kemp D. Stimulated acoustic emissions from within the human auditory system. J Acoust Soc Am 1978;64:1386–91
6. Stevens JC, Webb HD, Hutchinson J, Connell J, Smith MF, Buffin JT. Click evoked otoacoustic emissions in neonatal screening. Ear Hear 1990;11:128–33
7. Uziel A, Prion JP. Evoked oto-acoustic emissions from normal newborns and babies admitted to an intensive care baby unit. Acta Otolaryngolica 1991;482(Suppl):85–91
8. Kennedy CR, Kimm L, Dees DC, Evans PIP, Hunter M, Lenton S, Thornton RD. Otoacoustic emissions and auditory brainstem responses in the newborn. Arch Dis Child 1991;66:1124–9
9. White KR, Vohr BR, Behrens TR. Universal newborn hearing screening using transient evoked otoacoustic emissions: Results of the Rhode Island Hearing Assessment Project. Semin Hear 1993;14:18–29
10. Bonfils P, Uziel A, Pujol R. Screening for auditory dysfunction in infants by evoked otoacoustic emissions. Arch Otolaryngol Head Neck Surg 1988;114:887–90
11. Joseph JM, Herrmann BS, Thornton AR. Well-baby hearing screening using automated ABR. American Speech–Language–Hearing Association, Anaheim, November, 1993.
12. National Institutes of Health Consensus Statement. Early identification of hearing impairment in infants and young children. 1993;11:1–24
13. Maxon AB, White KR, Behrens TR, Vohr BR. Referral rates and cost efficiency in a universal newborn hearing screening program using transient evoked otoacoustic emissions. J Am Acad of Audiology 1995;6:271–7
14. Joint Committee on Infant Hearing. 1994 Position Statement. AA0-HNS Bulletin 1994;12(12):-insert
15. Kemp DT, Ryan S, Bray P. A guide to the effective use of otoacoustic emissions. Ear Hear 1990;11:93–105
16. Kemp DT, Ryan S. Use of TEOAE in screening. Semin Hear 1993;14:30–44
17. Eysholdt U, Schreiner C. Maximum length sequences—a fast method for measuring brain-stem evoked responses. Audiol 1982;21:242–50

APPENDIX A

The National Center for Hearing Assessment and Management (NCHAM) has assembled the following summary of information from research studies and clinical experience in an effort to help programs select appropriate equipment.

Issue	AABR	DPOAE	TEOAE
1. Cost of equipment (These figures are based on suggested retail prices by the manufacturer and include all necessary equipment to conduct newborn hearing screening. In those cases where the screening equipment is sold but requires a computer to operate, we have included the cost of a moderately priced computer. The cost for a printer is not included.)	Natus ALGO II $15,500 ALGO-E $ 9,000 Intelligent Hearing Systems Smart Screener $11,850	GSI 60 $10,500 Bio-logic $12,750 Virtual $10,000 Mimosa $ 9,000	Otodynamics ILO88 Echoport $9,000
2. Cost of supplies (Included here is the cost of all necessary supplies and reoccurring expenses [e.g., calibration] for doing screening. It does not include supplies for communicating the results of screening with parents or pediatricians, printing educational materials, or other ancillary materials. Costs are estimated per baby based on reported usage by typical programs with 1000–4000 births per year.)	$8.50–10.00 per baby includes the costs of disposable earphones and electrodes	$.50–1.50 per baby includes the costs of disposable tips for the probe assembly, calibration, and probe replacement	$1.00 per baby includes the costs of disposable tips and for the probe assembly and replacing the probe assembly every 750 babies
3. Initial training of screening technicians (Although it is possible to start any program by reading the literature that comes with the equipment and teaching yourself, most programs find that hands-on, competency-based training by someone who is already experienced with that particular equipment and has used it successfully is the best way to begin a program. Estimated times are based on the experience of operational programs and include only the initial training of screening technicians. Regular supervision with additional upgrading of skills should be included in addition to this initial training.	2 h	4 h	4 h

4. Time to do screening per baby

(This is often misunderstood because the term "screening time" is used by people to refer to different aspects of the screening process. As used here, it is the total amount of time devoted to screening babies and includes getting the baby ready for screening, talking to the parents if necessary, setting up the equipment, conducting the screening, recording information about the baby so results can be retrieved later, etc. "Screening time" is best computed by taking the total number of hours worked by screening technicians and dividing that time by the number of babies screened during that period. Numbers for each device are based reports of well-established programs.)

4. Time to do screening per baby	20–40 min per baby	15–30 min per baby	10–20 min per baby

5. What is being measured?

(None of the devices is a direct measure of hearing. Instead, each one measures slightly different physiological mechanisms which are related to hearing. Issues related to this are discussed below.)

5a. What degree of hearing loss is likely to be detected?

As used in most programs, the ALGO II uses a 35 dB-nHL click and, consequently, would probably miss children with very mild sensory hearing losses (25 or 30 dB). An alternative mode for the ALGO II measures 40 dB and 70 dB and, thus, would also miss such children.	Although there is not unanimous agreement, most researchers believe that DPOAEs will only be detected when hearing is better than 40 dB nHL. Thus, children with mild losses would be missed.	There is substantial agreement that TEOAEs will be detected if hearing threshold is 25 dB nHL or better. Thus, children with mild losses would generally be detected.

Issue	AABR	DPOAE	TEOAE
5b. Is frequency-specific information available? (In addition to indicating whether or not a child has a hearing impairment, some people are interested in knowing at what frequencies that hearing impairment is likely to occur. Others argue that the purpose of a screening test is not to provide detailed information about the nature of the loss, but to identify those children who need further diagnostic tests, during which information about frequency and severity of hearing loss can be determined.)	The ALGO II only provides information about whether or not a hearing loss is likely. No frequency specific information is available.	DPOAEs have the best potential for providing frequency-specific information, and some argue that it may even be possible to use DPOAEs as a diagnostic tool. However, this has not been sufficiently demonstrated. There is general agreement that DPOAEs provide more information about the higher frequencies (6–10 kHz) than do TEOAEs, but most would agree that the improved information in these higher frequency areas is not critical for hearing screening.	TEOAEs provide information about the frequencies at which emissions are detected between 1 and 5 kHz. However, the absence of an emission at a particular frequency with neonates does not always correspond to a hearing loss at that frequency.
5c. What is being measured?	The AABR provides information about the auditory pathway up to the brainstem (including the middle ear, the inner ear, and the VIII nerve).	DPOAEs provide information only up to and including the cochlea. Hence, infants with central auditory processing problems would not be discovered. Although definitive prevalence data are not available, most experts agree that this represents less than 1% of all children with hearing loss, or less than 3 children per 100,000 in the general population.	TEOAEs provide information only up to and including the cochlea. Hence, infants with central auditory processing problems would not be discovered. Although definitive prevalence data are not available, most experts agree that this represents less than 1% of all children with hearing loss, or less than 3 children per 100,000 in the general population.

6. Scoring criteria and ease of interpretation (Because DPOAEs and TEOAEs produce a wave form for each infant, users must decide what constitutes a pass or a refer. Because the widespread use of these techniques is fairly recent, there is not universal agreement on what criteria should be used. In practice, however, this lack of agreement affects a small number of infants, because in most cases emissions are clearly present or clearly absent, and it is only the relatively small number of infants around the cut point where disagreement occurs.

The ALGO II equipment uses a predetermined algorithm, which is interpreted by the computer based on the data gathered. Thus, interpretation is easy, and there is no argument abou what the pass criteria should be. Studies that have compared the results of the ALGO II with expert scoring of conventional ABR have found agreement ranging from 83 to 98%.

DPOAEs are the most recent of the techniques, and, not surprisingly, there is a lot of disagreement about what constitutes a pass or a refer. Most people have tended to use fairly conservative pass criteria until more data are available. The numerical criteria are easy to interpret, and most programs use technicians to make this determination in less than 1 min per baby.

Although they have been used extensively since the early 1990s, there are still many different pass/refer criteria being used in TEOAE-based newborn hearing screening programs. The most frequently used criteria recommended by NCHAM is a very conservative criteria. Using this numerical criteria, interpretation is straightforward and is done in most programs by technicians in less than 1 min per baby.

7. Flexibility of administration

Because it was intended to be a completely automated system, the ALGO II is designed to have little flexibility. This is viewed by most people as an advantage. It is possible to screen at either 35 or 40 dB and 70 dB, and it is possible to screen both ears simultaneously or each ear separately.

There is a lot of flexibility in how the test is administered. Unfortunately, there is little agreement about what parameters are best for screening. This is particularly true with respect to the different primaries to be used for f_1 and f_2 and the intensity of the stimulus. There is also little agreement on how many data points per octave are required for an adequate test.

Although there is a great deal of flexibility with regard to collecting TEOAE information, parameters used in screening programs are usually those recommended by NCHAM (e.g., QuickScreen, low frequency filter, 50 low-noise samples, peak stimulus between 78 and 83 dB SPL).

Issue	AABR	DPOAE	TEOAE
8. Referral rates (Screening is designed to identify a small group of at-risk infants who will require further diagnostic testing. As in all screening programs, it is expected that some children who have normal hearing will be referred for further diagnostic testing, but the lower this number is, the better.	Reported referral rates at the time the infant leaves the hospital for programs using the ALGO II equipment range from 1 to 10%, with an average of about 4%.	Reported referral rates at the time the infant leaves the hospital for DPOAE programs range from 4 to 15%, with an average of about 8%. Because most DPOAE programs do a two-stage screening process where those who do not pass before discharge from the hospital are rescreened before referring them for diagnostic testing, the percentage referred for diagnostic testing is about 1%.	Reported referral rates for infants at the time they are discharged from the hospital range from 3 to 12%, with an average of about 7%. Because most TEOAE programs are a two-stage screening program, with infants who are referred at the time of discharge from the hospital being screened a second time before being referred for diagnostic assessment, the percentage of infants referred for diagnostic assessment ranges from 1/2 to 1%.
9. Screening in noisy situations. (Noise that interferes with screening can come from the external environment or from the baby. Because hospitals in general [and newborn nurseries in particular] can be quite noisy, many people have questions about the effects of noise on newborn hearing screening procedures [this is especially true for intensive care nurseries.])	The ALGO II manual recommends that babies be in a "deep quiet sleep" for screening to be done. An artifact reject system stops collecting data when ambient noise is >50 dB SPL at 2000 Hz. Thus, the equipment can be used in noisy settings, but data collection is slower.	The key to screening in noisy situations is achieving good probe fit. Not all DP equipment provides feedback regarding adequacy of probe fit. Most DP units have artifact reject systems which exclude noisy data from averaging. Thus, the equipment can be used in noisy settings, but data collection is slower. Because DPOAEs measure one frequency at a time, they are more susceptible than TEOAEs to a response at that frequency being obscured by noise. Babies do not need to be asleep, but a noisy baby will slow data collection substantially.	The key to screening in noisy situations is achieving good probe fit. The ILO88 provides excellent real-time information to monitor probe fit and has an artifact reject system, which excludes noisy data from averaging. Thus, the equipment can be used in noisy settings, but data collection is slower. Babies do not need to be asleep, but a noisy baby will slow data collection substantially.

10. How many children with hearing loss will pass the screen?

(These children are often referred to as false-negatives and reported as a measure of the test's sensitivity. It is important to minimize the number of infants in this category. While no screening test is perfect, ideally, as few children as possible should be in this group. This does not refer to children who have late onset losses, but instead is only concerned with those children who have impaired hearing at the time of the test and still pass the screen.

Infants with very mild losses (25 to 30 dB) will likely pass the screening as will infants with high-frequency losses, reverse slope losses, or precipitous losses.

Children with hearing losses less than 40 dB, as well as children with reverse slope losses and neural or central auditory pathology.

Children with neural or central auditory pathology or children having reverse slope losses.

11. Cost per infant screened

(Although there has been numerous reports in the literature and anecdotal reports about the cost per baby screened in newborn hearing screening programs, most of these analyses are based on gross estimates of time devoted to different tasks, or have been incomplete [e.g., have ignored fringe benefit costs for personnel, indirect costs, supervisory costs] or costs associated with supplies and equipment. How the program is organized can also have a big impact on the cost per baby. Because of such factors, people trying to interpret reported costs should be very cautious and remember that cost per baby is primarily a function of how long it takes to do the tasks, coupled with the hourly rate of people doing the work and the cost of supplies, equipment, and facilities.

Reported costs range from $15 to $75 per baby.

We are unaware of any reports of costs per baby, but expect that they would be similar or a little bit higher than those reported for TEOAE.

Reported costs range from $8 to $30 per baby.

APPENDIX B
SOURCES FOR ADDITIONAL INFORMATION AND TO PURCHASE OAE SYSTEMS AND AUDITORY EVOKED POTENTIAL SYSTEMS

1. Bio-logic Systems Corp.
   One Biologic Plaza
   Mundelein, IL 60060
   708-949-5200, 800-323-8326
2. EarCare Products
   40 Glen Street
   Glen Cove, NY 11542
   800-229-4634
3. Grason Associates, Inc.
   23 South Street
   Box 277
   Berlin, MA   01503
   508-838-2124
4. Grason-Stadler, Inc., A Welch Allyn Co.
   One Westchester Dr.
   Milford, NH 03055
   603-672-0470
5. Intelligent Hearing Systems
   10689 N Kendall Drive, Suite 315
   Miami, FL 33176
   305-595-9170
6. Madsen Electronics
   5600 Rowland Rd.
   Minnetonka, MN 55343
   612-930-0804, 800-362-3736
7. Maico Hearing Instruments, Inc.
   7375 Bush Lake Road
   Minneapolis, MN 55439
   612-835-4400, 800-328-6366
8. Mimosa Acoustics
   P.O. Box 1111
   Mountainside, NJ 07092
   908-518-0711, 800-805-7515
9. NASED—National Association of Special Instrument Distributors
   P.O. Box 870923
   Stone Mountain, GA 30087-0024
10. Natus Medical Inc.
    1501 Industrial Road
    San Carlos, CA 94070
    415-802-0400, 800-225-3901

11. Nicolet Biomedical, Inc.
    5225 Verona Blvd.
    Madison, WI 53711-4495
    608-273-5000, 800-356-8088
12. Otodynamics, Ltd.
    32-38 Beaconsfield Road
    Hatfield, Herts, AL 108BB
    England, UK
    +44-1707-267540,800-659-7776
13. SonaMed Corp.
    68 Harvard Street
    Brookline, MA 021436
    617-232-6499

6

The Normal Newborn Nursery

GRACE ROWAN

Introduction

The newborn nursery is unique in that it is the one place in the hospital where a patient's arrival is a joyous event. This "healthy patient," nevertheless, requires specialized and coordinated care and handling to help him or her make a successful transition into the world. The audiologist and hearing screener participate in this important process by virtue of their role in the evaluation of the newborn. It is essential, therefore, that the audiologist and screening technician be familiar with the nature, characteristics, and behavior of these small patients. In addition, insight into the emerging relationship between infants and their parents will help to guide the screener to interact appropriately with new parents. Because the screener must work within the nursery and coordinate his or her activities with other nursery personnel, it is also necessary that he or she be thoroughly familiar with the protocols, routines, flow, and dynamics of the newborn nursery. In this way, the screener can function as a knowledgeable member of the nursery team. The result will be an effective and smooth screening operation. The purpose of this chapter is to describe the normal newborn and the environment in which he or she will be cared for after birth. Throughout the discussion, practical suggestions for screeners working within the newborn nursery will be made.

After Delivery

In many hospitals today labor and delivery can occur in the same room, thus eliminating the inconvenience and discomfort of transferring laboring women from the labor room to a delivery room for the birth, as is the practice in the traditional setting. This single-room maternity setting is referred to as a Birthing Room, or LDR Labor Delivery Recovery. This setting allows parents and other family members to become acquainted with their new family member and is conducive to providing a family-centered care approach. In this setting a nurse can perform the newborn system assessment as well as educate the parents/grandparents about the unique characteristics of their newborn, and assure the new family of a caring, secure and safe environment. Depending on the institution and space allocated for the hearing screen, the screening technician may perform the hearing screen in the room in the presence of the family. This allows the screener an opportunity to observe family dynamics.

> If the screening technician "feels" something just is not right with a witnessed interaction between mother and baby, he or she should bring it to the attention of the primary nurse.

In the traditional setting, the normal full-term newborn is transferred from the delivery room to the admission nursery shortly after birth. Depending on the protocol of the hospital, the newborn may go to the nursery in the mother's arms or via transporter crib. The father usually accompanies the newborn to the nursery, a practice that encourages the father–infant attachment. Upon arrival in the nursery, the newborn is placed under a radiant warmer. At this time, the newborn nurse and the labor and delivery nurse perform the following tasks:

A: check the identification bands to verify name, spelling, identification number.
B: verify sex of the newborn.
C: verify the official weight and length.
D: place a temperature probe on the newborn.
E: report is then given relating pertinent prenatal history of the mother, labor history, delivery information, postdelivery care of the newborn.

The "first" bath is usually given within the first hour after birth if the newborn temperature is stable.

Next to establishing respirations, heat regulation is most critical to the newborn's survival. From the moment of birth, the initial focus is assisting the newborn in temperature regulation. Newborns are prone to heat loss because they have a large surface area in relation to body weight. Newborns have less adipose tissue for insulation, thinner skin, and blood vessels in close proximity to the skin surface allowing them to experience a greater transfer of heat to the external environment. The newborn's mechanism for producing heat is primarily through increased metabolic processes. Cold stress significantly increases metabolism, thus requiring an increase in oxygen and calorie consumption. Heat loss in the newborn is decreased by vasoconstriction of blood vessels. Shivering, a major mechanism of heat production in the adult, is rarely seen in the newborn. To increase heat production the newborn will increase his or her metabolic rate and muscular activity. This is evidenced by an increase in respiratory rate. Non-shivering thermogenesis (temperature regulation), is the main method of heat production in the newborn. To prevent cold stress, or what is commonly referred to as hypothermia, the newborn is placed in a heated environment (under a radiant warmer), or in a heated isolette, until he or she is able to maintain thermal stability (Table 6–1).

Just as cold stress can effect the newborn's oxygen and calorie consumption, so can overheating. A neutral thermic environment is the ideal. The newborn will respond to an increased temperature by dilating blood vessels to dissipate

Table 6–1.   Signs of Hypothermia

Pallor
Mottling
Tremors
Cool skin

heat. This is referred to as hyperthermia. A full-term newborn is capable of per-spiring and may then lose heat through evaporation. A sign of hyperthermia is increased perspiration. As in hypothermia, the metabolic rate and oxygen consumption will increase. The newborn's temperature is assessed on admission to the nursery and then at least every hour for the first 4 h of life. After that, temperature is assessed once per shift as long as a normal body temperature is maintained.

At all times, newborn care and procedures must take place in a draft-free environment. Be sure that the location of the hearing screen is free of drafts and takes place in a neutral temperature. If any of the signs of hypothermia or hyperthermia are observed, if the newborn feels unusually warm or cold to the touch, or appears to be breathing rapidly, the nursery personnel must be notified immediately.

Transition

The newborn requires a thorough skilled observation to ensure a satisfactory adjustment to extrauterine life. The time period immediately after birth is referred to as transition and may last anywhere from 4 to 8 h. During transition, a complete systems assessment and the estimation of gestational age of the newborn is performed by the nursing staff.

Vital signs (VS) are checked every h for the first 4 h. If at any time the VS are not within the normal range they are checked more frequently and the pediatrician is notified. The bottled fed infant is offered either water or formula approximately 3–4 h after birth, but if the mother is breast feeding she usually begins in the LDR, immediately after birth.

Nursery Routines

Although each institution may vary somewhat, newborn nursery routines are basically the same in all hospitals. The newborn requires observation, assessment, nutrition, and care. The first 2–8 h after birth are the most crucial to adaptation to extrauterine life. How the newborn responds during this initial time period is an excellent indicator of how he or she will be during hospitalization. If the newborn is responding well (i.e., he or she maintains thermal stability, color, respiration and heart rate within normal limits), the newborn can be brought to the mother's bedside for feeding, interaction, and continued bonding[1]. Private pediatricians are notified of the newborn's arrival shortly after the birth and usually examine the newborn within the first 8–12 h of life, but many nurseries today have house staff or nurse practitioners available to assess the newborn immediately upon arrival.

Newborn Characteristics

Each newborn is an individual with unique characteristics and capabilities. The following briefly reviews the appearance and characteristics of the normal newborn.

Head: The newborn head is disproportionately large in relation to the rest of the body. The average head circumference is 13–14." This is in direct response to the birth process, and the molding that takes place during the birth process. Swelling is normal and it will subside in several days. One noticeable difference between the vaginally delivered newborn and the cesarean newborn is that the head of the vaginally delivered newborn is sometimes misshapen. Sometimes swelling occurs on either side of the top of the head of a baby delivered vaginally. The head of the cesarean newborn is well rounded, not molded by the birth process. The neck muscles of the newborn are weak, and the newborn head is heavy. Therefore, it is important that the head be supported at all times when the baby is lifted. The forehead is usually large and prominent.

Of great concern are the "soft spots," or fontanels. The anterior fontanel is diamond shaped and is located on the top of the head. The posterior fontanel is triangular shaped and is located toward the back of the head. These are areas in the skull where the bones are not joined, but instead are held together by membranes. They allow for molding during the birth process, and also for further growth of the skull. The anterior fontanel should not appear indented or bulging. One might notice pulsation, which is normal.

Eyes: The eyes should appear clear, without redness. However, pressure during birth may cause the rupture of a capillary resulting in a small subconjunctional hemorrhage. This will absorb in 2–3 weeks. The color of a baby's eyes is usually gray or dark blue. Because the lacrimal ducts are not fully developed, the baby will cry without tears. Newborn babies will blink at bright lights. Many times they appear cross-eyed. This is because the eye muscles are not fully developed.

Newborn babies are able to see objects at a distance of 12–15" from them. When newborns are quiet and alert, they can focus on objects. They prefer to look at human faces, complex patterns, and slow moving objects.

Ears: Even before birth the newborn can hear. A newborn will respond to a familiar voice in the delivery room by turning toward the sound. Hearing becomes more acute several days after birth as the amniotic fluid in the middle ear space and ear canal is completely absorbed. Vernix, a cheesy white protective skin covering, may also be present in the ear canal. This takes several hours to absorb. For this reason, it is best to do the hearing screening *at least* 6 h after birth. The external ear of the newborn is soft and bends easily.

> It is important to check the alignment of the ear when positioning the baby on his or her side to avoid bending of the pinna.

Nose: The nose sometimes appears large for the face, small "white heads" may be noted on the nose which are referred to as *milia*. These are immature oil glands and will disappear without treatment. Newborns have a refined sense of smell. They can recognize differences in smells and can differentiate between the smell of their own mother's milk and that of another mother's milk. The activity of the newborn will increase in the presence of strong odors.

> It is important that staff working in the newborn nursery do not wear strong-smelling perfumes. Strong perfumes use up oxygen in the air and can affect newborn breathing and oxygen consumption.

Red spots may be noticed on the forehead, bridge of the nose, eyelids or nape of the neck, which are referred to as "stork bites or angel kisses." These are actually minute blood vessels that are close to the skin. They fade over time, however, they will appear more prominent when the newborn is crying.

Arms and Legs: A newborn's arms and legs are proportionately short for his or her body. You will note his or her arms are usually bent and held close to the chest with the hands in fists. The position of the legs may be tucked, similar to the position in utero and for this reason may appear bowed. This well-modulated posture is the hallmark of an infant in a calm and stable state[2] (Table 6–2).

Reflexes: Newborns do not consciously control their movements but they are equipped with certain protective reflexes. Newborns will sneeze to clear their nasal passages and blink when their eyelashes are touched or a bright light shines in their eyes. Newborns do feel pain and will pull away from painful stimuli (i.e., pinprick in the heel from blood work). Yawning is also considered a protective reflex.

Two very important protective reflexes are the gag reflex, which prevents choking, and the cough reflex, which expels mucous. The infant delivered by cesarean section usually has more mucous than the vaginally delivered newborn. This is due to the fact that the cesarean section newborn did not pass through the birth canal, which compresses amniotic fluid from the lungs.

> If newborns gag or appear to have mucous in their mouth, turn them on their side and pat the upper back gently. If gagging persists, summon help.

Table 6–2.   The Screener Can Help the Newborn Attain an Optimal State for Screening by Providing Physical Boundaries

Keep Newborn in Flexion:
1. Swaddling
2. Facilitate flexed hands to face
3. Facilitate tucking
4. Use supportive rolls
5. Tightly cradle newborn when holding

Adapted from Als 1982 from ref. 2.

Rooting, swallowing, sucking, and grasping are survival reflexes. The rooting reflex is evidenced by the newborn turning and opening his or her mouth in search of a nipple for nutrition, when the side of the cheek is touched. If the palm of the newborn's hand is touched he or she will grasp your fingers firmly and be able to hold on supporting some or all of his or her body weight. This is referred to as the grasp reflex.

Newborns are not born helpless. If an object is placed over the newborn's nose and mouth, he or she will twist away from it vigorously, or attempt to knock it off with his or her arms. A newborn lying on his or her stomach, will lift his or her head and turn to the side to avoid smothering. A healthy baby should remain on his or her back at all times.

Periods of Reactivity

In the period immediately after birth, the newborn progresses through a series of predictable behavior patterns known as periods of reactivity. The newborn may need specialized nursing care during each period because adaptations, especially respiratory and thermoregulation, are not always accomplished smoothly and in a timely manner. The first 30 min after birth finds the newborn alert, crying vigorously, possibly sucking on anything that comes in contact with his or her mouth, and generally appearing interested in the environment. This is the first period of reactivity. After this initial stage of interacting with the environment, the newborn enters a period of inactivity. At this time the newborn is relatively calm and eventually enters the sleep phase. An attempt to stimulate the newborn at this time will illicit a minimal response. This period usually lasts about 2–4 h. The heart rate, respirations, and body temperature will decrease. It is important to avoid exposing the newborn to cold stress (undressing or bathing) at this time.

When the newborn awakes from this deep sleep and begins to interact with the environment, it is a signal that the second period of reactivity, which can last anywhere from 4–6 h, has begun. During this time the newborn is once again somewhat interactive with the environment. Heart rate as well as respiration increases and temperature begins to stabilize. During this phase there may be a variation noted in respiratory and cardiac rates. There may even be period of apnea (no breathing), tachypnea (fast breathing), gagging, regurgitation of mucous, and transient cyanosis (blue color), alternating with periods of quiet sleep. In the second stage of reactivity, most healthy full-term newborns achieve a state of equilibrium. This means that the transition from intrauterine to extrauterine life has been accomplished successfully[3]. The hearing screening can be performed at this time.

Sleep Cycles

After adjusting to the new environment after birth, a newborn will sleep anywhere from 4–6 h. Sleep cycles are often associated with how often the newborn eats. Six states of sleep have been identified in the infant: deep sleep, light sleep, drowsy, quiet alert, active alert, and crying. Each state has specific characteristics. The movement from state to state varies with each newborn. Some move gradually while others make abrupt transitions.

Properly identifying the sleep state can help identify the best time to perform the hearing test.

Deep sleep: The newborn is very quiet in this state. Breathing is rhythmic and with a regular pattern. An occasional sucking movement may be made with his or her lips and the newborn may also startle (jerk). The newborn cannot be roused during the state of deep sleep. He or she may awaken for a moment, then resume the state of deep sleep. This is the best state in which to do the hearing screen (Fig. 6–1).

Light sleep: In this state the newborn will have his or her eyes closed, but movement may be seen behind the lids. In light sleep the breathing is irregular. In this state the newborn moves, makes noises, sucks, and grimaces. He or she will respond to noises during this state.

Drowsy: In this state the newborn breathes irregularly and responds to sensory stimuli in a lethargic way.

Quite alert: Breathing is regular. In this state the newborn lies still, will look at objects calmly with bright wide eyes, and will focus attentively on what he or she hears or sees.

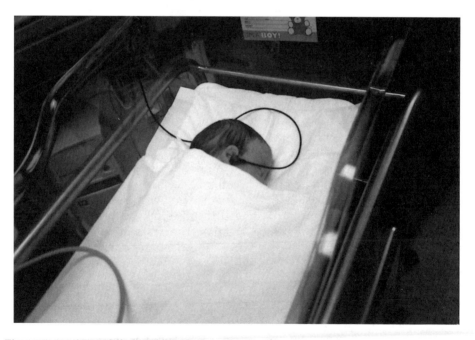

Figure 6–1. A swaddled and blanketed infant in the newborn nursery undergoing transient otoacoustic emissions screening. An infant in deep sleep is in the optimal state for hearing screening.

Table 6–3.   What to Watch for in the Newborn

1. Color—normal pink
   • hands and feet may appear blue due to the newborn's immature circulation system or being cold.
   • a blue ring may appear around the mouth. This is called **circumoral cyanosis** and should be reported. In some cases, this may be normal and will disappear upon stimulation of the newborn (i.e., crying).
   • Tongue and gums should be pink, if blue report immediately.
2. Breathing may be irregular at times—this is normal
   • sounds—breathing should be quiet. If breathing is noisy, especially on expiration, this should be reported.
   • rate—normal rate is between 40–60 breaths per minute. Notice of nasal flaring must be reported.
   • apnea—Periods of *no* breathing-lasting longer than 15 sec. Stimulate the newborn and call for help.
3. Mucous in the mouth is normal
   • Keep the newborn on his/her side, (use of a rolled blanket behind the newborn's back will keep him/her properly positioned), the mucous will drain from the mouth and will cause no distress in the infant.
   • The newborn should be positioned on his/her right side after a feeding. This encourages escape of air from the stomach and minimizes risk of regurgitation.
   • to avoid the risk of mucous occluding the oropharynx, do not place an unattended newborn in a supine position.
   • gagging—call for assistance, turn the infant to his/her side, pat or rub the back. Ask to be shown how to use bulb syringe.
4. Thermal neutrality
   • reduce potential for hypothermia or hyperthermia.
   • Heat loss increases metabolism and oxygen consumption.

It cannot be overemphasized that all significant changes in the newborn status and behavior must be reported promptly. This allows for quick assessment and treatment if necessary.

Active alert: Now, the newborn does not lie still; he or she is readily affected by hunger, fatigue, noise, and too much handling. Breathing, at this time, will be irregular. This is the time he or she needs comforting. If acted on immediately, one may be able to calm the baby and prevent him or her from entering the crying state.

Crying state: Crying is a signal that tells us that the newborn is tired, wet, hungry, lonely, etc. The newborn at this time will move around actively, making faces and breathing irregularly (Table 6–3).

Bonding

There is wonder, excitement, and a sense of relief when a baby is born. The birth of a baby stirs more emotion than any other event in our life experience. The impact that a newborn has on all who come in contact with him or her is magical and awe-inspiring when one thinks how little we have consciously done to create this perfect person. Meeting and greeting this new individual for the first time requires a "private" period of time. This special time is referred to as bonding. Bonding has been defined as the initial phase in a relationship thought to be characterized by strong attraction and a strong desire to interact.[4] Bonding is a process of rapid attachment that takes place after birth. Not all mothers, however, feel instantly close to their newborn. The relationship begins in the delivery room and continues to develop over time, as does any relationship between two human beings who have just met for the first time.

The acquaintance process can be observed through maternal and newborn interactions and behaviors. Babies arrive in the world with a special fascination for their parents' faces. Newborns have the ability to make eye contact with their parents right after delivery. This spontaneous visual curiosity draws the parents to their newborn and is not only rewarding for the parents, but also fosters the attachment process. The attachment process is a reciprocal relationship that must be mutually satisfying to both participants who must gain a sense of comfort with each other.[5]

Maternal touch has been described in detail by Klaus and Kennell.[6] A mother touching her newborn for the first time, touches only small portions of the newborn's body, using her fingertips ever so gently. As she becomes more comfortable with herself as a mother, she will use her hand in a stroking manner over larger portions of the newborn's body. Eventually as familiarity and comfort increase, the mother will enfold the newborn in her arms and hold the newborn close to her body.

Fathers initially tend to remain in awe and at a physical distance from the newborn in the delivery room, while staring at the infant maintaining a face-to-face position. One may describe this as being engrossed or all-consumed with the newborn. Along with an unusual sense of excitement, a hovering, protective behavior is observed. Touching the infant immediately is not common, but embrace behaviors will increase with encouragement. Positive father–newborn interaction can be promoted by pointing out the newborn's unique capabilities and characteristics. Fathers are usually "hooked" when they learn that newborns are interactive with the environment and possess special unique abilities and are capable of social responses.

Events during the early hours and days following birth can effect the parent–newborn acquaintance. Prolonged separation and the events preventing initial newborn contact are factors that can have an influence on the parent–newborn relationship. Giving praise, providing information, encouraging interaction, and providing time alone are all ways to enhance this special developing relationship.

> The screener should keep the bonding process in mind when he or she takes the newborn away from the nursery or the mother's bedside for the screening. The mother needs to know where the infant will be at all times and that the infant will be safe.

The Newborn Nursery

Most hospitals provide mothers the opportunity to keep their newborns with them in their hospital room. This arrangement known as *rooming-in*, allows the mother and newborn to have continuous contact 24 h a day. Mothers who room-in with their newborn may also have access to a central nursery. This central nursery may be used during visiting hours or by the mother when she desires a period of uninterrupted rest. Today, in most institutions, there is a limited time when all newborns are in the nursery.

In newborn nurseries, infants are cohorted. A cohort usually consists of all well newborns born during the same 24- to 48-h period. These neonates remain assigned to this single room for the duration of their stay. When necessary, the newborns are moved as a group to the next open nursery room. This process allows for adequate cleaning and preparation of the room for the next group of newborns or cohort.

Each nursery is equipped with a patient finder board. The name of the newborn is listed under that room designation. At night, if not rooming-in, the newborn is returned to the assigned nursery. To accommodate the pediatricians, some hospitals will designate certain time periods when all newborns must be returned to the nursery for evaluations, exams, blood work, hearing screen, etc. Some institutions, on the other hand, perform all these activities at the mother's bedside.

Safety and Security

Security and identification of the newborn is of utmost importance in all institutions. The staff at each hospital must be completely familiar with the identification policy and security system in the institution. It is imperative that staff know where the newborn is at any given time of the day or night.

> Personnel working in the newborn nursery, such as a phlebotomist, photographer, technicians, and audiology staff, MUST be aware of the security policy and practice for the hospital. Discretion must also be used when giving out information regarding the newborn they are caring for.

The newborn must be identified with the mother each time the newborn is brought to the mother. Each newborn wears two bands, one on the wrist and one on the ankle. The newborn should never be handed to the mother or father without first checking the identification bands of the infant and parent. The identification of the infant should also be checked before the infant is examined by the nurse, physician, or technician. The crib is also identified with a name tag, which should be checked against the identification bands to ensure that the newborn is in the proper crib.

Performing the newborn screening on every newborn requires collaboration and a team effort. The screening technician must be aware of the safety and security system of the unit he or she is working in as well as be familiar with the unit philosophy and everyday routine. In many institutions, the hearing screen will be done throughout the day with little disruption to the unit. This is often the case when a separate area has been designated to perform the procedure. The newborn can be taken from the mother's room after an introduction and explanation of the procedure and brought to an area for the test. The family should be given the option of accompanying the newborn and the technician to the test area.

> It is very important that the new family feel safe in turning their newborn over to this total stranger—the hearing screener. It is helpful for the screener to wear some sort of

identifying badge or uniform that identifies him or her as part of the screening staff. The screener can then be easily identified and recognized as "official" hospital personnel with whom parents can entrust their infant.

A newborn should never be removed from the newborn nursery or the mother's bedside without the mother's and staff's knowledge. A mechanism must be instituted within the institution to inform the staff and mother of the newborn's location at all times.

Documentation

Chart: The newborn chart is usually kept at the main desk area of the newborn nursery. Flow sheets attached to the crib, however, permit easy charting at the cribside when recording intake, output, temperature, and teaching of the parents. The completion and the results of tests are recorded on the progress note section of the newborn chart. Documentation that the hearing screening was performed can be entered on the flow sheet which will become part of the permanent medical record for the infant.

> A specially designed stamp that indicates that the hearing screening was performed is a time-saver and acceptable for documenting the screening in the newborn's chart. The imprint should be signed and dated by the person performing the test.

Log Book: This vital book records the name of every newborn admitted to the hospital. The following information will be found in this book: (1) last name of the newborn, (2) medical record number, (3) date of birth, (4) sex and weight of the newborn, (5) name of the mother, (6) type of delivery, (7) blood type of mother, (8) name of pediatrician and obstetrician, (9) date of newborn screening, and (10) a comment section.

It is useful to record the hearing screening in the nursery log. This allows for a quick check to ascertain which infants have been screened, when the screen was performed, and which newborns are still in need of screening.

Infection Control

Handwashing: Upon entering a newborn nursery all personnel working or handling the newborn must scrub at the start of their shift or activity to minimize transmission of disease. An antiseptic soap-filled brush is provided for this scrub. Minimal amount of jewelry may be worn, but should be removed for the antiseptic scrub. Between touching or handling the newborn, hands must be washed thoroughly with soap and water. Disposable gloves may be used but are not necessary.

> Handwashing is the primary method of infection control. It is important to check the infection control book within the institution for other requirements.

Equipment: The sharing of equipment leads to the spread of infection. Therefore, there should never be any sharing of equipment, clothing, or blankets between babies. To prevent this, each newborn crib is completely stocked with all the items needed to care for that infant. If a blanket or other item falls to the floor, it should be replaced with another.

Attire: Usually staff working on the maternity/newborn units wear scrub attire. This is not mandated in all institutions, each hospital has its own dress code for postpartum and newborn nursery personnel. Those who perform tests or examine infants should be sure that their clothing does not touch the newborn. Some institutions require the wearing of cover gowns or use of a barrier when handling the newborn in the newborn nursery. However, this type of covering has not been confirmed as an effective method of infection control.[1]

Personnel: Anyone with an infection (sore throat, herpes simplex, upper respiratory infection, gastrointestinal infection, or skin lesions) should be excluded from working with either the mother or baby.

Summary

The screener needs to exercise care in the performance of the hearing screen, keeping in mind the needs of the newborn, the family, and the rest of the nursery staff. It is important that the screener respect the role of the nurse who will ultimately determine when a baby is ready to be screened. As was pointed out above, the newborn's status is labile throughout transition. The nurse caring for the newborn is in the best position to assess the readiness of the newborn for the hearing screen.

The mission of the screening technician, to ensure that every newborn receives a hearing screening before discharge, must be carried out with little or no disruption to the newborn nursery routine. This is a challenge and can only be accomplished through cooperative efforts among the staff. The screener must be sensitive to the needs of the newborn, family, and nursery staff. To maximize the potential for a positive experience, it is of utmost importance that the roles and responsibilities of the nursery staff be defined and adjusted to meet the needs of all involved.

References

1. American Academy of Pediatrics and American College of Obstetricians and Gynecologists. *Guidelines for Perinatal Care* (3rd ed). Elk Grove Village, IL, American Academy of Pediatrics, 1992
2. Als H. Toward a synactive theory of development: Promise for the assessment and support of infant individuality. Infant Mental Health J 1982; 3:229–43
3. Pelleteri A. *National Child Health Nursing* (2nd ed). Philadelphia, Lippincott Co., 1995
4. Klaus M, Klaus P. *The Amazing Newborn.* Menlo Park, Addison-Wesley, 1985
5. Bolton IJ. *When Bonding Fails: Clinical Assessment of High Risk Families.* Beverly Hills, Sage, 1983
6. Klaus MH, Kennel JH. *Maternal–Infant Bonding* (2nd ed). St. Louis, C.V. Mosby, 1982

7

The Neonatal Intensive Care Unit

KATHI SMILLIE

Introduction

The Neonatal world is a very delicate and fragile one. Over the years it has evolved into one of the most technical, sophisticated areas of health care dedicated to the care of the sick newborn. It is an organized world of routines, procedures and protocols carried out by highly trained personnel with one goal in mind: to dramatically improve each infant's outcome. Hearing impairment is of major concern in the neonatal intensive care unit (NICU), as these infants are at high risk for this condition. Providing hearing screening for these newborns will significantly improve their outcome as it relates to developmental milestones such as hearing, speech, and social skills.

Organization of the NICU

Physical facilities for perinatal care in hospitals are categorized into three levels. Level I facilities provide areas for resuscitation, admission, observation, normal newborn care and parent-neonate visitation. Infants cared for here are generally normal full-term or preterm neonates who weigh more than 2000 grams at birth and have adapted well to extrauterine life. Additionally, some of these Level I nurseries can provide continuing care for neonates with relatively uncomplicated problems that do not require more advanced services.

Level II facilities provide the same services as Level I hospitals, however, they are capable of handling sick neonates who may not require intensive care, but who require additional nursing care hours. The care is more complex than the care rendered in a Level I setting and the equipment required is more technical, i.e. incubators, radiant warmers, ventilators, cardiac monitors, infusion pumps, etc.

Level III facilities, also called tertiary care facilities, provide high-tech care for severely ill infants who require constant nursing care and continuous cardiopulmonary support for survival (Fig. 7–1). Because emergency care is provided

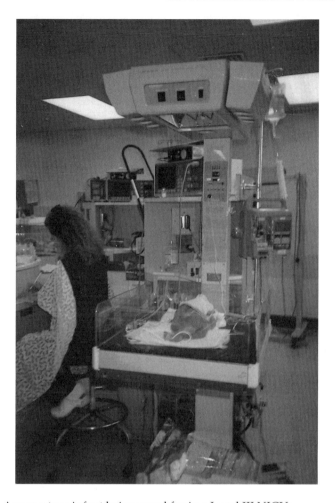

Figure 7–1.   A premature infant being cared for in a Level III NICU.

here, laboratory and radiological services are available 24 h a day as well as complete consultative services. There is also a greater number of nursing, medical, and surgical personnel required, as well as a greater amount of high-tech equipment and supplies to provide Level III care. Level III facilities also provide high-risk infant transport bringing sick infants from the community hospitals to the tertiary care center for intensive care (Table 7–1).

Many Level III units will transport their convalescing babies back to their Level I and II nurseries of birth. Some neonatal intensive care nurseries have intermediate care areas or continuing care areas within their facility to which they transfer their inborn babies when they no longer require intensive care or higher levels of care. The infants who would meet criteria and be eligible for hearing screening are those infants who require intermediate care or less. These infants

Table 7–1. Perinatal Care Facilities

Level of Care	Type of Service	Staffing Ratios
I	Routine care of normal full-term or preterm neonates who have adapted successfully to extrauterine life	1:6–8
II	More complex care of the sick neonate *not* requiring intensive care, but requiring more nursing hours per day	1:3–4
III	Severely ill infants requiring constant nursing care and continuous cardiopulmonary monitoring and support	1:1–2

are generally those who are older and ready for discharge within the next several days.

Intermediate Care Nurseries (ICNs) are open rooms with the capacity to hold a number of growing newborns. Each infant is individually assigned to a nurse or caregiver based on the feeding schedule, complexity of care, and number of diagnostic tests needed to be performed that would require transport to another department or area within the hospital. All of these factors impact on the daily routine of each infant and ultimately, on the availability of each infant eligible for hearing screening. The staff nurse assigned to each infant must work closely with the audiologist to coordinate an optimal time for the screening to be performed.[1]

Nursing Staff

The different patient populations, protocols, and demands of the newborn nursery and the neonatal intensive care unit (NICU) require different training on the part of nurses who staff these two areas.

The newborn nursery nurse is a Registered Nurse (RN) who completes training and orientation in the care of the well newborn. Training also addresses assessment and identification of an infant in distress. Being alert to subtle signs and symptoms of an infant who may be getting sick is an integral part of caring for the well newborn.

A neonatal nurse is an RN who completes an additional 16 weeks of specialized training and orientation in the care of the very sick infant. This training includes certification in basic life support (BLS), as well as neonatal advanced life support (NALS). NICU nurses are also trained to go out on transport to area hospitals to pick up critically ill infants and bring them to a tertiary level facility for high-risk care. They are trained to handle any and every aspect of intensive care for the very sick, critical infant.

Continuing the care of high-risk infants requires close observation and monitoring of their vital signs and their needs in relation to nutrition, cardiopulmonary support, infection control and elimination, as well as their developmental needs and the physical environment that surrounds them. Staffing in the ICN is maintained at 1:3 or 1:4 depending on acuity and complexity of care.[1] A modified primary nursing model is practiced in most nurseries where the registered nurse is responsible for the "total" care of an infant during his or her shift. Often, there are two or more nurses in each ICN room caring for their assigned infants. Additionally, there may be physical therapists, respiratory therapists, neonatologists, developmental team members, ophthalmologists, social workers, speech pathologists, and ancillary personnel present, each carrying out specific roles throughout the day. Good communication between the staff nurse and the screener is vital to identify the infants eligible for hearing screens, as well as to identify an appropriate time for each infant to be tested. The screener must also understand that delays and changes may be made based on certain occurrences or an emergency situation that may arise at any given time.

Unit Routines

The nursing care in the ICN focuses on continuous assessment and observation of the neonate. While providing daily care and feeding, nurses are constantly assessing the infant for temperature instability and change in activity (including any change or refusal of feeds), any unusual change in skin color, abnormal cardiac or respiratory rate or rhythm, or any alteration in elimination patterns. In turn, they are also concerned with the physical environment in the nursery. Excessive stimulation should be avoided especially since these are growing premature or chronically ill neonates. Noise levels should be lowered and low-level lighting is all that is needed for adequate observation. Unit activities and routines, such as monitoring vital signs, care and feeding, and tests and procedures, should all be altered or "clustered" to allow for diurnal cycles and rest or nap intervals. It is important that the screener and the RN collaborate to determine the best time to perform the hearing test on each infant.

As mentioned before, routines are often based on the feeding schedules in the ICN. Each infant is fed every 3 to 4 h and care rendered accordingly. The audiologist/screener should perform the hearing screen no sooner than 1 h after the last feeding so that the risk of aspiration is minimal.

The nurse assesses each baby's vital signs (i.e., temperature, pulse, respiration, and blood pressure), as well as measures the infant's abdominal girth every 3 to 4 h before feeding and reports any unusual findings to the physician before starting feeds. The screener must understand that the nurse's assessment before and during feeding to determine an infant's feeding tolerance may affect whether he or she will release an infant for a hearing test. If the nurse determines that an infant is lethargic, having frequent periods of apnea, or "just not acting right," it may be in the infant's best interest to delay the test until further observation and examination can be made. Additional stress for the infant could prove detrimental at this point. The nurse and the screener need to communicate well so all aspects of the baby's care can be coordinated to include the required tests and procedures.

Special Equipment

Because constant nursing and continuous cardiopulmonary support is provided in the NICU and the ICN, equipment and supplies are highly technical and should be part of the orientation for anyone having direct patient contact.

Each room and patient station is supplied with multiple outlets: electrical outlets, oxygen outlets, compressed air outlets, and suction outlets. These outlets are connected to regular and auxiliary power in case of an emergency outage situation.

Every infant in the ICN is housed in either an open bassinet where they are dressed and blanketed or in an enclosed incubator used for thermal regulation (i.e., temperature control). Each infant is attached to a cardiac monitor with chest leads and to an oximeter via a probe to measure the oxygen saturation. The screener must learn how to disconnect the wires and probes so the crib can be rolled into the screening room. Also, if the infant is still in an incubator, the screener must ask a nurse to transfer the infant into an open crib for transport to the screening room.

Often the infants in the ICN are "learning" to nipple and trying to grow. During this course, they may require enteral feeding via a nasal or orogastric tube. These are thin feeding tubes that are taped to the nose or mouth for intermittent feeding purposes. The screener should never disturb this tube and should notify the RN if the tube dislodges, or if the infant gags. The infant may also be sucking on a pacifier, as non-nutritive sucking is encouraged for infant development.

Many infants in the ICN require antibiotic therapy or fluid therapy that is infused via intravenous (i.v.) lines. The intravenous catheter or butterfly can be found in an infant's hand, arm, foot, and sometimes even the head. Great care must be taken not to dislodge these lines as i.v. access of these infants is usually very difficult.

Some infants may have a central line in place (i.e., Broviac) and may be going home with this line intact for fluid/medication/chemotherapy purposes. Great care and gentle handling should be practiced if an infant has such a line because they are "surgically" implanted and dislodging them would require further surgical intervention. It is important that a nurse must be notified immediately if this line is leaking or accidentally dislodged.

All i.v. lines are connected to an infusion pump. Most units use infusion pumps or auto-syringe pumps. These pumps run on battery so they can be disconnected, then reconnected following the test. A nurse should be available to do this. Again, it is imperative that a nurse be immediately notified of any incident involving a pump or an i.v. line.

Proper care of the equipment during procedures is vital. Never leave pumps on top of other equipment, and make sure all equipment is reconnected and properly plugged in when the infant is returned to the nursery.

Developmental Behaviors

High-risk infants communicate through certain behaviors and cues that are recognized as vital to each infant's development. The NICU nurse coordinates the

Table 7–2   Signs of Infant Stress

- Decreased heart rate
- Decreased respiration
- Constant sucking
- Dilated pupils
- Infant turning toward stimuli
- Fingers stretched out toward object
- Eyes fixated
- Suck searching
- Hands to the mouth
- Hand clasping

infant's care and daily interventions with the infant's awake states, giving special attention to behaviors indicating that the infant is stressed or overstimulated.

Recognition of these behaviors and stress reactions by the hearing screener can be helpful in obtaining a more accurate test result and influence infant development. Some examples of these behaviors or "cues" include signs of attention, such as a decrease in heart rate or respiration, constant sucking, dilated pupils, turning toward the stimuli, fingers stretched toward an object, eyes fixated in an alert and inactive state, suck searching, hands to the mouth, and hand clasping (Table 7–2). Behaviors indicating fatigue may include decreased muscle tone, increased respirations, yawning, tongue thrusting, closed eyes or gaze aversion (Table 7–3). Signs of overload (Fig. 7–2), or too much stimulation, can be detected with a change in color, finger splaying, extension of extremities, a worried frenetic stare, irregular heart and respiratory rates, even gagging or vomiting (Table 7–4).

As was mentioned previously, reducing detrimental stimuli such as decreasing noise levels and lowering light levels, as well as avoiding sudden position changes or movement, will assist with maintaining an optimal developmental state for the neonate. Providing appropriate developmental interventions is vital. This is achieved by limiting stimulation and paying attention to positioning, such as flexion of the extremities and using blanket rolls to create boundaries and contain arms and legs.

Gentle swaddling of the infant enhances positioning that promotes motor development and reduces stress. Respect for the infant's sleep–wake cycles is achieved by providing a calm and relaxing visual and auditory environment.

Table 7–3.   Behaviors Indicating Fatigue

- Decreased muscle tone
- Increased respirations
- Yawning
- Tongue thrusting
- Closed eyes
- Gaze aversion

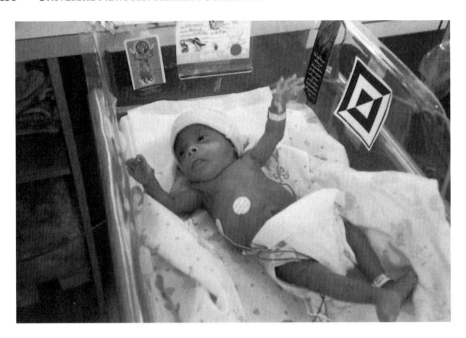

Figure 7–2. An NICU infant showing signs of overstimulation.

Encouragement of non-nutritive sucking is a soothing practice that has positive developmental implications. It has been linked to facilitating earlier bottle or breast feeding, increasing weight gain, and increasing oxygenation of the preterm infant.

Every member of the health-care team requires some knowledge of the premature baby's developmental needs. Tending to these needs through assessment and application of appropriate interventions will help these preterm infants avoid depleting their already limited physiological reserves, and will not only assist the hearing screener with obtaining a quicker, clearer, and more accurate test result, but assist nurse and screener with determining the best time to perform the test.

Table 7–4.   Signs of Overstimulation

- Color change
- Finger splaying
- Extension of extremities
- Worried frenetic stare
- Irregular heartbeat and respirations
- Gagging and/or vomiting

Common Problems

Respiration

Every premature infant has a "normal" respiratory pattern of periodic breathing. This is described as short, recurring pauses in respiration of 5- to 10-sec duration. However, many premature infants experience a complete cessation of respirations greater than 10- to 15-sec duration, which is known as "apnea." An apneic episode or spell may also be accompanied by other physical changes such as circumoral cyanosis, bradycardia, or hypotonia. Very often, diffuse tactile stimulation, such as tapping the infant's foot, will stop the spell if begun immediately. A mask and ambu bag should be set up in the testing area in case its use is required (Table 7–5).

Within 10 to 15 sec after the onset of apnea, the infant's heart rate may start to drop below 100 beats per minute. This is known as bradycardia. Because the infants are often removed from monitors prior to being tested, this condition may be undetectable during the screening test. It is important to alert the primary nurse immediately when sign of an apneic spell or episode is observed (Table 7–5). The nurse will respond by using the mask and ambu bag if necessary or by placing the infant on a cardiorespiratory monitor to appropriately and accurately record the event.

It is important for the screener to know that apnea and bradycardia can be indications of more serious problems, such as hypoglycemia, mild dehydration and temperature fluctuation, to name a few.

Temperature

Temperature control (thermoregulation) of all infants is an important concern. Infants do not have the ability to regulate body temperature as well as older children and adults. Brown fat, a substance that can be quickly metabolized to generate heat, is lacking in the preterm infant. This presents a greater challenge to the caregiver in promoting thermoregulation.

Normal body temperature for neonates ranges from 35.5 to 36.5°C. Factors effecting the neonate's ability to maintain normal body temperature include evaporation, convection, conduction, and radiation. Chilling and cold stress brought on by these environmental factors can result in increased metabolism and oxygen consumption and depletion of glycogen stores. Caregivers must be certain to modify environmental factors, adjusting room temperature and preventing drafts. Infants typically wear caps to prevent heat loss from the head. As

Table 7–5.   Apnea of Prematurity

- Cessation of respirations >10- to 15-sec duration
- Circumoral cyanosis
- Bradycardia (heart rate drops below 100 bpm)
- Hypotonia

Table 7–6.   Situations in Which an RN Must be
Notified Immediately

- Any dislodged or leaking tube (oral, nasal, or intravenous)
- Any blood backed up into a tube
- An alarm sounding on any piece of equipment
- Any color change
- Absence of respirations
- Choking or gagging

---

neonates advance along the gestational continuum toward full term, maturing and gaining weight, their ability to regulate body temperature improves.

Feeding

Awareness of the signs and symptoms of feeding intolerance is important for the screener working with preterm infants. Apnea and bradycardia after feedings can be a sign of fatigue for the infant learning to nipple feed. Breathing problems, anemia, and the inability to coordinate the suck, swallow, and breathing mechanism simultaneously can necessitate tube feedings. Infants with respiratory problems cannot breathe as easily on a full stomach. Indeed, the screener will note the practice of elevating the head of the crib, which is done for most babies after feedings to facilitate breathing. Vomiting can result in aspiration of gastric contents into the lungs, which can lead to pneumonia. The screener should report any signs of distress to the nurse immediately (Table 7–6).

Bilirubin Levels

Hyperbilirubinemia is a condition in which the level of bilirubin in the infant's blood rises and causes the skin to look yellow (jaundice). Phototherapy treatment of infant jaundice includes the use of blue and white fluorescent lights, which have been shown to help the body break down bilirubin. The infant is placed naked under the lights in a heated isolette to expose as much skin as possible to the lights. The eyes are covered with a patch. Infants coming out of phototherapy for feedings and procedures need to be dressed and covered in a blanket.[2]

Documentation

Accurate recordkeeping is an important aspect of any screening program. The hearing screen supervisor keeps a log book of each infant's name, date and type of screen performed (e.g., otoacoustic [OAE], auditory brainstem response [ABR]). The primary nurse, as part of the discharge planning process, informs the parents of the importance of the hearing test and that it is noninvasive, takes a short period of time, and will assist in determining if their baby is at risk for hearing impairment. A pamphlet entitled *A Hearing Test For Your Newborn* is included in the neonatal unit parent information packet on admission to Schneider Children's Hospital and it answers common questions that a parent may have regarding hearing screening. The audiology supervisor is also available to field any questions or concerns that may arise.

The hearing screener documents the infant's pass–fail status in the log book. If an infant fails the initial OAE, a second screening test known as an ABR is performed. The screener records the results of the screening test in the patient chart and on the Neopath Caremap in the designated area by initialing the appropriate box. A "red dot" is then placed on the infant's isolette or crib to indicate that a hearing screen has been performed. This enables the hearing screener to do a perfunctory check in each ICN to identify any babies that may have been missed.

Infection Control

All nursery personnel having any significant contact with a neonate should be free of any transmissible disease. All screeners are required to be cleared by Employee Health Services to ensure they have clean health records and to report any illness they may have. Any time a screener has a rash, open lesion, exposure to chicken pox, or any audible active respiratory condition, he or she should be removed from patient care and not handle patient care equipment until the condition resolves (*Guidelines for Perinatal Care,* p. 117).

As mentioned in the previous Chapter, the most important means of preventing the spread of any infection is careful and thorough handwashing. In the NICU, at the beginning of each shift, before handling a neonate, all personnel should wash their hands and arms to a point above the elbow. An antiseptic (antimicrobial) handwashing agent should be used and a 3-min scrub using a scrub brush from fingertips to elbows is recommended. After washing, hands should be rinsed thoroughly and dried with paper towels. The 3-min scrub is only required at the beginning of the shift; a 15-sec wash—without a brush, but using soap with vigorous rubbing—is required before and after handling each neonate and after touching objects or surfaces likely to have been contaminated. It is imperative that all personnel involved in direct patient contact understand and adhere to the rigid handwashing practices described above.

All screeners with direct patient contact should wear a short-sleeve cover gown or other type of barrier clothing to avoid contact between the newborn and their clothing. Most importantly, any information about an infant with a communicable disease or potential infection (i.e., HIV, hepatitis, and TB) should be communicated to the screener. If an infected or potentially infected neonate is to be handled outside the bassinet, a long-sleeve gown should be worn over the screener's clothing and discarded after use. Nonsterile gloves should be used as a barrier in any infected or potentially infected case.

Nosocomial infections are difficult to define in newborns. The most useful definitions exclude those infections that develop within 24 to 72 h of birth because many of these organisms are acquired from the mother rather than from the hospital environment. Once a nosocomial infection is identified, surveillance and analysis by hospital infectious disease personnel is vital to prevent clustering and a potential outbreak. Cohorting infants can be established to minimize transmission of microorganisms or infectious diseases among different groups of neonates. This is accomplished by keeping all infants possibly infected with the same organism colonized or in a single room for their entire hospital course. Although it is possible to schedule the same personnel to care for these infants, this is often not practical in an NICU setting. Once discharged, the room must be cleaned and disinfected prior to admitting another neonate from a different group. If neonates are placed in cohort for a potential epidemic situation, the hearing screener should be made aware of the situation and should adhere to and follow established practices.[1]

Safety

Maintaining a safe environment is a key element in any NICU. This begins with proper identification of each infant by checking the ID band prior to testing. The screener should identify himself or herself to the parent or caregiver at the bedside and give a brief explanation for their presence while coordinating a "best time" with the infant's nurse.

Although each screener is taught how to disconnect an infant from a cardiac monitor and an oximeter, it is wise to ask the nurse if he or she prefers to perform this task.

When transporting an infant in an isolette or crib, the screener should never leave the baby unattended. The head of the bed should always be in the flat position during movement of a crib. All isolette doors and latches should be secured during transportation and during the testing period when possible. Wheels are to be locked into place when not moving the crib or isolette. The hearing screener should never touch any dials or switches on the isolette. A nurse should be immediately notified if a dial or switch is accidentally touched, or if the alarm sounds.

Occasionally a baby may be going home on a cardiorespiratory (apnea) monitor. If so, the infant can never be removed from the monitor even for the few minutes it takes to do the hearing screening. The screener should attempt to perform the test at the baby's bedside, or ask the nurse to move the equipment with the baby attached and remain within earshot to listen for an alarm.

All equipment is to be plugged into the appropriate outlets. Any wire fraying or broken plugs, etc. should be reported to the nurse immediately. It is also good practice to be gentle with the handling of any equipment (Table 7–7).

Education

As stated elsewhere in this book, education of the entire neonatal nursing and medical staff about the importance of having a hearing screening program for high-risk patients is essential. Nurses and physicians working in the NICU need to understand that they play a key role, not only in protecting the hearing ability of their neonatal patients, but also in taking an active role in establishing and participating in a hearing screening program.

Multiple in-services should be provided to all NICU staff, focusing on education related to types of hearing loss, the benefits of early detection, and the types

Table 7–7. Safety Measures in an NICU

Baby:	• Properly identify each infant by checking the ID band
	• Latches on isolette doors should always be closed
	• *Never* leave babies unattended
	• *Never* walk or turn away from open isolettes
Equipment:	• Know the use and care of equipment
	• Never leave pumps or monitors on top of isolettes
	• Make sure all equipment is plugged in properly
Electrical:	• Do not use water on babies with i.v. in place and a pump plugged in
	• Have spills mopped up promptly
	• Make sure all equipment is properly grounded

of screening methods available to detect hearing loss in infants. Details of the hearing screening programs should be added to the neonatal nursing orientation program so that new nurses can immediately incorporate this most beneficial program into the basic care of the neonate, as well as help increase parents' awareness of the importance of early identification of hearing loss. New fellows and residents should also be apprised of the importance of having a hearing screening program and its benefits for high-risk neonates.[3]

Nursing Point of View

In an NICU, dealing with helpless infants whose parents are often traumatized by the shock of a premature birth, nurses often take over and become the infant's gatekeeper. Introducing a new program that will affect or change already established practices and protocols in an NICU is a difficult process, to say the least. Acceptance of a new program by the staff is a slow process of in-depth education and implementation of a well-thought-out, organized program that is easy to follow with minimal disruption to their everyday care.

The nursing and medical staff must believe that they play an important role in protecting the hearing ability of their patients, as well as a vital role in helping to implement the screening program to buy into it. Their understanding must include helping to educate parents about hearing loss, language and speech milestones, as well as the importance of hearing screening and appropriate and timely interventions implemented when needed. Support and encouragement from the nursing and medical staff will be helpful to parents trying to process all the information they receive throughout their baby's illness.

Cooperation with hearing screening personnel is important and key to the program's success. Nurses tend to follow routines and activities of daily living on a strict schedule. When faced with heavy assignments and diminishing resources, their perception of an added test (no matter how brief) is that it is disruptive to their normal routine. Learning to work with hearing screening personnel as a member of the health-care team is imperative. Proper introductions and establishment of a positive working relationship are important. Each nurse and screener must develop mutual trust in their relationships with one another, as well as respect for and understanding of the importance of the hearing test, and that it is everyone's responsibility to ensure that the test is done on every baby.

References

1. American Academy of Pediatrics and American College of Obstetricians and Gynecologists, *Guidelines for Perinatal Care* (3rd ed.) American Academy of Pediatrics, Illinois: Elk Grove Village, 1992

2. Klaus M, Fanaroff, A. *Care of the High Risk Neonate.* 3rd ed. Philadelphia, W.B. Saunders Company, 1986

3. Letko MD. Detecting and preventing infant hearing loss. Neonat Net 1992;11:33–7

8

Practical Medical Issues When Screening Normal Nursery and Neonatal Intensive Care Unit (NICU) Infants

BETTY R. VOHR

Introduction

The rationale for infant hearing screening is well established; sensorineural hearing loss is a serious morbidity, there are appropriate diagnostic tests available and intervention will diminish the devastating effects.[1,2] Developing and successfully carrying out a comprehensive hearing screen program, however, requires a team approach with the involvement and collaboration of health-care professionals, paraprofessionals, and the family. This chapter will address some of the day-to-day important medical issues and decisions that must be considered when developing a new hearing screen program, or when updating an ongoing program to meet current standards.

Who Should Be Screened?

In any screening program, it is important to identify the population at risk. Recommendations for hearing screening in the 1980s to l990s have gradually shifted from recommending screening of specific populations of infants with "at-risk" factors to screening of all infants.[3–5] In 1993, the National Institutes of Health (NIH) Consensus Panel recommendation stipulated that all infants be screened for hearing impairment within the first 3 months of life.[4] In addition, the Joint Committee on Infant Hearing in 1994 recommended that all infants be identified by 3 months of age and receive habilitation by 6 months of age.[5] This shift in policy was based, in part, on the fact that several investigators had identified that approximately 50% of children with sensorineural hearing loss do not have an established risk factor and would be missed by programs screening only those infants with risk factors.[6,7] It has been estimated that 10 to 12% of neonates have

Table 8–1.   High-Risk Neonatal (Birth to 28 Days) Indicators Associated with Sensorineural and / or Conductive Hearing Loss

1. Family history of hereditary childhood sensorineural hearing loss
2. In uetero infection such as the TORCH (toxoplasmosis, rubella, cytomegalovirus, syphilis, and herpes)
3. Craniofacial anomalies, including those with morphological abnormalities of the pinna and ear canal.
4. Birth weight less than 1500 g.
5. Hyperbilirubinemia requiring exchange transfusion.
6. Ototoxic medications, including but not limited to the aminoglycosides, used in multiple courses or in combination with loop diuretics.
7. Bacterial meningitis.
8. Apgar scores of 0–4 at 1 min or 0–6 at 5 min.
9. Mechanical ventilation lasting 5 days or longer
10. Stigmata or other findings associated with a syndrome known to include a sensorineural and or conductive hearing loss.

an established risk factor,[8] and using these risk factor criteria, 2.5 to 5% of these neonates with at least one risk factor have sensorineural hearing loss.[8] In an effort to make the "risk factor" approach more inclusive, the Joint Committee on Infant Hearing increased the number of established risk factors from 5 (1972)[9] to 7 (1982)[10] and then to 10 in 1990.[3] The list of 1994 neonatal risk factors is shown in Table 8–1. These risk factors are to be used for hearing screening when a universal screening program cannot be accomplished. They are also used to determine which infants need follow-up despite a normal screen.

All of the above risk factors are either congenital (existing at birth) or acquired (occurring after birth), and likewise sensorineural hearing loss may be divided into categories of congenital (existing at birth) and acquired. Congenital sensorineural loss has a genetic origin in approximately 50% of the cases.[11,12] This means that there is a defect in a gene (the basic unit of inheritance). Thousands of genes link together and are the basic components of chromosomes. Humans have 23 pairs of chromosomes or a total of 46 chromosomes consisting of 22 pairs of autosomal chromosomes and 1 pair of sex chromosomes. Most of the genetic hearing abnormalities are caused by a defect of one gene or a pair of genes. An acquired hearing deficit, on the other hand, is secondary to an intervening event such as infection, asphyxia, or hyperbilirubinemia. Each of the congenital and acquired risk factors listed in Table 8–1 will be discussed in greater detail.

Family History

Risk factor #1 is a family history of childhood onset of sensorineural hearing impairment.[11–13] Syndromes associated with deafness are classified as inherited either as a recessive, a dominant, or an X-linked trait. Figure 8–1 shows the inheritance patterns for an autosomal dominant trait and an autosomal recessive trait. In situations of autosomal dominance (only one gene of a pair necessary for ex-

INHERITANCE PATTERNS

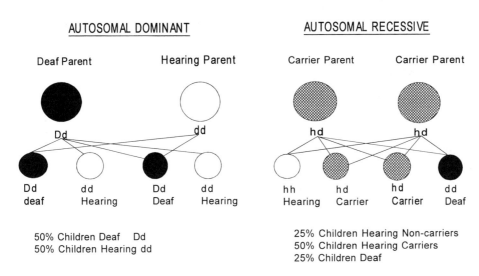

Figure 8–1.   Inheritance patterns.

pression of the defect), 50% of the children will be deaf. In contrast, in autosomal recessive inheritance, the gene is expressed only if there are a pair of genes present. As seen in Figure 8–1, 25% of the children will have normal hearing, 50% will be carriers, and 25% will be deaf. The inheritance with sex-linked (X-linked) is somewhat more complicated. The type of inheritance is usually X-linked recessive. Therefore, the mother will carry a dominant gene for hearing on one X chromosome and a recessive gene for deafness on her other X chromosome. A mother who carries the recessive gene will, therefore, pass it on to 50% of her children. Because daughters have two X chromosomes, they will either be carriers (inherited their mother's recessive gene for deafness) or noncarriers (inherited their mother's dominant gene for normal hearing) and have normal hearing. Sons, however, who receive the mothers recessive gene, will be deaf because they have only a single X chromosome. The risk of deafness goes up significantly with a deaf sibling, a sibling with a syndrome known to be associated with deafness, or a deaf parent. Consanguinity (parents are first cousins) also increases the risk of hearing impairment. An attempt should be made to obtain family history information by chart review and parent interview. Obtaining detailed family history and outlining a transgenerational family tree are the optimal approaches to unraveling the inheritance puzzle. The hospital geneticist is an excellent resource.

In-utero Infection

In utero infection is risk factor #2. Specific infections that occur in the mother prior to her pregnancy (antepartum) or during pregnancy (intrapartum) may have significant neurosensory and physical effects on the fetus and newborn. Screening for the TORCH infections is done with appropriate blood and urine cultures and titers for Toxoplasmoses,[14] rubella,[15] cytomegalovirus (CMV),[16–21] syphilis,[22] and herpes simplex virus (HSV).[23] Routine screening for these infections, however, does not occur because it is not cost-effective. Specific tests will be ordered by the physician in charge based on a combination of the maternal history and the clinical findings in the neonate at the time of birth. Prior to widespread immunization, Rubella was the most common viral infection resulting in serious hearing impairment.[13] As part of the immunization schedule currently recommended in the United States, most children routinely receive rubella vaccine. Not all women of childbearing age, however, have been immunized. The rubella vaccine, however, is highly effective and produces few side effects in women of reproductive age. Rubella screening and vaccination of susceptible women are part of the marriage application process in many states and has resulted in the near elimination of this disease. Outbreaks may, however, still occur in college students, other groups in their 20s or 30s, or new immigrant populations.

Although all the TORCH diseases are of concern, it is currently estimated that CMV is the most prevalent virus causing hearing loss in the neonate.[16–21] CMV infection is estimated to occur in 1% or 30,000 to 40,000 infants born in the United States each year.[16] Primary CMV infection in pregnancy is usually asymptomatic but the probability of transmission of the infection to the fetus is about 50%. Routine serological testing of pregnant women is currently not recommended because it does not specifically identify intrauterine infection, and the incidence is extremely low. About 90% of infants with CMV infection are asymptomatic at birth. Hearing impairment is more common[16] in infants with clinical signs including petechiae, jaundice, hepatosplenomegaly, and central nervous system findings, including abnormal computed tomographic scans. Although hearing impairment occurs in 20 to 65% of symptomatic infants, it is also found in about 7 to 13% of the asymptomatic population.[18] Primary maternal infection during the pregnancy is associated with the most severe sequelae including hearing loss.[17] CMV has also been shown to be associated with temporal bone abnormalities, including a short malformed cochlea.[20] It has been suggested that a significant number of hearing-impaired infants with no known risk factor for hearing loss may actually have CMV infection.

Infants delivered vaginally to mothers with an active primary genital HSV lesion have a 50% chance of getting the disease.[23] If the mothers' infection is secondary, the transmission rate is 0–8%. Most infants with HSV infection, however, are delivered from mothers without an active lesion and with a negative history. Infants suspected of the diagnosis are treated with Varicella-zoster immune globulin (VZIG). Human immunodeficiency virus (HIV) infection in the neonate remains uncommon but varies depending on the geographic area. This population of infants is, however, increasing in number and should be considered at risk for hearing loss. TORCH infections are more common in HIV-infected infants. A recent report identified late onset sensorineural hearing loss in a patient with clinical AIDS.[24]

Syphilis is caused by a spirochete, Treponema pallidum.[22] The incidence of syphilis in the United States, since the 1980s has increased in at risk populations. Routine prenatal care includes serological testing for syphilis in the first trimester. Identified mothers are then aggressively treated with antimicrobials. In untreated mothers, congenital syphilis can occur through transplacental infection or direct contact with infectious lesions during delivery. Infants with the disease are treated with antibiotic therapy based on their serological tests, cerebrospinal fluid and radiographic findings.

Toxoplasmosis is caused by exposure to the parasite Toxoplasma gondii.[14] This parasite infects many warm blooded species including cats. It is transmitted by eating poorly cooked food or accidentally ingesting the oocysts (germ cell) from soil. The infected neonate may manifest a rash, enlarged liver and spleen, enlarged lymph nodes, jaundice, and thrombocytopenia. Cerebral calcifications may be present on computed tomography (CT) scan and are a consequence of intrauterine meningoencephalitis. The sequelae may include mental retardation, vision impairment, learning problems, and hearing deficit. The diagnosis is confirmed by the detection of specific Toxoplasma IgM or IgA titers. Treatment with Pyrimethamine and sulfonamides is effective. Infants with congenital HIV infection have an increased susceptibility to Toxoplasmosis.

Craniofacial Abnormalities

Risk factor #3 is the presence of craniofacial abnormalities.[25] To better understand the variety of combinations of craniofacial abnormalities that can occur, it is important to be aware of the basic development of the embryo's craniofacies in the first 8 weeks of conception and the concurrence of events.[26,27] During the 4th week of gestation, the mesoderm of the ventral foregut becomes segmented and forms 5 bilateral swellings called the branchial arches. The first branchial arch pair is the precursor of the jaws, the maxilla, and the mandible. In addition, a component of the 1st arch, known as Meckel's Cartilage, forms major components of two ear ossicles, the malleus and the incus. The second branchial arch (the hyoid) forms the third ear ossicle, the stapes, but also contributes to the malleus and incus. Further, the muscles of the hyoid are all innervated by the facial (VIIth) nerve. The third branchial arch contributes to the body of the hyoid bone, the fourth branchial arch forms the thyroid cartilage, and the fifth and sixth contribute to the thyroid, laryngeal, and cricoid cartilage. Close proximity of the branchial arches to one another in the context of similar timing in embryological development and shared insults contributes to the many syndromes with various forms of mandibulo facial dysostosis, abnormalities of the mouth, tongue, as well as the middle, inner, and outer ear which may occur in conjunction with anatomical or sensorineural hearing impairment. Fusion of the three embryonic components of the palate occurs at 8 weeks of gestation and insults occurring at this time may result in a variety of cleft defects. Cleft palates may be unilateral or bilateral and involve the hard and or soft palate. Cleft lip and or cleft palate occur in a rate of 9.7 per 10,000 births. The highest incidence is in Native Americans, and the vast majority of these infants have associated middle ear effusion. In addition, ophthalmological abnormalities may also be associated with craniofacial stigmata. The eyes form from lateral expansions of the forebrain remain connected to the brain via optic nerves and migrate from a lateral to a medial position between 5 and 9 weeks of development of the embryo. There is, therefore, a temporal relationship in the early development of the facial structures. An abnormality such as an ear tag, may, however, be found alone, in association with other stigmata or with a specific syndrome.[11] The most common craniofacial anomalies are abnormalities of the pinna, ear tags, ear canal abnormalities, cleft lip, cleft palate, and low set ears. Minor stigmata, such as an ear tag, will be described in the physician's newborn physical exam in the medical record, whereas complex diagnoses will be made after specific X rays, blood, urine, and chromosome studies are ordered and results reported in the record. In summary, insults to the embryo between 4 and 9 weeks can cause disruption in components of the development of the ears, mouth, palate, and eyes.

Very Low Birth Weight

Many studies[28–34] have reported the risks of hearing impairment associated with very low birth weight (VLBW) (<1500 g), risk factor #4. One percent of infants born in the United States are VLBW. The prevalence rates of severe to profound hearing loss in this group of infants have ranged from 9 to 17%. The vast majority of these infants are cared for in a neonatal intensive care unit (NICU) and have many additional risk factors such as jaundice, amino glycoside medications, infection, assisted ventilation, asphyxia, etc. Survival of micropremies (<800-g birth weight) has resulted in a subgroup of infants at even greater risk of sensorineural hearing impairment. Screening and follow-up of VLBW infants are of prime importance because of their known increased risk, the occurrence of multiple risk factors, and the risk of late onset hearing loss.

Hyperbilirubinemia

Although risk factor #5, hyperbilirubinemia, has clearly been shown to be associated with neurological abnormality, including the development of choreoathetotic cerebral palsy and sensorineural hearing loss[35]; jaundice requiring exchange transfusion has become a relatively uncommon finding in the newborn nursery in the United States in the 1990s. Preventive treatment of the mother with Rh-immune globulin (Rhogam) and aggressive treatment during pregnancy with in utero transfusions have lessened the risk for severe neonatal jaundice (>20 mg/dL) requiring exchange transfusion. The finding of kernicterus (staining of the basal ganglia with bilirubin) on autopsy is now extremely rare. Mild jaundice, however, is a common finding which occurs in 2 of 3 infants in the newborn period. Bilirubin is formed by the breakdown of red blood cells and is then disposed of by the liver. Newborns are susceptible because of a shortened life span of red cells and immaturity of liver function. Breakdown of 1 g of hemoglobin results in the production of 35 mg of bilirubin. Bilirubin exists in two different forms in serum. One is indirect bilirubin, which is unconjugated to glucuronic acid and the second form is direct bilirubin which has been conjugated in the liver. Once conjugated in the liver, bilirubin can be rapidly excreted. It is the indirect unconjugated bilirubin at levels that approach or exceed 20 mg/dL that places the infant at risk for neurosensory insult. At greatest risk for pathological indirect hyperbilirubinemia are infants with fetal maternal blood group incompatibility (Rh, ABO, etc). Several reports have shown the effects of low levels of bilirubin on the prolongation of the ABR latency, abnormal cry characteristics, and atypical neonatal behavior.[35,36] Health professionals must remain vigilant to the effects of hyperbilirubinemia in view of recent reports of severe jaundice developing in breast-fed infants after early hospital discharge. Fortunately, recovery of the auditory brainstem response (ABR) in response to early exchange transfusion has been well documented.[36]

Ototoxic Medications

Specific medications commonly used in the NICU have been shown to have ototoxic effects (risk factor # 6). Salamy et al.[29] studied the effects of multiple neonatal risk factors on the development of sensorineural hearing loss in VLBW infants. He reported that increased amounts of furosemide (a diuretic) administration for extended periods or in conjunction with amino glycosides (an antimicrobial) was statistically associated with hearing loss. Amino glycosides including gentamicin, kanamycin, amikacin, tobramycin, netilmycin, and streptomycin have been shown to be associated with ototoxicity characterized by auditory and vestibular dysfunction. Proposed mechanisms of injury include alterations in the endolymph and destruction of the cochlear hair cells. Ototoxicity including high-frequency hearing loss may become apparent during treatment or 4 to 6 weeks posttreatment. Infants at greatest risk of amino glycoside toxicity include premature infants, infants with renal problems (decreased clearance), and infants receiving other ototoxic drugs. These medications are frequently prescribed for VLBW infants and the sickest infants with other neonatal complications are the ones most likely to have prolonged courses of these medications. More recently, chemotherapeutic agents, such as Cisplatin, which may be used in children, have been shown to have transient and progressive effects on sensorineural hearing.[37]

Bacterial Meningitis

Bacterial meningitis is risk factor #7. Bacterial meningitis is an infection with inflammation of the meninges (the membranes that surround the brain and spinal fluid). Hristeva et al.[38] reported on the 7-year incidence of neonatal meningitis. The rate of bacterial meningitis was 2.5 per 10,000, viral meningitis was 1.1 per 10,000, and the rate of fungal meningitis was 0.2 per 10,000. Group B *Streptococcus* was the most common cause of early onset meningitis and gram-negative organisms accounted for the majority of late onset meningitis. Twenty-seven percent of the infants had neurological sequelae. Bacterial meningitis in the neonatal period is currently stated to be the leading cause of acquired deafness in childhood.[8] Group B *Streptococci* and *Escherichia coli* account for approximately 70% of neonatal meningitis. The overall incidence rates in neonates range from 2 to 4 per 10,000 infants. The peak incidence in childhood occurs between 6 and 9 months of age. A recent study of children age 1 month to 13.8 years with bacterial meningitis revealed a mortality rate of 4.3% and permanent neurological morbidity rate of 25%. The most frequently reported sequelae of bacterial meningitis was hearing impairment, which occurred in 9% of children.[39]

Apgar Scores

Low Apgar scores (risk factor #8) or other indications of asphyxia, such as acidosis, have been associated with sensorineural hearing loss.[40–42] Apgar scores are routinely recorded in the delivery room at 1 and 5 min of age. The score is based on 2 points for heart rate, 2 points for respiratory effort, 2 points for muscle tone, 2 points for reflexes, and 2 points for color. A perfect score is 10. Although guide lines have been established for a low score at 1 and 5 min, in cases of severe asphyxia, the Apgar Score will also be recorded at 10 min. A low 10-min Apgar Score (0–6) is highly predictive of neurosensory abnormality. It is of interest that animal studies have shown that the combination of asphyxia and hyperbilirubinemia is associated with sensorineural hearing loss.[28] Infants with severe perinatal asphyxia with multiorgan (heart, liver, kidney, and brain) involvement and seizures are at increased risk of sensorineural hearing impairment.

Mechanical Ventilation

The risk derived from mechanical ventilation (risk factor #9) has more recently been associated not only with prolonged duration of assisted ventilation, but with specific medical diagnoses and specific types of ventilation.[43–46] Specifically, persistent fetal circulation,[43] also known as persistent pulmonary hypertension,[44] jet ventilation,[45] and Extra Corporeal Membrane Oxygenation (ECMO)[46] have been associated with sensorineural hearing loss. Infants who require assisted ventilation most often have hypoventilation or respiratory distress with hypoxemia (decreased oxygen) and carbon dioxide retention. Respiratory distress may be due to:

1. Primary lung disease (respiratory distress syndrome [RDS], Meconium aspiration, or Pneumonia).
2. Obstruction (such as subglottic lesions or vocal cord paralysis).
3. Poor respiratory effort.
4. Space occupying lesions (pneumothorax, diaphragmatic hernia, and tumors).
5. Retained fluid.
6. Paralysis of the diaphragm.

The most common protracted respiratory abnormality in premature infants is RDS, which can develop into a form of chronic lung disease, referred to as bronchopulmonary dysplasia (BPD). Infants with chronic lung problems are more likely to have prolonged oxygen and ventilation requirements, prolonged or chronic hypoxemia with decreased delivery of oxygen to body tissues, cardiovascular instability with episodes of hypotension and hypertension and repeated exposures to ototoxic drugs such as the amino glycosides and furosemide.

Associated Syndromes

Risk factor #10 refers to a constellation of physical findings known to be identified with hearing loss, which if taken together, are referred to as an association or a syndrome.[25] There are over 200 syndromes known to be associated with varying degrees of severity of deafness, including early onset, late onset, or progressive deafness. Most of the syndromes are extremely rare and it is impossible for the clinician to be familiar with each one. It is recommended, therefore, that the newborn nursery clinical staff have a syndrome reference book available. If the findings of a careful physical exam or the family history suggest a syndrome, a genetics computer program should be accessed and a genetics consult obtained. Eight syndromes that are more common will be discussed.

1. *Branchio-oto-renal Syndrome (BOR).* This syndrome is characterized by abnormalities including branchial cleft defects, malformations of the pinnae, preauricular pits, and renal anomalies. This disorder has an autosomal dominant inheritance pattern. There is variable expression of this syndrome, however, and the severity with which it is manifested in families varies from minimal to severe. The prevalence is approximately 1 per 40,000, and 75% of the patients will have a significant hearing loss.

2. *CHARGE Association* is characterized by the following findings C (coloboma), H (cardiac abnormalities), A (choanal atresia), R (retarded growth), G (genital abnormalities), and E (ear abnormalities or deafness). Approximately 85% of the patients will have a mixed hearing loss.

3. *Pendred Syndrome* is a disorder characterized by the presence of a thyroid goiter in association with subtle or pronounced hypothyroidism. The sensorineural hearing loss ranges from mild to severe and is progressive in about 20% of children.

4. *Usher Syndrome* manifests itself by retinitis pigmentosa in conjunction with sensorineural hearing loss. It is the most common syndrome, which has an association between sensorineural hearing loss and eye abnormalities.

5. *Neurofibromatosis Type II* is associated with café au lait spots, subcutaneous neurofibromas, acoustic neuromas, and other types of neural tumors. The incidence is about 1 in 50,000 newborns. Sensorineural hearing loss is present in 45% of patients and it is bilateral in 90% of the cases. It is frequently progressive and may lead to complete deafness. Surgical removal of the acoustic neuromas is difficult and not always successful.

6. *Goldenhar Syndrome* is also referred to as Oculo-Auriculo-Vertebral (OAV) syndrome. The ocular abnormalities include anophthalmia and microphthalmia, the auricular abnormalities are pinnae defects or anotia and may oc-

cur in association with defects of the middle ear. The vertebral findings usually involve the cervical spine. Facial asymmetry of varying degrees is a common component. Fifty percent of patients have a sensorineural, conductive, or mixed hearing loss.

7. *Wardenburg Syndrome* is characterized by hypertelorism, high nasal bridge, synophrys, and hypoplastic alae nasi. It is more often recognized because of pigment abnormalities including a white forelock, partial albinism, hypopigmentation of the fundi, blue irises, and premature greying. It may be associated with dystopia canthorum and lateral displacement of the lacrimal ducts. The incidence is 1 in 40,000 births. Sensorineural hearing loss is either unilateral or bilateral.

Limitations of Risk-Based Hearing Screening Programs

There are several pragmatic issues that must be considered when using the risk-factor approach to screening. The first is that not all infants with a risk factor will be cared for in a NICU or Special Care Nursery. In fact, most infants with family history, clinically inapparent in utero infection, mild craniofacial abnormalities, and specific syndromes (i.e., Wardenburg, Down, etc.) may be cared for in normal nurseries. This fact indicates that hospitals using the risk-factor approach must develop surveillance protocols to identify at-risk infants in the normal nurseries. This would involve two important components. First, chart review of the physical examination and test results including blood, urine, or radiographic by a health professional familiar with medical terminology is necessary. In addition, in most hospitals risk factor number 1 (family history of sensorineural hearing impairment) is not routinely requested or recorded in most neonatal hospital records. Therefore, a mechanism of either an appropriately worded and informative questionnaire or direct interview of the mother must be established to obtain reliable information. Hospitals must then cope with the issue of language barriers and literacy. For example, before hearing screening became a standard of care at Women and Infants Hospital of Rhode Island, it was necessary to print the informed consents for a universal hearing screen study in eight languages. Effective screening using risk factor #1 would necessitate developing a process for providing interpreters for all necessary languages to ensure that the parent understands the information requested. Obtaining reliable family history data is not easy to implement on a universal basis.

Several states have developed "birth certificate registries," a registry for tracking purposes.[7,47,48] At-risk information is collected from the hospital record and parent interview, entered into a database (birth certificate) and provided either to the primary-care provider or the health department and the parents, informing them that a follow-up audiological evaluation is recommended. The interview method, however, can be time consuming (15–20 min per family) and may not be accurate. Other limitations of using the interview as a screen method include lack of availability of the mother due to illness or fatigue, language barrier, or early discharge. Difficulties in tracking families after discharge and poor compliance for follow-up evaluations have limited the success of the birth certificate registry. As stated earlier, 50% of infants with sensorineural hearing impairment do not have an established risk factor.[7]

Late Onset and Progressive Hearing Loss

The second area of concern is risk factors associated with progressive loss or late onset loss as shown in Table 8–2. These factors are to be used between 29 days of age and 2 years of age. Infants at risk for late onset hearing loss are infants who have a risk factor and a normal neonatal hearing screen and, therefore, must be scheduled for follow-up by 6–8 months of age, or infants who develop an at risk medical condition between 28 days of age and 2 years of age.

A small percentage of infants who do not pass their newborn screen are actually "false-positives" and pass when retested 1 month to 6 months later. This result may be secondary to temporary blockage of the ear canal, middle ear fluid, or transient abnormalities in brainstem conduction secondary hyperbilirubinemia, asphyxia, or neurological abnormality. In contrast, infants with other etiological factors, including hereditary hearing disorders, viral infections including CMV, and prolonged assisted ventilation, especially jet ventilation and ECMO, may have negative findings or a mild abnormality at the time of the discharge hearing screen, but subsequently develop hearing loss or have progressive loss.[30,49–51]

Two of the risk factors for ages 1 month to 2 years deserve additional discussion. The first is parental concern about the child's hearing status or development of speech and language (risk factor #1). In the past, it has not been unusual for parents of children with hearing loss to complain that they had voiced their concerns repeatedly to health professionals; often pediatricians reassured them or ignored their complaints. Health-care providers in the 1990s should be more aware of early childhood language milestones and more responsive to parent observation. Because the health-care provider has only brief opportunities to observe the child during provider visits, he or she must, therefore, rely to a certain degree on parent observation and report and respond accordingly. Basic screening for speech and language milestones should be a routine component of the well-baby visit.

Table 8–2.   Risk Factors for Hearing Loss between 28 Days and 2 Years of Age

1. Parent/care giver concern regarding hearing, speech, language, and/or developmental delay.
2. Bacterial meningitis and other infections associated with sensorineural hearing loss.
3. Head trauma associated with loss of consciousness or skull fracture.
4. Stigmata or other finding associated with a syndrome known to include a sensorineural or conductive hearing loss.
5. Ototoxic medications, including but not limited to chemotherapeutic agents or amino glycosides, used in multiple courses or in combination with loop diuretics.
6. Recurrent or persistent otitis media with effusion for at least 3 months.

The second is risk factor #6, which is recurrent or persistent otitis media with effusion lasting greater than 3 months.[52-53] Otitis media is the most common medical problem seen in the pediatrician's office. There are several risk factors that have been identified for otitis media including male gender, bottle feeding, family history of otitis media, and daycare. Hispanic and Native American children, with chronic pulmonary disease, ex-premature infants and immunocompromised infants are also at increased risk. In addition, the earlier the first occurrence of otitis media, the more likely it will recur. It has been reported that 50% of children who have their first episode of otitis before 12 months of age will have 6 or more episodes by 2 years of age. Although otitis media occurs until 7 to 8 years of age , the peak occurrence is during the first 3 years of life, a critical period for speech and language development. Hearing loss with effusion has been shown to range from mild to moderate and to impact on the development of language skills. The Boston Otitis Media Study reported significant effects on developmental outcome of children with middle ear effusion for greater than 120 days.[54]

Specific Medical Considerations Regarding Selection of Screen Population

Current Joint Committee and ASHA guidelines recommend the implementation of universal screening in the United States. The current economic constraints, however, imposed in part by the emergence of managed healthcare in the United States have placed limitations on the ability of many hospital pediatric and audiological programs to implement universal hearing screen programs. The hearing screen recommendations were made at a time before capitation issues rose to the forefront. Therefore, despite legislative mandates, and the well-intentioned plans of health professionals in a number of states, the lack of availability of hospital resources and limitations on the availability of third-party reimbursement have all affected the types of programs emerging throughout the country. Table 8–3 shows the possible types of populations served in hearing screen programs and range from the most comprehensive (universal) to the least comprehensive (referral basis only). Many tertiary care centers have implemented universal screening of their NICU populations, considering that all infants admitted to a

Table 8–3.   Populations Served in Hearing Screen Programs

Population	NICU Nursery	% Screened	Normal Nursery	% Screened
Universal	Yes	100	Yes	100%
NICU Admissions	Yes	100	No	None
Risk Factor Total	Yes	<100	Yes	Small %
Risk Factor Total	Yes	100	No	None
Risk Factor Partial	Yes	<100	No	None
Risk Factor Partial	Yes	<100	Yes	Small %
Referral Basis	Yes	Variable	Yes	Variable

Table 8–4.   Indicators for Delayed Onset of Sensorineural Hearing Loss 6 Months to
3 Years of Age Infants Who Require Periodic Monitoring

1. Family history of hereditary childhood hearing loss.
2. In utero infection, such as cytomegalovirus, rubella syphilis, herpes, or toxoplasmosis.
3. Neurofibromatosis Type II and neurodegenerative disorders.

Indicators of Conductive Hearing Loss
1. Recurrent or persistent otitis media with effusion
2. Anatomic deformities and other disorders that affect eustachian tube function.
3. Neurodegenerative disorders.

NICU have some degree of risk. A total risk factor screen program may screen NICU and normal nursery infants for medical risk factors and family history or it may be utilized only in a NICU. A partial risk-factor program may have one of two screen protocols. It may (1) screen the NICU and normal nursery populations for all the established medical risk factors and not include family history or (2) screen only NICU infants with medical risk and family history risk factors. The final screen approach of physician referral on an individual basis is least optimal and is dependent on the individual attending physician's bias. The goal of all programs currently should be universal screening. If there are hospital financial constraints that prevent universal screen implementation, it is recommended that a plan be developed to systematically expand the program in stages over a period of 12 to 24 months. For example, in the initial phase the program would screen only infants with risk factors in the NICU; during phase 2, all NICU infants would be screened; during phase 3, normal nursery infants with risk factors would be added; and during phase 4, universal screening would be implemented. During these stages of development programmatic issues such as staffing, data management, and reimbursement would need to be developed (Table 8–3).

A final group of risk indicators is used for infants from 6 months through 3 years of age. These infants have risk factors for delayed onset or progressive sensorineural hearing impairment and it is recommended that they be evaluated every 6 months until 3 years of age. Risk factors for delayed onset are listed in Table 8–4.

When Should Infants Be Screened?

Early discharge guidelines developed within the past few years have resulted in term infants being discharged as early as 8, 12, 18, and 24 h of age. This means that all the examinations, procedures, and maternal education that previously took 3 to 4 days must now be completed in a specific shortened period of time. One method to address the issue of providing all necessary care is to implement the use of a tool called a CareMap.™ This tool uses a timeline to standardize and prioritize patient care. It monitors, documents and reviews patient care concurrently. Components of care which need to be included in an 18- to 24-h period include an admission and discharge physical assessment, and assessments of vital signs, feeding, voiding, stooling, and activity. It also includes administration of Vitamin K, the newborn metabolic screen, administration of Hepatitis B vaccine, other blood or urine studies when ordered, teaching sessions on breast-feeding or bathing, and the hearing screen. This mechanism, which is used in the Women and Infants' Hospital normal nurseries, facilitates the scheduling of all necessary neonatal patient care, and prevents missed tests, procedures, and education sessions within a discrete time frame.

The overall assessment for readiness for screening is the same for all types of screen procedures whether it is transient otoacoustic emissions (TOAE), automated ABR or standard ABR. For ABR screening, attention must be directed at skin preparation. The ABR should be attempted after the hospital staff has thoroughly washed the infant to remove vernix and debris from the skin surface. This will need to be followed by vigorous standard cleaning of the electrode sites to ensure optimal impedance at <5 ohms.

Readiness of Testing

THE FULL-TERM INFANT

Fortunately most full-term newborns are stable in terms of their cardiorespiratory status shortly after birth and presumably could have their hearing screened. Two other factors, however, middle ear fluid and ear canal debris, can interfere with obtaining a screen pass in an infant with normal sensorineural hearing. Middle ear fluid or negative pressure has been shown to decrease the transient evoked otoacoustic emissions (TEOAE) below 2 kHz.[55] It is fortunate that middle ear problems in normal full-term infants are relatively rare.[52] This is in contrast to the NICU where one study reported that 30% of infants, especially those who required assisted ventilation, had effusion at the time of discharge.[53] In our own study of the tympanic membranes of full-term newborns in the first day of life, we identified that 81 of 82 (99%) visualized tympanic membranes were considered to have normal landmarks and normal contour.[56] This is similar to the findings of Cavanaugh[57] in full-term infants. In our study we also performed otoscopic examinations to evaluate the ear canal for the presence of vernix caseosa or other debris or ear canal collapse. We identified within a sample of 82 ears that 48 of 82 (58.5%) ear canals had no debris, 27 of 82 (32.9%) had the ear canal partially occluded with debris and or collapse, and 8 of 82 (9.7%) were totally occluded. Partial occlusion was associated with a diminished OAE emission and total blockage was associated with a significantly lower emission or absent emission. After the ear canals were cleaned of debris under direct vision, the OAE was repeated and we demonstrated that the pass rate could be significantly improved. The improved response indicates that cleaning of the ear canal and in some cases, dilation of a collapsed canal in full-term newborns is an important part of the screening process. This is, therefore, an important issue for early newborn hearing screening. Many newborn screens, however, are completed by paraprofessionals who are not qualified to clean out ear canal debris by inserting an instrument into the ear canal.

We, therefore, looked for an alternate approach to clearing the canal, which could be completed by paraprofessionals. It had been observed both the insertion of a pediatric otoscope into the ear canal often resulted in the re-expansion of a collapsed canal and that debris often adhered to the otoscope when it was removed. It was also noted that the ILO-88 ear probe was the same size as the Welch Allyn, Inc., N.Y. otoscope tip and that debris also was noted to adhere upon removal of the ILO-88 tip. We then evaluated the effects of two simple procedures of (1) running the OAE, then viewing the ear canal with the pediatric otoscope, cleaning the probe tip of any attached debris and then repeating the OAE and (2) running the OAE, removing the ILO-88 tip, cleaning any attached debris, and then repeating then OAE.[58] We found that the otoscopic exam procedure and the refit procedure were effective in improving the TEOAE response. This is a cost-effective method for improving test results, which can be accomplished by paraprofessionals during routine screen protocols.

Early discharge (within the first 24 h of life) of infants cared for in the normal nurseries has been reported to increase hearing screen fail rates. Kok et al.[59] reported increasing screen pass rates with increasing age for infants tested with otoacoustic emissions. Seventy eight percent of infants less than 36 h of age had emissions compared to 99% of infants older than 108 h of age. The experience of the screen program at WIH, which currently has 24-h discharge for healthy infants in the normal nurseries is that a first stage screen fail rate of 7% can be maintained if standard refit procedures are used.[60]

Readiness for Testing

THE NICU INFANT

The hearing screener must rely on the NICU team members to learn when it is safe and feasible to test a NICU infant. There are several problems that can interfere with testing. Early transfer of infants to another facility is often sudden and unexpected. Critically ill infants may be hospitalized for extended periods of time and then may be transferred to other tertiary centers or to a level II nursery. If the infant is being transferred to another tertiary care center for surgery or ECMO, the infant is critically ill and not a candidate for a hearing screen at that time. It is important, however, to have a mechanism to track this high-risk infant so that he can be screened at a later date. It is often the sickest infants, who because of their multiple medical complications, miss their screen. Infants transferred on the weekend to a level II hospital because of a census problem can also be missed, and need to be recalled for testing.

Continued use of special equipment provides special problems when conducting screening. With the survival of infants with chronic medical problems who may be discharged on monitors, intravenous solutions, oxygen, or even on a ventilator, protocols must be set up for testing these medically at-risk infants. One approach is to test the infant in the NICU, making adaption for the noise and confusion of the NICU. Arrangements can often be made to test these infants after hours when the NICU is less chaotic. Another approach is to have the infants' primary nurse accompany the infant to the test site and remain in attendance during the testing. A third approach for infants who are stable but on a cardiorespiratory monitor is that they be brought to the test site with their monitor. The test site should, however, have an audio hookup with the NICU in case assistance is required. Guidelines need to be made for the amount of time that the infant is involved with the screen so as not to interfere with the feeding schedule or with temperature control.

Another factor that must be taken into consideration is the infant state during the screen. State is the infant's level of arousal and ranges from crying to awake to dozing to deep sleep. It has been shown that carrying out the TEOAE procedure while the infant is crying prolongs the test time and increases the fail rate. Optimal screen results are obtained if the infant is quietly awake, dozing, or asleep. This can best be accomplished by scheduling the screen after a feeding, a natural time for the infant to go to sleep. Additional methods for calming the infant include bundling the infant securely in a blanket, picking the infant up for a brief period and burping or patting, returning the infant to its mother for a feed, or giving the infant a pacifier. If the infant is about to be discharged and the state is nonoptimal, such as crying, the infant may have to be scheduled to be screened at a later date.

Where Should the Infants Be Screened?

The hospital is the obvious site for attempting to accomplish universal screening on a captive audience. There are, however, alternate sites within and outside of the hospital that are shown in Table 8–5. Several factors must be considered in choosing the hearing screen site including accessability, lack of barriers, safety, infection control measures, noise level at site, level of congestion, and efficiency of the process.

Low-risk infants, primarily full-term are cared for in "normal nurseries." These infants are usually brought to the nursery at specific times for nursing care or routine procedures. Performing the hearing screen during these established time periods allows the screeners to scrub, perform the screen procedure, and complete the necessary paperwork at a single site. This eliminates the additional time required to transport infants to and from a dedicated screen area and avoids the additional time and personnel needed for transport. In addition, nursing personnel are in constant attendance for an emergency. Any screen method must develop a mechanism to provide feedback to families that the screen was performed. At Women and Infants' Hospital, an informational brochure for parents about infant hearing screening is placed in the infants' crib

Table 8–5.   Sites for Conducting
Hearing Screening

Normal Nurseries
NICU
Dedicated Hospital Area
Audiologists' Office Clinic
Pediatricians' Office
Home
Mothers' Room

after the screen. Normal nursery infants are usually considered ready for screening when in an open crib. Exceptions are infants who are receiving phototherapy for neonatal jaundice who may be discharged within 12 to 24 h. It is recommended that rather than completely missing a late afternoon or early evening discharge, the screen be completed while the infant is still receiving phototherapy. The phototherapy lights may be turned off for the 5 to 30 min that it takes to complete the screen.

Another site for the healthy infant is the mother's room. More hospitals are moving toward 24-h rooming-in with the mother. The infant remains in the mother's room for all nursing care and screening procedures. This situation can be addressed with a portable screening unit. It is more time-consuming because the screener must move the equipment from room to room. It also takes more time because the screener must take more time to speak with the mother and explain the procedure. If an audiologist is performing the screen, immediate feedback can be provided to the parent; if, however, the screen is being completed by a paraprofessional, it must be explained that the results will be provided after the screen results are interpreted by the program audiologist.

Severity of illness or lack of cardiovascular stability often dictates that high risk infants are screened within the NICU.[61–64] A number of factors affect the efficiency of screening within the NICU. Noise levels in the NICU have been shown to range from 55 to 75 dB SPL.[62] This noise level has been shown to affect screen results. If noise is a problem, some adaptions can be made to lower the low-frequency background noise. Approaches to lower the background noise include screening on off hours (evenings or nights), use of acoustic tiles, room dividers, or testing infants in an enclosure such as an incubator.[63]

A third choice of test area is the dedicated site separate from the NICU, which maintains all the safety and infection control standards of the nursery including (1) scrub sink, (2) appropriate electronic hook-up to cardiovascular monitors and oxygen, and (3) audio hook-up with the NICU staff for emergencies. The dedicated site is ideally located immediately adjacent to the NICU, although other hospital sites may be used. To ensure safety, it is recommended that infants being discharged on cardiorespiratory monitors for neonatal apnea or bradycardia and infants with chronic lung disease (bronchopulmonary dysplasia) going home on oxygen be accompanied to the screen site by a primary-care nurse who remains for the duration of the screen.

Another option for a screen site is the private audiologist's office or the audiology clinic. This option could be considered feasible in centers where the audiology department is located in the same facility as where the primary care is provided. The disadvantage of this approach is that separate appointments would have to be scheduled, presumably prior to discharge. This would minimize the problems that arise secondary to language barriers, lack of a home phone, and lack of transportation. The advantages are that the screen would be carried out in older infants (several days to 3 months) with a lower false-positive rate, there could be immediate informational feedback from an audiologist, and an immediate diagnostic evaluation could be completed or at least scheduled.

A fourth choice for completing a hearing screen is the pediatrician's office or the pediatric clinic at the time of the 2-week or 4-week well-baby check-up. This is actually a pragmatic option because it is another mechanism for "capturing" the infant for a screen during a standard scheduled physician visit. It is also at an infant age when the false-positive rate is minimal. This approach, however, would involve pediatricians obtaining training for office staff and developing a new-screen protocol within the context of the well-baby visit. In recent years, tympanometry in the pediatrician's office has become a common procedure to assess middle ear status. This suggests that continuing developments in automated screen procedures would encourage the establishment of hearing screening within the context of pediatric primary care. This "one-stop shopping" approach would also facilitate accomplishing the rescreen. Procedures such as the Algo automated screener for brainstem auditory evoked response and the Echosensor for evoked otoacoustic emissions are possibilities.

The development of automated techniques would also benefit the concept of the visiting nurse completing the hearing screen as a component of the initial home visit. Some countries have reported successful behavioral screening as part of a home visiting program. The success of a neonatal screen being done at home would depend on a simplified automated approach that could easily be replicated.

Who Needs to Be Educated About Infant Hearing Screening?

Everyone, including professionals and lay personnel, involved in any component of hearing screening needs to be educated about the purpose of a new hearing screen program, the procedures involved, the referral mechanisms and the intervention services available (or needed). Groups targeted for education about hearing screening, hearing impairment, and early intervention for hearing impairment services are shown in Table 8–6.

Parents of a newborn infant will have many questions and anxieties about the routine and normal procedures occurring during the newborn hospitalization.[65] Therefore, it is important to begin the education process prior to hospitalization.

Table 8–6.   Groups Targeted for Education
on Hearing Screening

Parents
Physicians/House Staff
Hospital Nurses
Visiting Nurses
Community Childbirth Educators
Community Audiologists
Community Physicians/Otolaryngologists
Early Intervention Staff
Special Interest Groups (AG Bell)
Fund Raisers

Utilization of a preadmission brochure explaining screening, and introducing hearing screening into the prenatal course are two approaches to providing information prior to the hospitalization. Another method that has been found effective in Rhode Island is to have a 5-min teaching video on hearing screening available in every patients' room on the hospital cable TV network. A video on infant hearing screening is currently used in all the eight birthing hospitals in Rhode Island and has been distributed to childbirth educators throughout the state. Although the video has been personalized for each hospital relative to the introduction and the description of the protocol at that hospital, each version contains that same basic information on hearing screening and hearing impairments specifically focused for the new parent. Separate materials and protocols must be developed for informing the parents that their infant did not pass the screen. Receiving the information about a failed newborn screen can be stressful for parents and every effort must be made to have a trained and sensitive professional explain the screen results, to answer their questions, to provide the information to their pediatrician, and to facilitate the referral process for an audiological diagnostic assessment. The education process must expand and be ongoing for parents of infants who are diagnosed with conductive or sensorineural hearing loss. Information about types of hearing loss, amplification systems, options for communication, types of intervention available, and funding sources must be made available to parents.[66] A 1995 collaborative effort by Rhode Island agencies and parents produced a parent education booklet on hearing loss and hearing aids.[67]

Full-time hospital personnel, including attending physicians, house staff, and nurses, require in-depth in-service for a new program and repeat in-services on at least a yearly interval. Education methods may include a program brochure for professionals, in-hospital teaching videos, department conferences, grand rounds, and new house staff orientation sessions. Effective interagency and interdisciplinary communication is facilitated by distributing regular program updates to local pediatricians, otolaryngologists, audiologists, and early intervention staff.

Community education may be even more challenging because it involves outreach and making appropriate contacts with individuals, agencies, and organizations. Approaches include sending out informational letters, speaking to local groups, speaking on local radio and TV talk shows, and starting a newsletter. Also, providing opportunities for key individuals from funding agencies and local government to view the screening program and to become apprised of program updates will be advantageous.

References

1. Ross M. Implications for delay in detection and management of deafness. Volta Rev 1990;92: 62–79
2. Bess FH, Hall J. *Screening Children for Auditory Function.* Nashville, TN, Bill Wilkerson Center Press, 1992
3. Joint Committee on Infant Hearing Position Statement, 1990. ASHA 1991;33(Suppl. 15):3–6

4. National Institutes of Health (NIH) 1993 NIH Consensus Statement Vol. 11 No. 1. *Early Identification of Hearing Impairment in Infants and Young Children*, pp. 1–24

5. Joint Committee on Infant Hearing. Position statement, 1994. ASHA 1994;36:38–41

6. Kramer SJ, Vertes DR, Condon M. Auditory brainstem responses and clinical follow-up of high risk infants. Pediatrics 1989;83:385–92

7. Mauk GW, White KR, Mortensen LB, et al. The effectiveness of screening programs based on high risk characteristics in early identification of hearing impairment. Ear Hear 1991;12: 312–19

8. Epstein S, Reilly JS. Sensorineural hearing loss. Pediatr Clin North Am 1989;36:1501–19

9. Joint Committee on Infant Hearing Position Statement. American Speech–Language Association, 1972

10. Joint Committee on Infant Hearing Position Statement. American Speech–Language Association, 1982

11. Lalwani AK, Grundfast KM. A role for the otolaryngologist in identification and discovery of genetic disorders and chromosomal abnormalities. Arch Otolaryngol Head Neck Surg 1991;117: 332–5

12. Coucke P, Van Camp G, Djoyodiharjo B, et al. Linkage of autosomal dominant hearing loss to the short arm of chromasome 1 in 2 families. N Engl J Med 1994;331:425–31

13. Robillard TAJ, Gersdorff MCH. Prevention of pre- and perinatal acquired hearing defects: I. Study of causes. J Aud Res 1986;26:207

14. American Academy of Pediatrics. Report on the Committee on Infectious Disease. Red Book, 1994

15. Cooper LZ, Preblud SR, Alford CA. Rubella. In Remington JS, Klein JC (eds): *Infectious Diseases of the Fetus and Newborn Infant*. Philadelphia, W.R. Saunders Co., 1995

16. Williamson WD, Percy AK, Yow MD, et al. Asymptomatic congenital cytomegalovirus infection: Audiologic, neuroradiologic, and neurodevelopmental abnormalities during the first year. Am J Dis Child 1990;140:1365–8

17. Fowler KR, Stagno S, Pass RF, Britt WJ, et al. The outcome of congenital cytomegalovirus infection in relation to maternal antibody status. N Engl J Med 1992;326(10):663–7

18. Williamson WD, Demmler GJ, Percy AK, et al. Progressive hearing loss in infants with asymptomatic congenital cytomegalovirus infection. Pediatrics 1992;90:862–6

19. Peckham CS, Stark O, Dudgeon JA, et al. Congenital cytomegalovirus infection: A cause of sensorineural hearing loss. Arch Dis Child 1989;62:1233–7

20. Bauman NM, Kirby-Keyser LJ, Dolan KD, et al. Mondini dysplasia and congenital cytomegalovirus infection. J Pediatr 1994;124:71–8

21. Strauss M. A clinical pathologic study of hearing loss in congenital cytomegalovirus infection. Laryngoscope 1985;95:951

22. Ikeda MK, Jensen HB. Evaluation and treatment of congenital syphilis. J Pediatr 1990;117:843

23. Whitley RJ, Arvin A, Prober C, et al. Predictors of morbidity and mortality in neonates with herpes simplex virus infections. N Engl J Med 1991;324–450

24. Grimaldi LM, Luzi L, Martino GV, et al. Bilateral eigth cranial nerve neuropathy in human immunodeficiency virus infection. J Neurol 1993;240:363–6

25. Smith DW, Grahm JM. *Smith's Recognizable Patterns of Human Deformation*. 2nd ed. Philadelphia, W.B. Saunders Co., 1988

26. Winter RM, Baraitser M. *London Dysmorphology Database*. New York, Oxford University Press, 1990

27. Sperber GH, Tobias RV. *Craniofacial Embryology*. Boston, Wright & Sons Ltd., 1989

28. Duara S, Suter CM, Bessard KK, et al. Neonatal screening with audiometry brainstem responses: Results of follow-up audiometry and high risk evaluation. J Pediatr 1986;108:276–81

29. Salamy A, Eldredge L, Tooley WH. Neonatal status and hearing loss in high risk infants. J Pediatr 1989;114:847–52

30. Eavy RD, Bertero MC, Thornton AR, et al. Failure to clinically predict NICU hearing loss. Clin Pediatr 1995;34:138–45

31. Galambos R, Hicks G, Wilson MJ. Hearing loss in graduates of a tertiary intensive care nursery. Ear Hear 1982;3:87–90

32. Bergman I, Hirsch RP, Fria TJ, et al. Cause of hearing loss in the high-risk premature infant. J Pediatr 1985;106:95–101

33. Gorga MP, Reiland JK, Beauchaine KA, et al. Auditory brainstem responses from graduates of an intensive care nursery: Normal patterns of response. J Speech Hear Res 1987;30:311–8

34. Cox LC, Hack M, Metz DA. Brainstem evoked response audiometry in the premature infant population. Int J Pediatr Otolaryngol 1981;3:213–24

35. Keaster an CB, Hyman CB, Harris I. Hearing problems subsequent to neonatal hemolytic disease or hyperbilirubinemia. Am J Dis Child 1969;117:406

36. Vohr BR, Lester BM, Rapisardi G, et al. Abnormal brain-stem function (brain-stem auditory evoked response) correlates with acoustic cry features in term infants with hyperbilirubinemia. J Pediatr 1989;115:303–8

37. Kretschmar CS, Warren MP, Lavally BL, et al. Ototoxicity of pre-radiation cisplatin for children with central nervous system tumors. J Clin Oncol 1990;9:1191–8

38. Hristeva L, Booy R, Bowler I, et al. Prospective surveillance of neonatal meningitis. Arch Dis Child 1993;69:14–8

39. Kaaresen PI, Flaegstad T. Prognostic factors in childhood bacterial meningitis. Acta Paediatr 1995;84:873–8

40. Sinha SK, D'Souza SW, Rivlin E, et al. Ischaemic brain lesions diagnosed at birth in perterm infants: Clinical events and developmental outcome. Arch Dis Child 1990;65:1017

41. Eichwald J, Mahoney T. Apgar scores in the identifiation of sensorineural hearing loss JAAA 1993;3:133–138

42. Silver S, Kapitulnik J, Sohmer H. Contribution of asphyxia to the induction of hearing impairment in jaundiced Gunn rats. Pediatrics1995;95:579–83

43. Hendricks-Munoz K, Walton JD. Hearing loss of infants with persistent fetal circulation. Pediatrics 1988;81:650–6

44. Walton JP, Hendricks-Munoz K. Profile and stability of sensorineural hearing loss in persistent pulmonary hypertension of the newborn. J Speech Hear Res 1991;34:1362–70

45. Konkle DF, Knightly CA. Delayed-onset hearing loss in respiratory distress syndrome: Case reports. J Am Acad Audiol 1993;4:351–4

46. Megathan Haluschak M, Cheung P-Y, Finer NN, et al. Sensorineural hearing loss in survivors of neonatal extracorporeal membrane oxygenation (ECMO). Early Hum Dev 1996;44:225–33

47. Mahoney TM, Eichwald JG. Newborn high-risk screening by maternal questionnaire. JAAA 1979;5:41–5

48. Pappas DG. A study of the high risk registry for sensorineural hearing impairment. Arch Otolaryngol Head Neck Surg 1983;91:41–4

49. Finitz-Hieber T, McCracken GH, Roeser RJ, et al. Ototoxicity in neonates treated with gentamicin and kanamycin: Results of a 4 year controlled follow-up study. Pediatrics 1979;63:443–50

50. Brookhouser PE, Worthington DW, Kelly WJ. Fluctuating and or progressive sensorineural hearing loss in children. Laryngoscope 1994;104:958–64

51. Meyerhoff WL, Cass S, Schwaber MK, et al. Progressive sensorineural hearing loss in children. Otolaryngol Head Neck Surg 1994;110:569–79

52. Keith RW. Middle ear function in neonates. Arch Otolaryngol 1975;101:376–9

53. Balkany TJ, Berman SA, Simmons, et al. Middle ear effusions in neonates. Laryngoscope 1978;398–405

54. Teele DW, Klein JO, Rosner B, and Greater Boston Otitis Media Study Group. Epidemiology of otitis media during the first seven years of life in children in greater Boston: A prospective cohort study. J Infect Dis 1989;160(1):83–94

55. Kemp DT, Ryan S, Bray P. A guide to the effective use of otoacoustic emissions. Ear Hear 1990; 11:93–105

56. Chang KW, Vohr BR, Norton SJ, et al. External and middle ear status related to evoked otoacoustic emission in neonates. Arch Otolaryngol Head Neck Surg 1993;119:276–82

57. Cavanaugh RM. Pneumatic otoscopy in healthy full-term infants. Pediatrics 1987;21:191–204

58. Vohr BR, White KR, Brancia Maxon A. Effects of exam procedures on transient evoked otoacoustic emissions (TEOAE) in neonates. J Am Acad Audiol 1996;7:77–82

59. Kok MR, van Zanten GA, Brocaar MP, Wallenburg HCS. Click-evoked otoacoustice emmisions in 1036 ears of healthy newborns. Audiology 1993;32:213–44

60. Maxon AB, White KR, Behrens TR, Vohr BR. Referral rates and cost efficiency in a universal newborn hearing screening program using transient evoked otoacoustic emissions. J Am Acad Audio 1995;6:271–7

61. Lasky RE, Rupert A, Waller L. Reproducibility of auditory brain-stem evoked responses as a function of the stimulus, scorer and subject. Electroencephalogr Clin Neurophysiol 1987;68:45–57

62. Jacobson JT, Jacobson CA. The effects of noise in transient EOAE newborn hearing screening. Int J Pediatr Otorhinolaryngol 1994;29:235–48

63. Vohr BR, White KR, Brancia Maxon A, et al. Factors affecting the interpretation of transient evoked oteacoustic emission results in hearing screening. Semin Hear 1993;14:57–71

64. Johnson MJ, Brancia Maxon A, White IB, et al. Operating a hospital-based universal newborn

hearing screening program using transient evoked otoacoustic emissions. Semin Hear 1993; 14:46–56

65. Luterman D. *Counseling the Communicatively Disordered and their Families.* Boston, Little Brown & Co, 1984
66. Infant Hearing Resource. *Parent Infant Communication: A Program of Clinical and Home Training for Parents of Hearing Impaired Infants* (3rd ed). Portland, OR, Author, 1985
67. Rhode Island Department of Health Early Intervention Program. Office of Children with Special Needs, Division of Family Health, RI Department of Health. *Hearing Loss and Hearing Aids: A Guide for Parents of Children Birth to Three.* Providence, Rhode Island, 1995

9

Data and Quality Management for a Universal Newborn Hearing Screening Program

Patricia Moore

Introduction

A comprehensive infant hearing screening program requires a marriage of technology management and information management to maintain efficiency and cost-effectiveness. The purpose of this chapter is to discuss the component and practical aspects of information management, whether manual or automated. Information management must be rational and continuous to ensure efficient utilization of resources and to identify areas for improvement. Discussion is largely based on the initial 3 years of the Rhode Island Hearing Assessment Program (RIHAP), a statewide public health program. The two primary sections are data management and quality management. Practical aspects of data management from data collection, patient correspondence, to data security, will be discussed under the data management section. The quality management section describes how a comprehensive approach, emphasizing objective measures, can be developed from common data sources. Quality management per se must be relevant and must not produce irrelevant data that cannot be converted into useful information . Specific indicators will be discussed that have been useful in providing a means by which RIHAP has evaluated its operations and has identified new strategic directions.

Data Management

Long recognized as an integral part of any information system[1], data management is a key component of every hearing screen program. Complexity of data management is related to the size of the population base, the number and organization of hospitals participating, the number of demographic and risk variables collected, and the goals of the program. The key components of a data management program, including data collection, data entry, and data retention, will be discussed relative to experience in RIHAP.

RIHAP is a statewide public health program mandated by Rhode Island law.[2] Fully operational at eight community hospitals, the central coordination site is located at Women and Infants Hospital of Rhode Island, a tertiary care facility. The coordination site is responsible for providing training, audiological interpretation and oversight, equipment and supplies, and information management, including parent and provider correspondence. Table 9–1 provides an organizational summary of key coordination staff. The role of the individual hospital is limited to the core activity: infant hearing screening. Each hospital is responsible for identifying and screening all eligible infants in its own facility, providing demographic data and risk factors on every live birth, transferring the data weekly, scheduling rescreens when indicated, and communicating to the coordination site when programmatic issues arise.

Because of differences in hospital size and birth volume at the outlying hospitals, different staffing arrangements have been implemented for screeners at each hospital. The screening process is considered an integral daily routine in each hospital's nursery and although geographically decentralized, all hospitals follow a standard set of data collection and documentation protocols. The selection of screeners is determined at the individual hospital site; Registered nurses, licensed practical nurses, certified nurses assistants, or trained technicians represent the current screening staff in Rhode Island hospitals. Presently all hospitals screen within the nursery.

The challenge related to data management for any decentralized delivery system includes the development of a secured comprehensive, yet accessible, information system for personnel in various roles. The key functions of data management will be discussed with emphasis on data collection, data processing, feedback to individual sites, storage, and security. In concert with the actual screening process itself, data management provides a platform by which pro-

Table 9–1.   RIHAP Organizational Chart

RI Department of Health, Family Health Division
• Assistant Medical Director
• Chief of Office of Children With Special Health Care Needs

Rhode Island Hearing Assessment Program
Central Coordination Office at Women & Infants Hospital
• Medical Director
• Administrative Coordinator
• Audiology Coordinator
• Data Clerk
• Screeners
• Senior Secretary

Eight Rhode Island Birthing Hospitals

grams can remain efficient, responsive, and effective. During the development and planning stages of the data management system for an inpatient universal hearing screening program, efforts should be made to ensure collaboration among the audiologist, pediatrician, hospital administrator, fiscal manager, information services manager, nurse manager, and health information manager. Each participant will contribute skills and information necessary for effective and complete data management. In addition, an inventory of available data and technology resources, such as wide area networks (WANS) and local area networks (LANS), to increase connectivity and electronic data transfer from sites distant to the coordination office, should be completed.

Although small screening programs may continue to use manual methods for data collection, given the wealth of clinical and demographic information to be managed in a comprehensive program, automation outperforms any manual method in terms of efficiency and accuracy. The foundation of RIHAP's information system is its custom database (RITRACK ver. 2.2)[3] that serves as a data depository, tracking system, and report generator on screening and follow-up data. Using a commercial relational database software, its structure includes over 240 variables and more than 22 reports or letters, assigns a unique tracking number to each infant, and generates correspondence and analytic reports through a hierarchy of menus. Its five computer input screens are set up so that related data are grouped and displayed on the same screen. The computer screens follow the logic and sequence of the screening and referral processes. Each infant is assigned a unique number (RITRACK number) by the database and this becomes the unique identifier for system users in subsequent discussions and transactions. Any letter generated by the database inserts the RITRACK number within the address header. Another advantage of using a uniform numbering system is that it can be used as a basis for the hard copy file storage system. Data entry standards should be defined early on so that data is entered in a consistent and reliable fashion. The use of coded data is highly recommended; developing a coding scheme may be a labor-intensive effort but failure to do so could compromise the integrity of the output.[4] The database submenu architecture provides easy and immediate access to code tables at most fields; this ensures standardization of data entry and minimizes the need to clean up invalid data retrospectively.

Data collection at RIHAP is a combination of automation and manual recording, depending on the available local resources at each site. Data entry into the database from all sites, however, occurs on a daily basis and batch reports are run weekly. Transfer of data from outlying sites occurs on predetermined days so that data entry is predictable and staff assignments at the coordination office can be made easily and accurately.

Data Collection Process

In designing an information system, the first decision should be to define the output needed. This perspective will prompt the next step of defining input processes and data collection instruments that support the desired output or information needed. RIHAP defined its mission as twofold: (1) newborn hearing screening and (2) tracking diagnostic follow-up on specified infants. In keeping with those goals, RIHAP's data collection form ("Sound Beginnings") records patient demographics and screening results. A sample of the form is shown in Table 9–2. Variables recorded on this form are: patient name and demographics, date and time of birth, pediatrician name, description of baby state, screening type (initial, rescreen, and redo), risk factor check list, insurance information, hospital medical record number, scored and coded transient evoked otoaoustic

Table 9–2. Sound Beginnings

Child's Name:_____	Screener ID # _____
	Initial Screen? _____
Medical Record #:_____	Redo Screen? _____
	Rescreen? _____
Date of Test:_____	Signed Consent? _____

OAE	ABR	STATE	
____	____	Deep sleep, no mvment, regular breathing	Time of birth _____am/pm
____	____	Light sleep, eyes shut, some movement	Child's date of birth __/__/__ Child's first name _____ Pediatrician _____
____	____	Dozing, eyes opening and closing	Mother's name _____ Address _____
____	____	Awake, eyes open, minimal movement	_____ Telephone _____
____	____	Wide awake, vigorous movement	Alt. phone no. _____ Insurance _____
____	____	Crying	Comments _____
____	____	Sucking	_____

__:__ Time OAE begun   __:__ Time OAE completed

Risk Factors

__ family hx of congenital loss   __ congenital infection
__ <1500 grams birthweight   __ cranio-facial anomaly
__ Bacterial Meningitis   __ mechanical vent > 5 days
__ multiple courses ototoxic meds   __ apgar 0–4 1min or 0–6 5min
__ syndrome associated with HL   __ skin tags
__ exchange for hyperbilirubinemia   __ other

- -

OAE Screen Results		ABR Screen Results		Audiologist
right	left	right	left	Recommendation:
		30dB ____	____	Discharge ____
		60dB ____	____	Rescreen ____
____	____	85dB ____	____	Rsc W&I ____
				Behavioral ____
				Dx ABR ____
				Medical Monitor ____
Audiologist				fam hx ____ meds ____
Signature _____				infec.____ other ____

emissions (TEOAE) results, audiologist recommendation for discharge or follow-up, and audiologist signature line. A Sound Beginnings form is completed for every screening encounter. At the completion of a rescreen post discharge, a normal nursery infant with an initial failed screen would have at least two Sound Beginnings forms in his or her chart: one initial and one rescreen. The neonatal intensive care unit (NICU) population, on the other hand, undergoes a slightly different screening protocol. At the tertiary care facility any NICU infant, who fails the initial TEOAE screen, undergoes a screening auditory brainstem response (ABR) during that same screening encounter. This collapses the initial and rescreen process for NICU infants. RIHAP found this to be advantageous in addressing the needs of families facing the challenge of managing medically complex infants after hospital discharge, and to avoid conflict with other provider appointments. As a result of this modified screening protocol, NICU infants who fail the initial screen, have only one Sound Beginnings form completed with the TEOAE and ABR screen results recorded on the same form.

Identification of Eligible Infants—Manual or Automation

At the beginning of each shift, screeners create a master list from which all babies to be screened for that day are listed. It serves two functions: provides a means for communication among screeners who work sequential shifts (to note a need for a redo only on one ear, for instance), and it provides an easy checklist to match against the completed Sound Beginnings and TEOAE computer files at the end of each shift. For hospitals with a LAN, administrative databases can also be programmed to produce daily census lists of live births that can serve as a checklist as well. Although the occurrence of a missed infant is a rare event, the screening staff should note the need to follow-up on the master list. This would alert the data staff to register the infant in the database and to contact the parent for scheduling an appointment.

Three specific groups of RIHAP staff are involved routinely with the processing of Sound Beginnings for the NICU and normal nursery: screening staff, data staff, and the audiologist. The screening staff perform the primary task of data collection of demographics, baby state, and risk factors on the Sound Beginnings form. The data staff then uses the Sound Beginnings form as an initial data entry source to register an infant in RITRACK, except for 60% of the Rhode Island births whose demographic information are transferred electronically on a daily basis. During the scoring process, the audiologist refers to the information on baby state and risk factors, interprets the TEOAE results, and enters his or her score on the Sound Beginnings form.

Options for capturing basic patient demographics of name, address, gender, date of birth, hospital number, vary from an automated download to manual collection. Sixty percent of Rhode Island infants (those born at the tertiary care center) have their data transferred directly into RITRACK by a download from the hospital's administrative database in the mainframe computer; this decreases the time that the screening staff need to capture demographic information and can focus their efforts on identification of risk factors. Prior to any data being downloaded into the RIHAP database, the database runs quality control protocols to screen the incoming data for validity and compatibility of codes. From this downloaded information, the database can generate patient labels for each infant's forms and screening file folder. A second option is for the screening staff or data staff to use each infant's Addressograph plate to stamp the Sound Beginnings sheet obtaining the information that is then manually entered into the RITRACK system. A third option that some hospitals choose to use is the manual transcribing of all information onto the Sound Beginnings sheet for later data entry into the database. The benefits of electronic data transfer from an administrative mainframe database are clear: reduction of data entry time, reduction of transcription errors, and elimination of under identification of eligible infants.

Data Collection of Risk Factors

The risk factors used in RIHAP are based on the 1994 Joint Committee On Infant Hearing Position Statement.[5] Prominently displayed as a checklist on the Sound Beginnings form, the screener checks off those factors that the infant exhibits. During the "screening rounds" at the beginning of each shift, screeners review the nursing kardex in the normal nurseries and the NICU admission log for risk factors. If clarification is needed related to a kardex entry, the screener consults the maternal prenatal history or the admission history and physical documentation in the medical record to determine whether risk factors are present. If the kardex indicates either a parent with hearing loss or a family history, the screener may interview the parent to clarify what type of hearing loss is involved. Although this process has its limitation, it will "catch" the vast majority of "at-risk" infants. In addition, charts of all NICU patients are reviewed daily for risk factors by the audiologist. Developing a coding scheme for each risk factor is recommended because it facilitates data analysis that would be difficult if the risk factor remained in text form. The RITRACK standard report menu includes a risk factor summary report that can be run at any time.

Transfer of TEOAE Computer Files

Programs located at a single site will not have to deal with the important issue of data transfer. Mode of transfer from outlying hospitals to the coordination office will be influenced by economic, political, and technology factors. Currently, RIHAP receives clinical screen data on floppy disks and demographic and risk factor data on Sound Beginnings forms. The Rhode Island Department of Health and Women and Infants Hospital, however, are currently investigating options for electronic data transfer between the coordination office and the outlying hospitals. Some low-cost options to consider are (1) modem-to-modem transfer, facilitated by commercial software or (2) modem-to-LAN transfer at the coordination site facility. The sensitivity about ensuring the confidentiality of hospital-specific and patient-specific data makes it all the more compelling that local experts, such as information services, are involved from the beginning of program planning.

Quality Control and Interpretation of Screen Results

The coordination office is located within the tertiary care hospital so that the facility's data is transferred electronically daily. For outlying hospitals, however, all master lists of live births, their screen status, date performed, TEOAE computer files, and correlated Sound Beginnings forms are transferred to the coordination site for processing on a weekly basis. Incoming data is scheduled on a staggered schedule so that the coordination office work flow is constant. By staggering the incoming data on a predictable schedule, staffing can be better anticipated. The following steps are completed. The screening staff print out the TEOAE files, collate them with the Sound Beginnings sheets for each patient, maintain quality control of the incoming TEOAE files, and give the printed TEOAE files and associated demographic forms to the data clerk for data entry. RIHAP determined that within their program, screeners' familiarity with the ILO88 software made them the most appropriate staff to quality control the incoming clinical computer files for appropriate documentation of all test data points. The audiologist retains responsibility for final determination that screening parameters were met and for interpretation of the actual screen results.

Data Entry

Prior to data entry of the data from Sound Beginnings, the data clerk confirms that the form is complete and legible. If quality control issues, such as a missing address or illegible names, arise, the infant's hospital of origin is called to request clarification. Data entry for screen results at the tertiary care center is completed on a daily basis. Data entry of outlying hospitals is entered in weekly batches and the data staff run a patient label report. Patient address labels with the unique identifier (RITRACK number) are then attached to individual file folders. After the audiologist interprets them as a pass or refer, the data staff enters the scored data and generates an "Initial Screen Report" listing demographics and coded screen scores. On a weekly basis these reports are then sent to the outlying hospitals for their use; this allows the outlying hospital to maintain an accurate record of screening activity and to schedule patients when required. The weekly Initial Screen Report reflects all those infants registered in the database since the previous batch data entry. Upon receipt of this report, each hospital is responsible for calling parents to schedule missed initial screens, to reschedule incomplete initials screens (one ear only), or to schedule infants for rescreens. The report also serves as a quality control mechanism for the outlying hospital staff to confirm correct spelling of demographic information. If corrections are indicated, the outlying hospital contacts the coordination office by telephone or by commenting on the current master list. The unique RITRACK number is always used as a reference during discussions and transactions.

Correspondence and Report Generation

In planning the letter and report generation component of a screening program, factors, such as cost, staffing, patient demographics and characteristics, physician support, and patient volume, need to be considered. For the initial screen stage, letters are generated only for those infants who have failed or who were not screened prior to discharge. This decision to limit letters to less than 10% of the initial screened population was based on cost-containment. On an annual basis of 14,000 live births with a 7% initial fail rate, 980 initial fail letters are mailed to physicians, rather than 14,000 letters. Communication of rescreen results, however, is done on a universal basis; the rescreen results letter is sent to both parent and physician. For infants who failed the rescreen, depending on the audiologist's recommendation, the parent and physician will receive a referral letter for either a diagnostic ABR or a Visual Reinforcement Audiometry (VRA).

Generating correspondence letters is a labor-intensive effort, if not automated. The RITRACK letter menu offers more than 10 letter options. Two critical variables to consider when defining program correspondence are to define who will receive the letters and the delivery schedule. For most letters, both parent and physician receive a copy. As mentioned previously, all Rhode Island live births are registered in the database and are assigned a unique number. All correspondence includes this unique number; this provides an easy and quick reference if the physician or parent contact the coordination office for further assistance. Another time-savings feature of database-generated correspondence is that the letters are designed to be folded in such a way that their address header (the parent or physician address) is visible though the window of a number 10 envelope; this feature eliminated the need to use address labels on the envelope.

Letters are not the only means by which staff communicates the recommendations for scheduling a screen appointment, screen results, or audiological referrals. Associated telephone contact protocols vary from letter to letter. Typically before a letter is mailed on missed infants or on the initial failed infants, the staff attempt to telephone the parents. A summary of 11 RITRACK standard letters is provided in Table 9–3.

Converting data into information is a challenge for a solo screening site or a multiple site system. The power derived from coded information manifests itself particularly in the report generation function of RITRACK. From a report selection menu, the user is able to select 1 of the 22 report options. Prior to running the report, the user must specify the search conditions listed in the criteria selection menu. From this submenu, various levels of aggregation can be chosen: statewide, nursery type, specific hospital, date of birth, screen date, screen results, hearing loss type, and referral recommendation. Most reports also feature summary lines at the end of the report to display descriptive statistics, such as the mean age of amplification for the total number of infants analyzed in the report.

Another helpful feature is the ability to define the print destination: computer screen, printer, or computer disk; RITRACK allows the user to select fields for saving in American Standard Code for Information Interchange (ASCII) format. The ASCII format option allows the user to transfer the data to a statistical analytic software application for further analysis.

The mission of screening programs is not necessarily limited to screening and may include the tracking of diagnostic and intervention services as well. All programs need to determine the scope of its tracking mechanisms and plan com-

Table 9–3. Summary of Letter Options

Name	Function	Interval
Initial screen fail	To report fail results	weekly
Initial refusal	To confirm screen availability when parent refused	as needed
Initial miss/rescreen	To notify of need to screen	weekly
Rescreen pass results	Reports rescreen pass results	weekly
Diagnostic ABR referral	To refer for immediate diagnostic ABR after rescreen in normal nursery or NICU initial screen fail	weekly
VRA referral 6 months	To refer for VRA at 6 months of age. May relate to actual fail, medical monitoring, or incomplete screening	weekly
Refusal at rescreen	To confirm screen availability when parent refused	as needed
No show to rescreen	For families who did not show for appointment	as needed
Unable to contact at rescreen	To contact families after 3 failed telephone calls	as needed
VRA reminder	To remind parent of need to schedule VRA	5 months of age
2nd VRA reminder	To remind parent of 6-month VRA, if they did not respond to first attempt	6 months of age

puter and staff resources accordingly. Benefits of a tracking system, beyond screening, are twofold: (1) the program is alerted to families that may require assistance with access; (2) data can be evaluated for regional issues to be addressed. As part of a tracking system, a mechanism for obtaining patient consent to release information is critical. The program needs to define a consent process and create forms that address release of information of screening results to other health-care providers, as well as patient consent for release of health-care provider information to the screening program. Standard hospital consent forms should be evaluated for their utility. The Rhode Island experience confirms that attaching standard release forms to referral letters on infants who failed the screen facilitates screening program and health-care provider sharing of information. Diagnostic results are entered into the database when received. Reports can be run at predetermined intervals to identify families that may require further encouragement by the screening program to follow-up or trends. Finally, in developing an information system, the program should consider developing a tickler system to remind families of upcoming deadlines for recommended referrals, such as a VRA at 6 months.

Data Retention and Storage Issues

For single site screening programs or a multiple site system, data retention and storage issues should be anticipated. During the development and planning stage for designing storage processes and policies, consultation should be sought from the risk manager and health information management professional. Laws vary from state to state regarding medical record retention and confidentiality of health-care information; some screening systems may require newborn record retention for as long as 23 years because of state medicolegal regulations. Staff education is also an important feature to a sound risk management approach. Staff education includes training on confidentiality and hearing screening documentation standards during department orientation for new employees and on an annual basis.

Whether manually or electronically stored, information needs to be secured but accessible. A benefit of an electronic storage system is that infrequently used data, such as older infant cohorts, can be archived or stored in an alternative location on the computer disk. Archiving data increases the speed and efficiency of data processing and report generation, yet it is still easily accessed when needed. Large screening systems may wish to consider options for electronic storage media that offer a higher storage capacity than a paper-based system; options include optical disk, CD-ROM, tape, or microfiche. In planning a data storage strategy, screening programs should utilize the expertise of the information services department and the health information management department. Policies should be developed to ensure security of the database. A critical policy is backing up the database on a daily schedule. RIHAP, not only performs daily tape backups, but also stores a tape backup of the database offsite and replaces the offsite copy on a weekly basis. In addition to the daily backup, the program also performs a monthly backup on the first day of every month and stores this off site.

Reimbursement Implications of Data Management

When designing a data management system for either a solo site or a multiple site system, the interrelationship of standardization of documentation and automation of billing charges support the program's fiscal viability. In an era of a strong presence by third-party reviewers, it is recommended that screening staff understand the importance of documenting that a screen was performed clearly and concisely in the medical record. During retrospective fiscal audits, third-party reviewers may challenge fiscal charges for hearing screening if documentation is missing or unclear. Specific documentation in the newborn medical record to confirm that the service being charged was actually delivered by the hospital is necessary. Screener documentation such as "OAE done" may not be clear to the third-party reviewer; as a result of third-party feedback, RIHAP established the documentation standard that when a screen is completed, "hearing screen performed" is entered into the medical record. Placement of the note within the medical record is influenced by individual hospital documentation policies and procedures; most hospitals make only one entry to document screening completion in the medical record but the location of that note varies and may be located in the nursing flow sheet, the critical path sheet, or the progress notes.

The filing of third-party billing charges can be done manually or electronically. If a hospital has the infrastructure to file electronically, it is recommended that the charges be filed automatically on all newborns. In a universal hearing screening program with more than 99% of newborn infants being screened, it is advantageous to modify the hospital's billing charge system so that the screening or data staff cancels a patient billing charge, only if the screen is not performed. Currently the RIHAP system at the tertiary care center requires that all hearing screen charges be electronically filed at the end of the shift for hearing screens performed that day, and, although the usual filing time spent is no more than 1 min per newborn entry, it is not a judicious use of staffing time. As a result, the hospital plans to modify its electronic billing system for hearing screens so that the screening charges are filed automatically on all newborns. For the less than 1% of infants who are missed, screeners would access the charge system and would reverse or cancel the charge. Thus, the workload for screener fiscal charge data entry will be reduced from a 99% newborn population basis to a less than 1% newborn population basis.

Data management requires collaborative planning to ensure efficient data collection, data entry, and data retention. Whether a single site or multiple-site screening system, each program should complete an inventory of available data sources, staff, local technical experts, and technology resources. From that inventory, strengths and weaknesses are identified for intervention. RIHAP's experience indicates that a mixed environment of manual data capture and electronic data transfer supports a statewide hearing screening program. In summary, a comprehensive data management system that supports a codified data structure and multiple report generation, including user-specified data searches at different levels of data aggregation, paves the way for an efficient, reliable, and timely screening program.

Quality Management

Whenever a new service or program is implemented, program leaders must be in a defensible position to justify the initial investment and risk. Factors, such as heightened reimbursement management by third parties, changing patient demographics, and increased patient expectation for service delivery, compel managers to design programs with accountability, cost-effectiveness, and efficacy in a rational and deliberate manner. Regardless of the dynamic health-care political and economic climate, a program's commitment to effective infant hearing screening must be unshakable. An ongoing quality measurement system, which is comprehensive, objective, and continuous, is one means to support that commitment.

The purpose of this discussion is to describe the planning and management of a quality management system for a universal hearing screening program. The terms quality measurement, quality improvement, and quality magement will be used interchangeably. In developing a quality management system for a hearing screening program, the manager needs to address the following issues: (1) determination of key processes of the screening program, (2) selection of which dimensions of quality are most relevant to the program, (3) minimization of costs associated with data collection and analysis, (4) selection of measurements that address the spectrum of program activities, and (5) creation of a team-based strategy to ensure staff participation and support.

Quality Management—A Basic But Essential Strategy

A common management slogan is that if "you can't measure it, you can't manage it." The pressure for screening programs to prove effective organizational performance will continue to be strong. A program's strategy should include an objective measurement system that monitors system performance on an ongoing basis. Historically, regulatory review focused predominantly on structure and its presence or absence but quality theorist Donabedian stressed the interrelationship of structure, process, and outcome.[6] Despite the infancy stage of quality management and outcome research, health-care programs are expected to develop and implement a measurement system that tracks performance, measures outcomes, and provides a means of cross-organizational comparison. Finally, quality performance costs less. Research indicates that typically 20 to 30% of a program's expenses are avoidable and stem from the system itself: error, inefficiency, rework, labor redundancy, and untrained staff. Ten percent of revenues can be lost, as the result of compromised quality.[7]

Since the early 1980s literature on quality management has proliferated and several sources are available to the reader.[8–11] By the late 1980s, Laffel's[12] article on the application of industrial management science to health-care represented a more data-driven approach for the health-care sector, de-emphasized the tradition of individual case analysis, and proposed a prospective approach to quality management. A second significant trend in the quality management literature is the consideration of service quality and its use as a competitive strategy in building a loyal patient population.[13] A review of the literature indicates a spectrum of pragmatic guides to health-care evaluation and performance improvement methods and models. [7,14–17] More recent articles have addressed quality management and risk management issues, specific to universal hearing screening programs.[18,19]

Benefits of Quality Management

If done efficiently, the benefits of an ongoing quality monitoring system can be significant to an infant hearing screening system. Predictability of resource utilization and service performance is enhanced; staff time spent on crisis management is minimized. Problems are identified and addressed as they occur, rather than retrospectively. Ongoing data tracking and analysis of feedback ensure that for a multiple site system, the coordination office maintains its finger on the pulse of other sites' activity and is able to use feedback as a means to guide priority setting. Of course, the cost of the measurement system must not offset the benefits gained. A program's measurement system should be an integral part of a program's routine operations. Automated data collection and analysis should be utilized whenever possible. By integrating its quality measurement system with its information system, the hearing screening program can generate routine, as well as special, reports at various intervals as required, and, yet, at the same time, control its cost.

Definition of Indicator

The RIHAP monitoring system is largely based on a set of variables (indicators) that are tracked over time to identify patterns and trends for further investigation. Indicators, according to Decker and Sprouse[15], do not measure quality directly but provide a means by which to measure dimensions of quality and variability of system performance to identify trends and areas for intensive review and intervention. An example of an indicator is the parent refusal rate that measures the number of families who choose not to have their infant screened. A wide degree of variability might prompt the screen program to evaluate the adequacy of its patient and provider education materials. In addition, it could assess whether changing patient demographics were a contributing factor.

Indicator Selection—Where To Start

Effective programmatic evaluation requires that any quality monitoring effort be relevant to the screening program's key processes: critical inputs, work processes, and outputs. For RIHAP it was determined that hearing screening, the referral process, and the tracking of follow-up services were its key processes. The second step is to determine which dimensions of quality are most relevant and should be monitored. Dimensions such as access to screening, accuracy, efficiency, timeliness of screening, family perception, and continuity of care, were judged to be central to RIHAP's mission of universal screening. Third, indicators should reflect the dimensions of quality defined as a priority.

Selection Criteria For Indicators

Indicators should be relevant to key processes and not reflect some obscure or rare event. Furthermore, indicators should be selected that make a difference either to the patient, the staff, or the program's budget. For example, an initial screen fail rate indicator would be relevant to the patient, staff, and budget. Avoidable high fail rates create unnecessary parental anxiety and inconvenience, and increase variable costs, such as screening supplies and staffing hours . Capture of indicator data should be routine and ongoing, require little manual effort, and be easily retrievable. In light of the paucity of indicator research, conclusive research findings on indicator validity and sensitivity are not available at this time; hearing screen programs must select indicators on face validity alone. Evaluation cycles should be planned and may vary from indicator to indicator. RIHAP's information system permits a full range of evaluation cycles from a daily to a yearly basis, but monthly and quarterly are the most common intervals. Table 9–4 summarizes factors that should be considered when developing a comprehensive indicator set.

Measurement Considerations—Setting Thresholds and Measurement Units

As the indicators are selected, it is recommended that the program define what range of values is acceptable for each individual indicator. If the selected critical value (threshold) is exceeded, it needs to be determined if more intensive review should occur. Sources of thresholds vary from performance data from other

Table 9–4.   Selection Criteria For Indicators

1. Relevance to key processes
2. Significant to patient, staff, or budget
3. Ease in data collection and manipulation
4. Ease in retrieving data
5. Face validity

screening programs, the program's historical data, or control limits (based on the standard deviation) from statistical process control models. Another decision involves the selection of the measurement unit for each indicator. Generally, indicators are expressed in either percentages or are rate adjusted per 1000 infants; a standardized measurement unit allows for quick comparison and historical trending but should be appropriate to the indicator. It is recognized that measurement units such as percentages are limited in the sense that the use of percentages can imply that the program views the percentage as an acceptable failure level. For example, although a program's missed rate of infants may be statistically low, such as 0.5%, for the missed infant with a sensorineural hearing loss, the impact of an undetected hearing loss is significant and could have lifelong consequences. Sentinel events, those incidents that occur rarely but involve high risk, may be low in frequency but when they do occur, they need to be addressed immediately. Patient injury is a sentinel event and the program should set a zero tolerance level for this type of occurrence.

Sources for Indicator Data

Data sources exist within the department, within the institution, and the external environment. It is recommended that the majority of indicators be derived from the available information technology and to limit reliance on manual sources. The screening program's information system can be designed so that data collection, analysis, and report generation include indicator tracking. The hospital's administrative database provides a rich resource for demographics, financial and third-party data, and critical clinical information, such as principal diagnoses. Integration of hospital data collection and hearing screening software applications may also serve as an indicator source.[18] Manual sources, such as patient medical records, do have their place, despite their limitations of labor-intensive data abstraction and storage. Patient satisfaction surveys, distributed by the hospital, may include comments specific to the hearing screen program. Communication mechanisms need to be developed so that this information can be directed to the hearing program. RIHAP maintains a patient feedback log to summarize and track general hospital survey results and specific patient correspondence. For example, if a letter of complaint is received, the complaint is categorized by complaint type and the results of the investigation and action taken are summarized in the patient feedback log for trending. Logs can be either manual or automated but a simple database is preferred. For a multiple site screening program, a telephone log should be maintained to record all incoming telephone requests, excluding routine inquiries, made by the outlying sites. This permits an assessment of the types of inquiries and may indicate opportunities for staff training. The patient screening record should not be overlooked as another manual source. Inventory control logs record utilization of screen supplies, such as ear probes or disposable tips. Finally, external party reports, such as community audiologist diagnostic reports, insurer audits, and other agencies' reports, may also be useful for indicator development. Their limitation is that these sources are infrequent, depend on outside parties forwarding them to the screen program, and, therefore, it is not easy to predict their availability. Table 9–5 summarizes sources for indicator data that should be readily available or easily developed by a hospital-based hearing screening program.

Classification of Indicators By Key Process

Rhode Island's comprehensive set of indicators were derived from its key processes: screening, referral process, and tracking access to follow-up services. More than 90% of the 26 indicators are available through the program's information system or the hospital administrative information system. Determination of the number and complexity of the indicator set will be influenced by patient volume, the magnitude of interagency collaboration, information technology support, and whether the screening program is a single site versus multiple site. For smaller programs with a stronger reliance on manual data collection and analysis, it is advised that the program limit itself to a small set of indicators to contain costs associated with data collection and analysis.

Screening Indicators

Screening indicators represent the largest set of indicators because screening itself represents the greatest staff effort (screeners, audiology interpretation, and data clerks) and the highest patient volume. All programs need to define the eligible screening population because this raw number serves as a denominator for some indicators, such as missed infants. Another decision is to define at what organizational level each indicator should be tracked; options include regional, program, hospital, nursery type, or individual screener level. Finally, data collection and tracking should be continuous but the interval of analysis may range

Table 9–5.   Data Source for Indicators

Screening information system
Hospital administrative database
Screening software
Patient survey and correspondence
Telephone log book
Patient screening record
Inventory control logs
Diagnostic and agency reports
Third-party payer reports

Table 9–6.   Screening Indicators

Eligible infants
Screened rate
Rescreen return rate
Fail rates
Missed rates
Lost rates
Parent refusal rate
Invalid screen rate
Fiscal billing charge per screened infant
Probe consumption index
Patient feedback

from monthly, quarterly, to yearly. The purpose of this section is to outline some screening indicators and brief definitions that RIHAP has found helpful in its first 3 years of operation. Table 9–6 lists the screening indicators, which will be described in greater detail. Eligible Infants are defined as the number of infants in the target population. For RIHAP this is the annual number of live births at the eight Rhode Island hospitals plus the homebirth population. The Screened Rate is the percentage of eligible infants that received a Stage 1 bilateral screen and the Rescreen Return Rate represents the percentage of initially failed infants who returned for a Stage 2 screen.

Fail Rates are defined as the number of failed infants, stratified by screening stage, and are expressed as a percentage of the infants screened at each respective stage. The Missed Rate is the percentage of infants that were not screened in the hospital and the Program could not screen as outpatients because the parents did not respond to program telephone calls and correspondence. The Lost Rate is the percentage of infants with whom the program has lost contact because of the inability to locate infants, secondary to invalid demographic information. This may occur at Stage 1 and Stage 2. Some programs may choose to combine this subpopulation with the missed rate. The Parent Refusal Rate is defined as the percentage of families who refuse explicitly to participate, stratified by screening stage. These are not lost infants per se because the parents have chosen to opt out of the screening program. The Invalid Screen Rate represents the percentage of total screened infants whose hearing screens cannot be viewed as valid because of screening parameters not being met; some programs may use this as a means to measure the technical fail rate. The Lack of Fiscal Billing Charge represents missing billing information on screened infants. The hospital administrative information system can be programmed to identify all discharged infants without a billing charge for hearing on a daily basis. Utilization rates of equipment, such as probes, are important clinical and economic indicators. For example, the Probe Consumption Index tracks the number of probes signed out to replace inoperable probes and its standard unit of measurement is expressed as adjusted per 1000 screened infants. Historically, this indicator was critical in the early days of RIHAP in identifying utilization variances among different sites and led to the development of guidelines for equipment handling and storage. It also serves as a warning system for hardware-related issues, that if overlooked, are costly. Finally, the Patient Feedback indicator includes family complaints and compliments, which are tracked in a manual log and are classified by type on a quarterly basis.

Referral Indicators

Maintaining and improving an effective screening program represents only half the challenge; the other challenge is maintaining an effective and efficient referral process. Critics of universal screening programs cite over-referral as a barrier to cost-effectiveness and it behooves the program to anticipate that kind of concern by developing indicators that specifically track referral activity, efficiency, and interagency collaboration. For RIHAP this is critical because referrals for diagnostic evaluation are not limited to a failed screen; infants may also be referred for diagnostic evaluation because of a medical risk factor or an incomplete screen. Table 9–7 provides a summary of referral indicators.

The Referral Rate is stratified by reason and are divided into four groups: total referral rate, failed screen, medical monitoring for identified risk factor, or incomplete screen. These rates are expressed as *n* per 1000. The Total Referral Rate represents all referrals regardless of referral reason, that is failed screen plus medical risk factor plus incomplete screen, and is expressed as n per 1000. The Referral Reason By Recommendation Type is displayed in two ways. Referred infants are profiled individually by diagnostic referrals as *n* per 1000: this includes either stratification by immediate diagnostic ABR referral and VRA referral at 6 months. Medical Risk Factor Monitoring is tracked using the hospital administrative information system to identify discharged infants with diagnoses associated with a risk factor for progressive hearing loss; the selected list of diagnoses was developed by the audiologist and a computer program was created to scan all infant discharge diagnoses. This list serves as a safety net for any infant whose inpatient record did not list the diagnosis at the time of the inpatient screening. The Early Intervention Referral Rate represents the raw number of infants referred to regional Early Intervention Agencies. The Risk Response Referral Rate is the raw number of infants that were referred to the regional visiting

Table 9–7.   Referral Indicators

Total referral rate
Referral rate by reason
   failed screen
   medical risk factor
   incomplete screen
ABR referral rate
VRA referral rate
Medical risk factor monitoring
Early intervention referral rate
Risk response referral rate
   screened as a result of referral

---

nurse agencies that assist in locating infants in need of screening, after RIHAP has exhausted its efforts in locating lost families. The Screened as a Result of Referral indicator represents the percentage of those infants referred to Risk Response agencies that were eventually screened. This indicator measures the effectiveness of interagency collaboration and this statistic is routinely shared with other agencies.

Follow-Up Indicators

These indicators are surrogate measures for tracking whether infants receive the recommended evaluations, their diagnostic outcomes, and family compliance with the referral. The primary basis for this set of indicators are the clinical reports from community providers sent to RIHAP. Gaining access to provider reports requires cooperation of the parent, screening program, and the community audiologist, otolaryngologist, and hearing and speech clinic. To obtain parent permission for access to follow-up records, RIHAP routinely asks parents to complete a formal release of information form as part of its referral process. Table 9–8 lists follow-up indicators.

The first indicator is Diagnostic Outcomes. This includes hearing diagnoses classified by hearing loss type and degree of hearing loss. The sensorineural hearing loss rate is expressed as n per 1000. The Amplification Age indicator profiles infant age at amplification by minimum age, mean age, and maximum age in months for specified intervals. Access to diagnostic servcies is critical and the Family Compliance Rates are surrogate measures to define whether infants received services. The Family ABR Compliance Rate is the number of infants who underwent an immediate diagnostic ABR and is expressed as a percentage of eligible families for the interval.

Family Compliance VRA Rate is the number of infants who underwent a VRA at 6 months and is expressed as a percentage of eligible families for the interval. This indicator can also be stratified by referral reason: failed infants, infants who passed hearing screen but have a medical risk factor, and incompletely screened infants.

Staff Participation

Staff participation is critical to the success of any quality improvement program and requires that the program plan opportunities for staff participation, such as incorporating indicators as a formal agenda item at staff meetings, and by using a small team format to collaborate on specific quality issues requiring investiga-

Table 9–8.   Follow-Up Indicators

Diagnostic outcomes
   loss type
Age at amplification
Family compliance ABR rate
Family compliance VRA rate

tion. Posting run charts of key indicators, such as monthly fail rates, in the new-born nursery can serve as a visible reminder to all hospital staff of the screening program's commitment to quality improvement. RIHAP found that these simple graphs were a powerful tool to raise physician and nursing staff awareness about declining fail rates. On occasion quality improvement data may suggest that staff training is appropriate. Staff training should not be limited to technical screening issues and may include topics, such as infant development, interpersonal skills with new parents, infection control, patient confidentiality, and team-building skills.

Quality Improvement Plan

Screening programs are advised to develop a formal written plan that defines their approach to quality improvement, including assignment of leadership and team roles and responsibility, method and rationale for selection of indicators, analysis cycle and procedures for development of an action plan when needed, and an evaluation plan for the impact of any improvement efforts. This should be reviewed annually by the entire staff, updated as required, and signed by program leadership.

A well-organized quality monitoring system provides a rational basis for evaluating a screening program, impacted by internal and external events. Reliance on its information system and the hospital administrative information system enables the infant hearing screening program to develop a cost-effective and continuous monitoring system that tracks its critical components: screening, referral process, and follow-up care. Benefits are immediate and long-term: increased system predictability, feedback to guide priority setting, and strategic risk management.

References

1. Henderson JC, Treacy ME. Managing end-user computing for competitive advantage. In Watson HJ, Carroll AB, Mann RI (eds): *Information Systems For Management.* Plano, TX, Business Publications Press, 1987, pp. 366–85
2. Rhode Island and Providence Plantations, General Laws. Title 23, Chapter 13, Section 13, as enacted by Rhode Island General Assembly in January 1995. Titled "Testing for Hearing Impairment"
3. Moore P, DiCristoforo, D. Rhode Island Hearing Assessment Program. RITRACK USER Documentation. Version 2.1, 1995
4. Aronow DB, Coltin K. *Information Technology Applications In Quality Assurance and Quality Improvement, Part 1.* Joint Commission Journal on Quality Improvement 1993, 403–15
5. Joint Committee on Infant Hearing (1994). 1994 Position Statement. ASHA. 38–41
6. Donabedian A. Explorations in Quality Assessment and Monitoring, Vol. 1: The Definition of Quality and Its Approaches To Its Assessment. Ann Arbor, MI, Health Administration Press, 1980
7. Leebov W, Ersoz CJ. *The Health Care Manager's Guide To Continuous Quality Improvement.* Chicago, IL, American Hospital Publishing, 1991
8. Deming WE. *Out of Crisis.* Cambridge, MA, Massachusetts Institute of Technology, 1986
9. Walton M. *The Deming Management Method.* New York, Dodd Mead, 1986
10. Camp RC. *Benchmarking: The Search for Industry Best Practices That Lead to Superior Performance.* Milwaukee, WI, American Society for Quality Control Press, 1989
11. Juran JM. *Juran on Planning for Quality.* New York, The Free Press, 1988

12. Laffel G, Blumenthal D. The case for using industrial quality management science in health care organizations. JAMA 1989;262:2869–73
13. Clemmer J. *Firing on All Cylinders: The Service/Quality System for High-Powered Corporate Performance.* Homewood, IL, Business One Irwin, 1992
14. Scholtes, P. *The Team Handbook: How To Use Teams To Improve Quality.* Madison, WI, Joiner Associates, 1988
15. Decker MD, Sprouse M. Hospital surveillance activity. In Wenzel, RP (ed): *Assessing Quality Health Care.* Baltimore, Williams & Wilkins, 1992, pp 157–92
16. Ziegenfuss JT, McKenna CK. Ten Tools of Continuous Quality Improvement: A Review and Case Example of Hospital Discharge. Am J Med Quality 1995;10:213–20
17. Hand R, Plsek P, Roberts HV. Tutorial: Interpreting quality improvement data with time-series analyses. Quality Manage Health Care 1995;3:74–84
18. Pool KD. Infant hearing detection programs: Accountability and information management. Semin Hear 1996;17:139–51
19. Marlowe, JA. Legal and risk management issues in newborn hearing screening. Semin Hear 1996;17:153–64

10

Follow-Up

Larry E. Dalzell
Matthew S. MacDonald

Introduction

A chapter regarding follow-up may be logically placed at the end of this book, but considerable attention and planning regarding follow-up need to be done during early stages of development of a newborn hearing screening program. A common goal of newborn hearing screening programs is to identify all newborns with disabling hearing loss as early and as inexpensively as possible so that infants and their families can receive appropriate habilitation as early as possible.

Early identification of hearing loss requires an effective screening program and an effective follow-up program. An effective newborn hearing screening program requires that the population of interest be screened and that there are few false-positive and almost no false-negative results. An effective follow-up program requires that the infants who have failed the screening be evaluated accurately to determine whether they have hearing loss. Further, the infants with hearing loss need to receive timely and appropriate habilitation intervention. Successful follow-up requires timely diagnosis and habilitation.

A newborn hearing screening program with an effective inpatient screening program but an ineffective follow-up program will be a failure, because many infants will continue to be diagnosed with hearing loss and enrolled in habilitation programs at later ages as they would have been without newborn hearing screening. An ineffective inpatient newborn hearing screening program, for example, with many false-positive and false-negative results and with many infants who are not screened before discharge (misses), will doom any early identification program to failure.

Just as there is no single best model for a successful screening program, there is no single best model for a follow-up program[1,2]. The purpose of this chapter is to discuss various components that are important in a newborn hearing screening follow-up program. The discussion will contain a general description of factors that are important to achieve an effective and cost-efficient follow-up rescreening and diagnostic program as well as specific suggestions. This chapter will not contain a discussion of habilitative early intervention programs. Some examples will be given throughout this chapter and in the appendices to show procedures and documents that have been used successfully in follow-up programs. This chapter will describe how to achieve a high return rate for screening failures and misses so that infants with hearing loss are diagnosed and provided intervention at a young age. We will assume that newborn screening generally occurs before hospital discharge and that follow-up work (rescreening and diagnostic evaluations) generally occurs after hospital discharge.

Who Needs Follow-Up

Should all infants who have failed inpatient newborn hearing screening be recalled for outpatient testing as newborns regardless of whether the failure was unilateral or bilateral and regardless of the severity of the failure, for example, no auditory brainstem response (ABR) at 60 versus 35 dB nHL or no transient evoked otoacoustic emission (TEOAE) in only one or two frequency bands? Most newborn hearing screening programs appear to follow the same general recall protocol for all types of failures. However, some programs differentiate or prioritize among failure types to increase the positive predictive value and to reduce the costs associated with follow-up. For example, unilateral failures or less-severe failures may not be recalled, or may not be recalled as newborns. Rather, parents and primary-care physicians may be informed of the screening results with a recommendation to monitor the child's speech–language development and to have the child's hearing evaluated at a later age if warranted. The follow-up may be periodic written or verbal contacts with the parents and primary-care physicians rather than formal outpatient audiological rescreening. Because the positive predictive value is presumably greater for the bilateral failures and the more-severe failures, a program may choose to more aggressively recall these infants than the unilateral or less-severe failures.[3,4] Should all misses, that is, infants who were discharged without newborn screening, be recalled for outpatient testing as newborns regardless of whether the infant was at risk for hearing loss? Because the positive predictive value is only approximately 0.003 for not-at-risk infants,[5,6] some programs do not recall the not-at-risk misses. The at-risk misses typically may not be recalled either, because few programs obtain hearing loss indicator information for all infants because of the cost and complexity of obtaining complete, accurate, and current information. Although misses may not be recalled by some programs, the parents and the primary-care physicians should be informed that the infant's hearing was not screened. They should be encouraged to monitor the child's speech–language development and to have the child's hearing evaluated at a later date, if warranted.

Because the positive predictive value varies greatly and depends upon the inpatient screening results, a recall priority is warranted especially for the group that is difficult to recall. Our program currently recalls all inpatient screening failures (bilateral and unilateral) and all misses (with and without indicators), but we use the following general priority for the difficult-to-recall group.

Follow-up priority:

1. Bilateral severe failures.
2. Bilateral mild-to-moderate failures.
3. Unilateral severe failures.
4. Unilateral mild-to-moderate failures.
5. Misses with indicators for hearing loss.
6. Misses without indicators for hearing loss.

When to Follow-Up

Follow-up testing typically should occur within a few weeks of discharge to minimize the number of infants who do not return. The probability that an infant will return for follow-up testing decreases greatly after the initial few weeks of life. Parents may be lost because of address and phone number changes. Parents may return to work 6–8 weeks after the birth. Parents and physicians will begin to see that the infants respond to everyday moderate-level broad-frequency sounds, and they will interpret the responses to mean that an infant's hearing is normal (at all frequencies in both ears). Therefore, they will question the need to return for retesting and may refuse the retesting. When infants are retested as outpatients at approximately 4 weeks of age, most infants will remain quiet or fall asleep rather easily for OAE or ABR rescreening without sedation. Rescreening without sedation is much less expensive than diagnostic testing with sedation. Also, mother and/or father may be on maternity disability so they can return for retesting without missing work.

Previous communication with the parents and primary-care physicians may determine when an infant should return for retesting. For example, some programs schedule return outpatient appointments for retesting before the newborns are discharged from the hospital. Other programs wait 2–3 weeks post discharge before contacting the parent(s) to schedule rescreening to allow time for the primary-care physician to discuss the inpatient newborn hearing screening results with the parent(s).

The severity of the failure, for example, no bilateral ABR response at 60 dB nHL, may suggest that the infant should return for a diagnostic rather than rescreening ABR to estimate an audiogram so that hearing aids can be recommended.[7,8] In our program, we attempt to do the diagnostic ABR when the infant is approximately 3 months old, and obtain hearing aids, if appropriate. We routinely perform diagnostic ABRs with sedation, which allows traditional patient scheduling and a complete test within one session. Some audiology programs perform the diagnostic ABR for young infants (e.g., less than 6 months of age) without sedation. This requires creative scheduling and may require multiple visits to complete the test.

Outpatient retest appointments may be coordinated with other return pediatric visits. At times, outpatient retesting may be delayed because of the infant's medical condition.

Notifying Parents And/Or Physicians

Perhaps no other single aspect of follow-up in a newborn hearing screening program is more important than the notification of parents and physicians of the inpatient screening results and the recommended follow-up.[3] The notification of the inpatient screening results is often combined with the recommendation for follow-up.[3] Therefore, close coordination between the inpatient screening and outpatient follow-up is often required to have the desired continuity of care and high return rate. It is essential to have the support of parents and physicians to have a successful follow-up program with a high return rate for the infants who need retesting.

The educational information given to parents and physicians regarding newborn hearing screening in general and regarding the local newborn hearing screening program will affect the content of the report of screening findings and recommendations. Examples of parent and physician educational brochures are contained in Appendices A and B, respectively.

Parents may be notified of screening results and follow-up recommendations at various times and by various people. Some programs notify parents of results and recommendations at the time of test or prior to discharge. Although audiologists typically should interpret screening results, parent notifications at times are made by others, such as, screeners, nurses, or physicians. Other programs notify parents after discharge, for example, in person at the first newborn-outpatient visit when the infant is 2 weeks old or by telephone a few days or weeks after discharge. Parents of infants who did not pass the inpatient screening may often have questions that may need audiologist or physician response. Therefore, some programs require that audiologists or physicians notify parents of screening results and recommended follow-up.

The audiologist program coordinator and the physician and nurse leaders need to determine guidelines for parent and physician notification of screening results and recommended follow-up. Notification procedures may vary depending upon whether the infant is in the well-baby nursery versus the neonatal intensive care unit (NICU), who is the screener, and the type of screening done. When notifying the parent(s) that their baby did not pass the screening, it is important not to alarm them but to emphasize the need for retesting because their baby did not pass the screening. The positive predictive value of the screening may vary greatly depending upon the screener and/or screening test used across programs. Suggestions for text to notify parents are in Appendix A.

Physician notification of screening results and recommendations typically occurs with hospital-chart notes and written reports after discharge. Suggestions for physician reports are in Appendix B.

Audiologist referral and communication networks should be developed. This is especially important for hospitals without audiology departments, but it is also important for many communities because of today's provider-choice restriction with managed care. Regional pediatric audiologists should be identified.

Tracking Families

Accurate and complete identifying information is essential to track families.[9] The following information is needed.

Identifying information for follow-up:

- Name.
- Date of birth.
- Hospital I.D. number.
- Mother's name.
- Father's name.
- Parent's address and phone number.
- Language spoken by parent(s).
- Primary-care physician's name, address, and phone number.
- Relative's or friend's name, address, and phone number.

Any existing local tracking programs should be identified to help contact families, for example, in the hospital nursery or county health department. The Infant Child Health Assessment Program (ICHAP) in the county health department may be a valuable resource to help contact and encourage a return visit for hearing rescreening. An ICHAP referral form is shown in Appendix C. Our program has found that the primary-care physician is usually helpful to track and recall noncompliant families. Tracking letters for parents and physicians are shown in Appendices A and B, respectively.

Follow-Up Methods

Rescreening Versus Diagnostic Testing

Outpatient rescreening is generally the preferred initial retest rather than diagnostic testing, because most of the infants will pass rescreening. For example, if the incidence of sensorineural hearing loss in newborns is approximately 0.3% (3 per 1000), and if a good screening program fails 3% (30 per 1000) during the inpatient newborn hearing screening, 90% (27 of 30) of the failures will have normal hearing. If the outpatient rescreening is done at age 3–4 weeks, it is often possible to perform at least an abbreviated diagnostic test under natural sleep for those infants who have failed the rescreening, time permitting for the audiologists and parents. Parents and audiologists often wish to prevent the need for another visit.

A diagnostic test with sedation (if available) may be the preferred initial outpatient retest for infants who are more-severe screening failures, for example, no bilateral ABR at 60 dB nHL, or for older infants who will not remain sufficiently quiet for rescreening without sedation. Diagnostic testing also may be preferred over a rescreening test for infants that have been or may be difficult to recall as outpatients. As mentioned previously, our program prefers to perform rescreening at age 3–4 weeks and sedated diagnostic testing at age 3 months. A diagnostic data form for infants with hearing impairment is shown in Appendix C.

Test Procedures

Selection considerations for the outpatient rescreening test procedure are similar to those described in Chapter 6 for selection of inpatient screening procedure. Programs will often use the same test procedures for outpatient rescreening as were used for inpatient screening.

Diagnostic testing to estimate an audiogram typically includes tone-burst ABR testing and acoustic immittance testing. Some programs also perform OAE testing when ABR findings are abnormal. For the very few infants who have abnormal ABR findings but normal OAE findings, further investigation is warranted, for example, behavioral audiological testing and neurological consultation, before proceeding with hearing aid and habilitation recommendations.

Cost and Funding for Follow-Up

Follow-up costs will be determined primarily by the number of infants that need to be followed and by the type of outpatient testing done, that is, rescreening versus diagnostic. Rescreening is typically done by technicians, nurses, or audiologists. Diagnostic testing is done by audiologists. Recordkeeping and patient tracking are typically done by technicians, nurses, or audiologists with clerical assistance. Follow-up costs can be minimized if few infants fail the inpatient screening and if few infants are missed, that is, discharged without screening.

Parents incur significant costs, such as, transportation, parking, unpaid time away from work, babysitting for their other children, and for the retesting itself when it is not paid in total by their insurance. Physicians can incur costs to their practices if the patients have capitated insurance plans, that is, physician-practice incomes are reduced when referrals are made for hearing testing and other specialty services.

Follow-up costs are viewed differently depending upon who has to pay the costs. The hospital, the parents, the insurance company, and the primary-care physician each will view the follow-up costs from a different perspective.

Funding is typically available with most types of health-care insurance to help parents pay for the outpatient retesting. However, many types of insurance require copayments by the parents, and as previously mentioned, parents have other costs associated with the return visits, in addition to the hospital charge for the retesting. Medicaid will often pay for the retesting. The state's early intervention program is typically managed by the local county health department. This national entitlement program for children less than 3 years of age does not require a financial-means test to determine family eligibility for the retesting.[10] Some of these programs will provide transportation for the outpatient testing. Additional potential funding sources are local service organizations.

Summary

Early identification of hearing loss requires an effective screening program and an effective follow-up program. A newborn hearing screening program with an effective inpatient screening program but an ineffective follow-up program will be a failure because many infants will continue to be diagnosed with hearing loss and enrolled in habilitation programs at later ages as they would have been without newborn hearing screening. A high return rate for screening failures is critical to achieve a successful newborn hearing screening program.

In this chapter we have discussed various components that are important in a newborn hearing screening follow-up program, and we have included some examples in the appendices to show procedures and documents that have been used successfully in follow-up programs. We have suggested a follow-up priority ranging from bilateral severe screening failures (highest priority for follow-up) to misses without indicators for hearing loss (lowest priority for follow-up).

Close coordination between the inpatient screening and outpatient follow-up is often required to have the desired continuity of care and high return rate. It is essential to have the support of parents and physicians to have a successful follow-up program with a high return rate for the infants who need retesting. The audiologist program coordinator and the physician and nurse leaders need to determine guidelines for parent and physician notification of screening results and recommended follow-up. When notifying the parent(s) that their baby did not pass the screening, it is important not to alarm them but to emphasize the need for retesting because their baby did not pass the screening.

Follow-up testing typically should occur within a few weeks of discharge to minimize the number of infants who do not return. The probability that an infant will return for follow-up testing decreases greatly after the initial few weeks of life. Parents and physicians will question the need to return for retesting and may refuse the retesting regardless of the screening results when the infants are older and begin to respond to moderately loud everyday sounds.

Outpatient rescreening is generally the preferred initial retest rather than diagnostic testing because most of the infants will pass rescreening. However, a diagnostic test may be the preferred initial outpatient retest for infants who are more-severe screening failures or who have been or may be difficult to recall as outpatients.

Accurate and complete identifying information is essential to track families. Any existing tracking programs should be identified to help contact families. The primary-care physician is usually helpful to track and recall noncompliant families.

Follow-up costs will be determined primarily by the number of infants that need to be followed and by the type of outpatient testing done, that is, rescreening versus diagnostic. Funding is typically available for follow-up testing.

References

1. Mahoney TM. Early identification of hearing loss in the USA. Audiol Today 1993;5:27–30
2. Welsh R, Slater S. The state of infant hearing impairment identification programs. ASHA 1993;35:49–52

3. Brown DP, Taxman SI. Five years of neonatal hearing screening: A summary. Infant-Toddler Intervent 1993;3:135–53
4. Jacobson CA, Jacobson JT. Follow-up services in newborn hearing screening programs. J Am Acad Audiol 1990;1:181–6
5. Joint Committee on Infant Hearing: 1994 position statement. ASHA 1994;36:38–41
6. National Institutes of Health (NIH). Early identification of hearing impairment in infants and young children. NIH Consensus Statement 1993;11:1–24
7. Weber BA. Auditory brainstem response: Threshold estimation and auditory screening. In Katz J (ed): *Handbook of Clinical Audiology*, 4th ed, Baltimore, Williams & Wilkins, 1994 pp 375–386
8. White KR, Vohr BR, Maxon AB, Behrens TR, McPherson MG, Mauk GW. Screening all newborns for hearing loss using transient evoked otoacoustic emissions. Int J Pediatr Otorhinolaryngol 1994;29:203–17
9. Fowler BA, Fowler SM. Infant hearing screening: A practical approach. Semin Hear 1994;15:85–98
10. Early intervention program for infants and toddlers with handicaps: Final regulations. Federal Register June 22, 1989;54:26306–48

APPENDIX A
Verbal and written information for parents

Page(s)

196   Your baby's hearing is important. An informational brochure for parents regarding the hospital's newborn hearing screening program (English).

198   Your baby's hearing is important. An informational brochure for parents regarding the hospital's newborn hearing screening program (Spanish).

200   Verbal report by audiologist to parents of newborn who did not pass the inpatient screening.

201   Written report to parents of infants in the NICU (pass).

202   Written report to parents of infants in the NICU (fail).

203   Phone text to contact parents to schedule outpatient rescreening.

204   Answering machine message for parents of infants needing outpatient rescreening.

204   Rescreening appointment confirmation letter for parents.

205   Phone text to contact parents to schedule diagnostic testing.

206   Recall letter for parents of infants needing diagnostic testing.

207   Parent information. Auditory brainstem response hearing testing.

208   Parent information. Insurance coverage for auditory brainstem response testing.

209   Diagnostic auditory brainstem response confirmation letter for parents.

210   Letter to difficult-to-contact parents of infants who need retesting.

YOUR BABY'S
HEARING
IS
IMPORTANT

[space for photo or sketch]

WHAT *YOU* CAN DO...

If you suspect that your baby is not hearing normally, request that your baby receive a thorough hearing test from an audiologist.

Hearing testing can be done accurately at any age. The type of test varies with age. If hearing loss is found, assistance is available. **Do not delay! It is never too early to test your baby's hearing.**

If you have questions or would like more information about hearing and hearing loss, contact:

Audiology and Speech Pathology
Department

[your address and phone #]

MILESTONES IN BABY'S HEARING...

Birth to three months...
- Startles or jumps when there is a loud sound

Three to six months...
- Turns eyes towards interesting sounds
- Appears to listen

Six to twelve months...
- Turns head toward soft sounds
- Understand "no" and "bye-bye"
- Begins to imitate speech sounds, such as, "da da", "ma ma", and "ga ga"

Twelve months...
- Says first words
- Understands many words

Eighteen months...
- Uses many words

TO IDENTIFY HEARING LOSS EARLY...

Babies born at (Your Hospital) are screened for hearing loss. This hearing screening program is sponsored by the New York State Department of Health.

DO YOU KNOW THAT...

Approximately 2–3 babies out of every 1000 healthy newborns are born with hearing loss, although few babies are totally deaf.

Without newborn hearing screening, hearing loss is usually not identified until the child is more than three years old.

Late identification of hearing loss causes speech-language and learning delays.

HEARING SCREENING

Your baby's hearing will be screened using an Evoked Otoacoustic Emissions Test. The screening will be done by an audiology technician, and the results will be analyzed by an audiologist. **A report will be sent to your baby's doctor.**

The test is done in a quiet room in the nursery area. A soft earplug is placed in the outer part of the ear canal. A clicking sound is put into the baby's ear, and a response is recorded from the inner ear.

What happens if my baby does not pass the hearing screening?

If your baby does not pass the hearing screening, it does not necessarily mean that your baby has a hearing loss, but it does mean that your baby's hearing screening needs to be repeated. Some babies do not pass the newborn hearing screening because of newborn material in their ear canals or middle ears.

If repeat screening is needed, you will be contacted by the Hospital Audiology Department, and an appointment will be scheduled 3 to 4 weeks after your discharge from the hospital.

Concerns for hearing loss should not stop at birth.

Some babies pass the initial hearing screening and later develop inner ear hearing loss. Hearing loss also may be caused by middle ear fluid in infants and young children.

Even mild degrees of persistent hearing loss may interfere with normal speech-language development and learning.

[space for photo or sketch]

LA AUDICIÓN
DE SU BEBÉ

ES

IMPORTANTE

[space for photo or sketch]

LO QUE *USTED* PUEDE HACER

Si usted sospecha que su bebé no oye normalmente, pida que un audiólogo haga un examen completo de la audición de su bebé.

El examen de la audición puede ser hecho con exactitud a cualquiera edad. El tipo de examen varía con la edad. Hay ayuda disponible si se determina que hay pérdida de la audición. **No se demore! Nunca es demasiado temprano para examinar la audición de su bebé.**

Si tiene preguntas o si desea tener más información acerca de la audición y la pérdida de la audición, comuníquese con:

Audiology and Speech Pathology Department

[your address and phone #]

ETAPAS EN EL DESARROLLO DE LA AUDICION DEL BEBÉ

Nacimiento a tres meses. . .
- Se asusta o brinca cuando hay un ruido fuerte

Tres a seis meses. . .
- Voltea los ojos hacia los sonidos interesantes
- Parece escuchar

Seis a doce meses. . .
- Voltea la cabeza hacia sonidos apagados
- Entiende "no" y "adiós"
- Empieza a imitar sonidos del habla, tales como "dada", "mama", y "gaga"

Doce meses. . .
- Dice primeras palabras
- Entiende muchas palabras

Dieciocho meses. . .
- Usa muchas palabras

PARA LA IDENTIFICACIÓN TEMPRANA DE LA PÉRDIDA DE LA AUDICIÓN

Los bebés que nacen en el Hospital reciben un examen para determinar si hay pérdida de la audición. Este programa de evaluación de la audición es auspiciado por el Departamento de Salud del Estado de Nueva York.

SABÍA USTED QUE...

Aproximadamente de 2–3 bebés de cada 1000 recién nacidos saludables nacen con pérdida de la audición, aunque pocos bebés son completamente sordos.

Sin una evaluación de la audición del recién nacido, la pérdida de la audición por lo general no es identificada hasta que el niño tiene más de tres años de edad.

La identificación tardía de la pérdida de la audición causa atraso en el habla-lenguaje y el aprendizaje.

EVALUACIÓN PRELIMINAR DE LA AUDICIÓN

La audición de su bebé será evaluada mediante del uso de la Prueba de Emisiones Otoacústicas Evocadas. La prueba será administrada por un technico de audiología y los resultados serán analizados por un audiólogo. **Se enviará un informe al médico de su bebé.**

La prueba se hace en un salón sin ruido en el cuarto donde duermen los bebés. Se coloca un tapón blando en la parte exterior del canal del oído. Se administra un sonido como chasquido al oído del bebé y se anota la respuesta de la parte interior del oído.

Qué pasa si mi bebé no pasa la evaluación preliminar de la audición?

Si su bebé no pasa la evaluación preliminar de la audición, ésto no significa necesariamente que su bebé tiene pérdida de la audición, pero sí significa que la evaluación preliminar de la audición de su bebé deberá ser repetida. Algunos bebés no pasan la prueba debido a material depositado en los canales del oido o el oído medio.

Si es necesario repetir la evaluación preliminar de la audición, el Departamento de Audiología del Hospital se comunicará con usted y se fijará una cita para 3 ó 4 semanas luego de que usted sea dada de alta del hospital.

La preocupación por la pérdida de la audición no debe terminar con el nacimiento.

Algunos bebés pasan la evaluación preliminar de la audición inicial y más tarde desarrollan pérdida de la audición del oido medio. La pérdida de la audición también puede ser causada por liquido en el oido medio de los infantes y niños jóvenes.

Aun, una pérdida leve de la audición persistente puede interferir con el desarrollo normal del habla-lenguaje y del aprendizaje.

[space for photo or sketch]

Verbal Report by Audiologist to Parents of Newborn Who did not Pass the Inpatient Screening

We didn't get a good response on the hearing screening. This doesn't mean your baby has a hearing loss but it means your baby's hearing needs to be retested. You will be contacted in 3 weeks to make an appointment for the retest. (Parents will often have questions for the audiologist regarding hearing testing and hearing loss.)

Written Report to Parents of Infants in the NICU (Pass)

Date _____

Dear Parents:

Hearing loss is much more common in infants who have been in a Neonatal Intensive Care Unit (NICU) than it is for full-term healthy newborns. Hearing screening is performed for all NICU babies at (your hospital). Your baby's hearing was screened. Your baby passed the screening at this time. Sometimes it is recommended that babies be tested again before or after discharge from the hospital. If follow-up hearing testing is recommended, you will be contacted. If you have any concerns regarding your child's hearing, inform your doctor or call Audiology.

Audiology Department

(your address and phone #)

Written Report to Parents of Infants in the NICU (Fail)

Date _____

Dear Parents:

Hearing loss is much more common in infants who have been in a Neonatal Intensive Care Unit (NICU) than it is for full-term healthy newborns. Hearing screening is performed for all NICU babies at (your hospital). Your baby's hearing was screened. Your baby did not pass the first screening. This does not necessarily mean that your child has a hearing loss, but the test needs to be repeated. Audiology will attempt to repeat the testing before your baby leaves the hospital. Sometimes it is recommended that babies be tested again after discharge from the hospital. If follow-up hearing testing is recommended, you will be contacted. If you have any questions regarding your child's hearing, contact your doctor or Audiology.

Audiology Department

(your address and phone #)

Phone Text to Contact Parents to Schedule Outpatient Rescreening

Hello, I'm calling from the hearing clinic at (your hospital). I am an audiologist who tests the hearing of babies. My name is _____ .

Your baby had his/her hearing screened at (your hospital). I am calling to let you know that the hearing screening needs to be repeated. The hearing screening is repeated for some of the babies because we didn't get a good response while they were in the hospital. This doesn't mean your baby has a hearing loss, but it means that she/he needs to be rescreened to be sure that they have normal hearing.

This rescreening will be done in the Audiology Department at (your hospital). It is very important to find hearing loss as soon as possible if present.

(If parent asks why is the test being repeated: Explain that sometimes when babies are first born their ears canals or middle ears are not clear and that can interfere with the test or the baby was noisy or fussy during the test. It doesn't necessarily mean that your baby has hearing loss.)

The retesting can only be completed successfully if your baby is quiet, preferably asleep. Bring a bottle and pacifier (if your baby uses them) and also an extra diaper.

[Directions to your clinic]

Answering Machine Message for Parents of Infants Needing Outpatient Rescreening

I am calling as a follow up to the newborn hearing screening that took place at (your hospital). Please give me a call at (phone #) and ask for (Audiologist).

Rescreening Appointment Confirmation Letter for Parents

Dear:

As you know, your baby has been scheduled for a hearing rescreen in the Department of Audiology and Speech Pathology on (date) at (time).

When you arrive at (your hospital), [Insert information about parking, directions to your clinic, etc.]. If you have any questions regarding your appointment please call me at (phone #).

Sincerely,

(Audiologist)

Phone Text to Contact Parents to Schedule Diagnostic Testing

Hello, I'm calling from the hearing clinic at (your hospital). I am an audiologist who tests the hearing of babies. My name is_____.

Your baby had his/her hearing tested at (your hospital). I am calling to let you know that the hearing testing needs to be repeated. The hearing testing is repeated for some of the babies because we didn't get a good response while they were in the hospital. This doesn't mean your baby has a hearing loss, but it means that she/he needs to be retested. Some babies are born with hearing loss with no obvious cause, and some babies have hearing loss caused by illness that they or their mothers have had. This retesting will be done in the Audiology Department at (your hospital). It is very important to find hearing loss as soon as possible if present.

(If parent asks why is the test being repeated: Explain that the hearing testing is repeated for some of the babies because we didn't get a good response while they were in the hospital. This doesn't mean your baby has a hearing loss, but it means that she/he needs to be retested.)

I will mail you information regarding the auditory brainstem response testing.

[Directions to your clinic]

Recall Letter for Parents of Infants Needing Diagnostic Testing

Dear:

All babies born at (your hospital) have a hearing screening prior to going home. It is recommended that your baby have a follow-up hearing test called an auditory brainstem response (ABR) test. Information is enclosed regarding this testing and insurance coverage.

Please call the Audiology Department at (your hospital) at (phone #) to make an appointment for the follow-up hearing testing. Thank you.

Sincerely,

(Audiologist)

Enclosures

Parent Information

Auditory Brainstem Response Hearing Testing

An Auditory Brainstem Response Test is an accurate hearing test that can be done on infants and young children. It must be done while the infant sleeps. To obtain accurate results, a sedative medication called chloral hydrate is given. Chloral hydrate is given by mouth and works best on an empty stomach. Please do not give your child any formula or breast milk for 2 hours before the test. Clear liquids may be given up to the time of the test. Also, please try to keep your child awake prior to your appointment so that she/he will be tired and sleep during the test. For example, parents should try to keep the child awake in the car on the way to the test. If your child is on an apnea monitor, it is important that this piece of equipment be brought with you to the appointment. The testing will be done in the Audiology Department at (your hospital). Audiology is located [Directions to your clinic]. Please plan to arrive about 30 minutes before your scheduled appointment. The entire appointment will take 2–3 hours (including recovery time). The results of the test will be shared with you and will be sent to your child's physician.

Infants with a developmental age of greater than 6 months may receive a behavioral hearing test before the auditory brainstem response test. For behavioral testing, the infant is seated with a parent in a sound booth, and she/he responds to various sounds from speakers.

Parent Information

Insurance Coverage for Auditory Brainstem Response Testing

The hospital fee for Auditory Brainstem Response Testing (and/or behavioral hearing testing) is covered by nearly all health insurance policies, including Medicaid. If the patient is uninsured, if a policy does not cover the fee, or if the family's deductible has not yet been met, the (your state) State Health Department's Special Children's Services will/may cover the cost. The neonatal follow-up staff will process the application for this coverage.

If your insurance requires a copayment, you will be responsible for the copayment. If your insurance is (an HMO), please be sure that your child's physician has called a referral number to the Audiology Department at (your hospital). Audiology needs this number before the test can be administered. If you have any health-care-insurance coverage questions, you should contact the Benefits Office of your employer or your insurance company directly. If you have questions for Audiology at (your hospital), please call (phone #).

Thank you.

(Audiologist)

Diagnostic Auditory Brainstem Response Appointment
Confirmation Letter for Parents

Dear * ,

As you know, upon referral of Dr. * , your child, * , has been scheduled at * **a.m./p.m. on** * for auditory brainstem response (ABR) testing in the Department of Audiology and Speech Pathology of (your hospital). **Please plan to arrive 30 minutes before your scheduled appointment.**

Please do not bring other children to this appointment unless you bring another adult to care for them in the waiting/playroom. Other children are not allowed in the test room.

An ABR test is an accurate hearing test that can be done on infants and young children. It must be done while the infant sleeps soundly. To obtain accurate results, a sedative medication called chloral hydrate is given. Chloral hydrate is given by mouth and works best on an empty stomach. Please do not give your child any formula or breast milk for 2 hours before the appointment. Clear liquids may be given up to the time of the appointment. Also, please keep your child awake prior to your appointment so that she/he will be tired and sleep during the test. For example, parents should keep the child awake in the car on the way to the test. If your child is on an apnea monitor, it is important that this piece of equipment be brought with you to the appointment.

We look forward to seeing * at * on *. The entire appointment will take 2–3 hours (including recovery time) so please plan your schedule accordingly. If you are unable to keep this appointment, please let us know as soon as possible (at least 48 hours in advance) so that another patient may be scheduled.

Enclosed is a brochure outlining the location of the visitor/patient parking lot and directions to our office. As mentioned above, **please arrive at (your hospital) 30 minutes prior to your scheduled appointment to allow adequate time to park and to register.**

Sincerely,

(Audiologist)

Letter to Difficult-to-Contact Parents of Infants Who Need Retesting

(date)

Dear Parents of baby * ,

All babies born at (your hospital) have a hearing test prior to going home. I am writing to let you know that the hearing test needs to be repeated. The hearing test is repeated for some babies because we did not get a good response while they were in the hospital. This does not mean that your child has hearing loss, but it means that hearing retesting is necessary.

We have been unsuccessful in contacting you by phone to schedule the hearing retesting.

Please call the hearing clinic at (your hospital) so this retesting can be scheduled. The phone number is (phone #). Please ask to speak with (Audiologist).

Sincerely,

(Audiologist)

APPENDIX B
Information for physicians

Page(s)
212 Information for primary-care physicians regarding newborn hearing screening at (your hospital).
213 Technician's report for hospital record at time of screening.
214 Audiologist's report for hospital record at time of screening.
215 Inpatient newborn hearing screening test report for fail, unilateral, miss, or pass.
216 Inpatient newborn hearing test report for severe fails, for example, no response at 60 dB nHL with ABR testing.
217 Outpatient newborn hearing rescreening test report.
218 Recall letter to physician for newborn needing diagnostic testing.
219 Chloral hydrate order.
220 Quality assurance letter to physician to recall a child of any age.
221 Information for physicians regarding early identification of hearing loss.

Information for Primary-Care Physicians Regarding Newborn Hearing Screening at (your hospital)

The National Institutes of Health Consensus Statement, Volume 11, No. 1, March 1–3, 1993 entitled "Early Identification of Hearing Impairment in Infants and Young Children" has generated considerable discussion during the previous 4 years. Because the average age of identification in the United States remains close to 3 years, the panel concluded that (1) all infants admitted to the neonatal intensive care unit be screened for hearing loss prior to discharge, (2) universal screening be implemented for all infants within the first 3 months of age, (3) the preferred model for screening should begin with an evoked otoacoustic emissions test and should be followed by an auditory brainstem response test for all infants who fail the evoked otoacoustic emissions test, (4) comprehensive intervention and management programs must be an integral part of a universal screening program, (5) universal neonatal screening should not be a replacement for ongoing surveillance throughout infancy and early childhood, and (6) education of primary caregivers and primary health-care providers on early signs of hearing impairment is essential.

The Joint Committee on Infant Hearing 1994 Position Statement: (1) endorses the goal of universal detection of infants with hearing loss and encourages continuing research and development to improve techniques for detection of and intervention for hearing loss as early as possible, (2) maintains a role for the high-risk factors (hereafter termed indicators) described in the 1990 Position Statement, and modifies the list of indicators associated with sensorineural and / or conductive hearing loss in newborns and infants, (3) identifies indicators associated with late-onset hearing loss and recommends procedures to monitor infants with these indicators, (4) recognizes the adverse effects of fluctuating conductive hearing loss from persistent or recurrent otitis media with effusion (OME) and recommends monitoring infants with OME for hearing loss, (5) endorses provision of intervention services in accordance with Part H of the Individuals of Disabilities Education Act (IDEA), and (6) identifies additional considerations necessary to enhance early identification of infants with hearing loss.

When newborn hearing screening is not universal but based on high-risk criteria, approximately 30–50% of the children with congenital hearing loss are identified. In other words, 50–70% of children with congenital hearing loss are missed. Therefore, (your hospital) has begun to screen the hearing of all newborns before discharge.

The primary-care physicians are sent reports of the screening results for their patients. Infants who fail the in-hospital screening or who are discharged without being screened will be recalled for outpatient screening. Infants who fail the outpatient screening will be scheduled for diagnostic auditory brainstem response testing.

Questions regarding the newborn hearing screening program may be addressed to (Audiologist) in Audiology at (phone #).

Technician's Report for Hospital Record at Time of Screening

AUDIOLOGY (Phone#)

_____   _____   _____

Date   Time   Location

HEARING SCREENING COMPLETED
WITH EVOKED OTOACOUSTIC
EMISSIONS TESTING

Report to follow.

_____

Audiology Technician

Audiologist's Report for Hospital Record at Time of Screening

AUDIOLOGY (Phone #)

Date

HEARING SCREENING WITH EVOKED OTOACOUSTIC EMISSIONS/AUDITORY BRAINSTEM RESPONSE TESTING

☐ Pass   ☐ Did Not Pass

☐ Needs Retest Pre/Post Discharge

☐ Report to Follow

_____

Audiologist

Inpatient Newborn Hearing Screening Test Report for Fail, Unilateral, Miss, or Pass. Report for Hospital Chart and Mailed to Primary-Care Physician at Discharge

Audiology (Phone #)

Date _____   Location _____

Results of Newborn Hearing Screening with Evoked Otoacoustic Emissions/Auditory Brainstem Response Testing

☐ **Pass—Right ear**   ☐ **Pass —Left ear**

☐ **Did Not Pass—Right ear**   ☐ **Did Not Pass—Left ear**

☐ **Did Not Test**—Discharged before test could be completed.

☐ Parents will be contacted by Audiology approximately 3 weeks after discharge to arrange for hearing screening/rescreening.

☐ No recommendations at this time. An audiologic re-evaluation is recommended if child receives ototoxic medications, including but not limited to aminoglycosides, used in multiple courses or in combination with loop diuretics, or if child has an in utero infection, such as, CMV.

cc:

Inpatient Newborn Hearing Test Report for Severe Fails (e.g., No Response at 60 dB nHL with ABR Testing). Report for Hospital Chart and Mailed to Primary-Care Physician at Discharge

Audiology (Phone #)

Date _____   Location _____

Results of Newborn Hearing Screening with Evoked Otoacoustic Emissions/Auditory Brainstem Response Testing

☐ **Pass—Right ear**   ☐ **Pass —Left ear**

☐ **Did Not Pass—Right ear**   ☐ **Did Not Pass—Left ear**

☐ **Did Not Test**—Discharged before test could be completed.

☐ Recommend patient return at 3–4 months of age for diagnostic auditory brainstem response (ABR) testing.

☐ No recommendations at this time.

CC:

**Outpatient Newborn Hearing Rescreening Test Report.
Report for Hospital Chart and Mailed to Primary-Care Physician**

Audiology (Phone #)

Date _____

**Results of Outpatient Newborn Hearing Rescreening with Evoked
Otoacoustic Emissions/Auditory Brainstem Response Testing**

☐ **Pass—Right ear**   ☐ **Pass —Left ear**

☐ **Did Not Pass—Right ear**   ☐ **Did Not Pass—Left ear**

☐ An appointment has been scheduled for diagnostic Auditory Brainstem Response testing in the Department of Audiology and Speech Pathology.

☐ No recommendations at this time.

cc:

Recall Letter to Physician for Newborn Needing Diagnostic Testing

Re:

DOB:

Dear Dr.:

Your patient, * , was discharged recently from the Well Baby Nursery (WBN) or Neonatal Intensive Care Unit (NICU) of (your hospital). At the time of discharge, it was recommended that she/he have follow-up audiological testing, because she/he did not pass the auditory brainstem response (ABR) test in the WBN/NICU.

The procedure of choice to rule out disabling hearing loss in an infant is the ABR test. Audiology will be contacting the family to arrange for this follow-up evaluation. Because this test needs to be done while the baby is quiet, chloral hydrate is given to ensure sleepiness. We have enclosed a chloral hydrate order form for you to complete and return to the Audiology Department in the enclosed envelope.

The fee for the ABR testing is covered by many health insurance policies, including Medicaid. If a policy does not cover the fee or if the family's deductible has not yet been met, the (your state) State Health Department's Special Children's Services Evaluation Program will/may cover the cost. Our office staff will process the application for this coverage. For babies who are covered under an HMO, would you please arrange to secure a referral number prior to the date of this examination. Please have the referral sent to Audiology at (your hospital). The ABR test results will be sent to you.

If you have questions, please feel free to call Audiology at (phone #).

Sincerely,

CHLORAL HYDRATE ORDER

Dear Dr.   RE:

                                            DOB:

Your patient, *, has been scheduled for Auditory Brainstem Response Testing at (time) on (date) in the Department of Audiology and Speech Pathology of (your hospital).

It is essential that the patient remain very still during this testing. Therefore, a young child must be sedated to complete the test. A chloral hydrate dose of 50 mg/kg of body weight is the recommended initial dose given to help the child sleep. If the child fails to fall asleep in 20 minutes, a repeat dose of 25 mg/kg may be given × 2 to equal a total dose of 100 mg/kg, not to exceed 2 grams. **If there are any contraindications to the administration of this medication, please inform us**. Please complete the physical exam, sign the order below, and return it to the Department of Audiology in the enclosed stamped self-addressed envelope as soon as possible. You will receive a report of the findings in 7 to 10 days.

Sincerely,

(Audiologist)

PHYSICIAN'S EXAMINATION FORM

_____   _____ kg
Patient's Name   Weight

I have examined the above named patient and have found him/her to be in satisfactory condition to receive chloral hydrate. If any problems arise before or after the administration of chloral hydrate, I can be contacted at _____(telephone number).

Physical Exam:

PMHx: _____

Active Health Problems: _____

Abnormal Physical Findings: _____

Current Medications: _____

Physician's Order: [50 mg/kg × __ kg = __ mg chloral hydrate PO (maximum 2 grams)]

Please give __ mg chloral hydrate P.O. prior to Auditory Brainstem Response testing. If necessary, may repeat __ mg (25 mg/kg) chloral hydrate × 2 at 20-minute intervals to equal a total dose of 100 mg/kg, not to exceed 2 grams.

_____
Physician's Signature   Date

If the child's weight differs from the above stated weight by more than 10%, or for significant health concerns on the date of testing, the audiology nurse will contact you. Please call (phone #) for any concerns or questions.

Thank you.

Quality Assurance Letter to Physician to Recall a Child of Any Age

Physician

RE: Patient's name

DOB: 00/00/00

Dear Dr.:

During recent quality assurance activities, your patient, *'s chart was reviewed. * was last seen on (date) in the Department of Audiology at (your hospital).

*** DELETE ANY/ALL OF THE FOLLOWING SENTENCES THAT DO NOT APPLY***

- **Based on our results, we have not been able to rule out a significant hearing loss.**
- **Although * was found to have normal hearing, we would like to see him/her back for follow up due to family history of progressive hearing loss.**
- **At that time, further testing was recommended following any indicated treatment for middle ear effusion.**
- **At that time, further testing was recommended in (time period) to further define/confirm the hearing loss.**
- **We have attempted several times to recall * but have been unsuccessful at having him/her return for follow up.**

"OTHER"

Would you please notify us if * is receiving audiological care elsewhere. If she/he has not received follow-up audiological testing, we would be happy to see him/her again upon your referral. An appointment may be scheduled at (phone #). If we do not hear from you, we will assume that * is receiving audiological care elsewhere.

If * is not your patient, or if the family has moved, would you please notify us. Thank you for your assistance.

Sincerely,

(Audiologist)

INFORMATION FOR PHYSICIANS REGARDING EARLY
IDENTIFICATION OF HEARING LOSS

Most hearing-impaired children can hear some speech, but the speech is not clear because of hearing loss in the higher frequencies. This causes late identification of hearing loss, because most hearing-impaired young children alert/respond to everyday sounds. Few hearing-impaired children have complete hearing loss.

Hearing aids help most hearing-impaired children. All hearing-impaired children (hard-of-hearing or deaf) need special education started as soon as possible.

Disabling hearing loss needs to be identified by 6 months of age for treatment to be most beneficial. The Joint Committee on Infant Hearing says that hearing aids should be fitted and special education initiated by that age. Yet, most infants are much older than 6 months at time of identification causing lost potential.

Formal audiological evaluations are necessary to rule out less-severe but equally disabling degrees of hearing loss. Unfortunately, late identification of hearing loss often occurs even for children with known risk factors. It is not appropriate to follow infants at risk for hearing loss waiting for signs of hearing loss to appear. Many hearing-impaired children will not have an obvious speech–language delay until 2, 3, or even 4 years of age.

An evoked otoacoustic emissions test or an automated auditory brainstem response test may be performed to screen hearing of newborns. The auditory brainstem response test is the diagnostic test of choice for infants less than approximately 6–9 months of developmental age.

Visual reinforcement audiometry is the diagnostic test of choice for infants greater than 6–9 months of developmental age. During visual reinforcement audiometry, an infant is conditioned to associate a lighted toy with a low-level frequency-specific stimuli.

Therefore . . . because **hearing loss needs to be detected early** and because **office clinical examinations often miss hearing loss,** we urge you to refer high-risk patients or anyone with a question of hearing problems for formal audiological evaluations.

APPENDIX C

MISCELLANEOUS FORMS

Page
223   Infant Child Health Assessment Program (ICHAP) assistance request or notification form.
224   Diagnostic data for infants with hearing impairment.

Infant Child Health Assessment Program (ICHAP) Assistance Request or Notification Form

AUDIOLOGY ICHAP REFERRAL FORM

Date _____

☐ Parent could not be contacted to schedule an outpatient rescreen.

☐ Child failed OAE outpatient rescreen and did not return for diagnostic ABR.

☐ Diagnostic testing confirmed hearing loss.

Comments:

_____
Audiologist

DIAGNOSTIC DATA FOR INFANTS WITH HEARING IMPAIRMENT

Name _____ DOB _____

Date of Inpatient Screening _____

NICU _____   Non-NICU _____

1. Age at diagnosis _____

2. Test(s) for Diagnosis-ABR and/or conditioned behavioral response

   _____

3. Diagnosis

   Unilateral or Bilateral _____

   Type (sensorineural, conductive, mixed) _____

   Severity (mild, moderate, severe, profound) _____

   Indicators for hearing loss from 1994 Joint Committee on Infant Hearing
   Statement (list risk factors) _____

   _____

   Age at hearing aid fitting _____

   Type of hearing aid fitting (monaural or binaural) _____

   Age at EI notification _____

   Age at EI enrollment _____

   Age at referral to ICHAP _____

   Age at enrollment in other special programming outside of EI _____

   Statement regarding infant's general development and health _____

   _____

   Other comments _____

   _____

11

Newborn Hearing Screening in the United States: Is It Becoming the Standard of Care?

Karl R. White
Gary W. Mauk
N. Brandt Culpepper
Yusnita Weirather

Introduction

> Hearing is perhaps our most versatile and valuable sense. . . . [I]t personalizes or decodes much of the world in which we live. It reaches behind, under, above, around corners, through walls, and over hills, bringing in the crackling of a distant campfire, the bubbling of a nearby stream, the closing of a door, the message of a voice, the myriad of sound which identifies much of our experience. Hearing (decoding) the sounds of his environment enables an individual to spin a web of language during his early childhood.[1]

Downs[2] has asserted that no other group has more to gain from early identification than do children with a hearing loss. Therefore, it is not surprising that the importance of identifying congenital hearing loss as early as possible has been recognized for more than 50 years.[3] For at least the last 30 years, many governmental commissions, task forces, and advisory groups have recommended finding ways to reduce substantially the average age at which congenital hearing loss is identified.[4–6]

The reason so much emphasis has been placed on early identification of hearing loss is the fact that the period between birth and the time at which most hearing loss is discovered at 2–3 years of age is the most valuable time for language development. Unfortunately, unrecoverable time is lost when identification of hearing loss occurs later.[7–9] Additionally, as pointed out by the Department of Health and Human Services[10] (p. 460), the late identification of hearing loss affects more than just language development:

The future of a child born with a significant hearing impairment depends to a very large degree on early identification (i.e., audiological diagnosis before 12 months of age), followed by immediate and appropriate intervention. If hearing impaired children are not identified early, it is difficult, if not impossible, for many of them to acquire the fundamental language, social, and cognitive skills that provide the foundation for later schooling and success in society.[11–14]

When early identification and intervention occur, hearing impaired children make dramatic progress, are more successful in school, and become more productive members of society. The earlier intervention and habilitation begin, the more dramatic the benefits.[15,16]

The Current Status of Universal Newborn Hearing Screening in the United States

To determine what types of hospital-based universal newborn hearing screening (UNHS) programs had been developed since the NIH Consensus Conference in March 1993, the National Center for Hearing Assessment and Management (NCHAM) located at Utah State University conducted a nationwide survey in the first quarter of 1996. The goal of the survey was to identify all UNHS programs operating in the United States. A UNHS program, for purposes of this survey, was defined as a hospital-based screening program in which at least 85% of the babies born or admitted to that hospital were screened for hearing loss prior to discharge using some type of physiological measure. To identify such programs, letters were sent to the following groups, asking them to nominate hospitals which they thought had a UNHS program:

- State Directors of Speech and Hearing Programs.
- Local Chapters of the American Speech–Hearing–Language Association (ASHA) and the American Academy of Audiology (AAA).
- Manufacturers of automated auditory brainstem response (AABR) and evoked otoacoustic emissions (EOAE) newborn hearing screening equipment.
- Coordinators of previously identified UNHS programs.
- Directors of State Maternal and Child Health (MCH) Programs.

Responses were obtained from one or more of these groups in 46 of the 50 states. For each hospital suggested as having a UNHS program, a telephone interview was conducted with someone associated with the program at that particular hospital to determine if it met the survey's criteria for being a UNHS program and to collect information about the nature of the program (e.g., the screening protocol and procedures used, the percentage of babies screened and referred for further diagnostic evaluation, and information related to financial, data management, and referral and follow-up procedures).

The Growth of Universal Newborn Hearing Screening Programs

At the beginning of 1996, 120 different hospitals, located in 31 different states, had implemented UNHS programs (see Table 11–1). Interestingly, the number of programs using EOAE- and ABR-based techniques for the initial screen are

Table 11–1.   Operational Universal Newborn Hearing Screening Programs
in the United States

Initial Screen Method	Number of Hospitals	Annual No. of Babies Screened	Average Births Per Year in Each Hospital
TEOAE	55	118,500	2155
DPOAE	9	18,500	2056
Autoated ABR	54	69,900	1294
Conventional ABR	2	7,000	3500

about evenly split, with 53% using EOAE and 47% using ABR. Of the EOAE techniques, transient evoked otoacoustic emissions (TEOAE) are used most frequently, while distortion product otoacoustic emission (DPOAE) techniques comprised about 8% of the total number of programs. The relatively small number of DPOAE programs is probably attributable to the fact that commercially available equipment for DPOAEs has been available for a much shorter time. Reports from hospitals who had purchased equipment and were working toward universal status suggest that the number of DPOAE-based programs will increase rapidly over the next several years. It is also interesting to note that in spite of the widespread opinion that conventional ABR is too expensive to implement in UNHS programs, two very successful programs based on conventional ABR have been operating since before the NIH Consensus Development Conference.

Table 11–1 also shows that OAE-based programs have generally been implemented in larger hospitals than have ABR-based programs. However, this should not be interpreted to mean that AABR programs are difficult to conduct in larger hospitals. Actually, the number of births per year in each hospital for AABR-based programs ranges from 81 to 4500, while the range for OAE-based programs is from 250 to 9500. Thus, it is clear that both OAE- and ABR-based programs can be conducted in hospitals of all sizes.

Figure 11–1 shows the rate at which UNHS programs have been established during the years prior to and following the National Institutes of Health (NIH) Consensus Conference.[36] At the time of the NIH Consensus Conference, there were only 12 UNHS programs. In the 3 years following the NIH Consensus Conference, there was a sixfold increase in the number of operational programs, with the rate of increase being most rapid for EOAE-based programs. If the rate of increase that has existed since the Consensus Conference continues, we will have nationwide universal newborn hearing screening by the year 2000. Of course, sustaining that rate of growth will require a great deal of effort.

Universal Newborn Hearing Screening Protocols

The NIH Consensus Panel recommended a two-stage screening protocol (Fig. 11–2) in which babies were screened initially with EOAE prior to hospital dis-

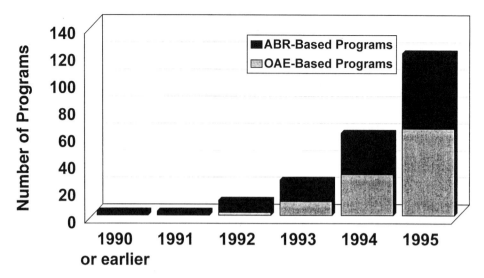

Figure 11–1. Universal newborn hearing screening programs in the United States by year of implementation.

charge, and those who did not pass were then screened with ABR (the Consensus Panel was not specific about whether the second stage should happen before or after the baby was discharged from the hospital). As shown in Table 11–2, the screening protocol followed by most hospitals (83 of 120) is consistent with the NIH Panel recommendation that it be a two-stage screening process. However, 37 hospitals use only a single-stage protocol, and even among those with two-stage protocols, there is a great deal of variation in the technology used and the timing of the two stages. In the most frequently used protocol, TEOAE screening is done prior to hospital discharge, and those babies who do not pass this first-stage screen are then rescreened with TEOAE, and those who still do not pass are screened with ABR.

The main lesson that should be learned from the information presented in Table 11–2 is that a wide variety of UNHS protocols are being used successfully. If any one of the 11 different protocols presented in Table 11–2 was clearly superior to the others, more people would adopt it because all screening programs have the same goal—minimizing the number of false alarms while maximizing the number of true positives, and still maintaining cost and effort as low as possible. The fact that so many different protocols continue to be used demonstrates that no one protocol is clearly superior to the others in all situations. Factors such as personal preferences about equipment, how difficult it is to get families to return for rescreens, reimbursement policies, etc. all have an influence on which protocol hospital staff decide to use.

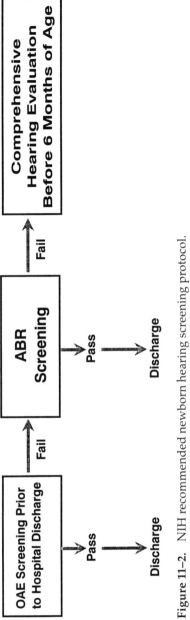

Figure 11–2.   NIH recommended newborn hearing screening protocol.

Table 11–2.   Protocols Used in Universal Newborn Hearing Screening Programs

Screening Procedure		
Before Hospital Discharge	*After Hospital Discharge**	
TEOAE	TEOAE and ABR†	44
DPOAE	DPOAE	5
AABR	AABR	24
AABR	TEOAE	2
TEOAE and ABR†		5
TEOAE and AABR†		2
DPOAE and ABR†		1
TEOAE		4
DPOAE		3
AABR		28
ABR		2

*Only those screening techniques used *prior* to referral for a diagnostic evaluation are listed here.
†The second technique listed in these categories is only done if the infant does not pass the first technique.

Percentage of Babies Screened and Referred

As shown in Table 11–3, OAE- and ABR-based UNHS programs are able to screen the vast majority of babies successfully before they are released from the hospital. Although many people worried that with earlier and earlier discharge times it would be impossible to accommodate newborn hearing screening programs in the busy atmosphere of a newborn nursery, that has obviously not been the case. Reflective of the national trends, the majority of these hospitals were averaging 24- to 36-h stays at the time these data were collected at the beginning of 1996. Therefore, it is clear that finding a way to integrate newborn hearing screening into the busy routine of a newborn nursery has not been nearly the problem that many people anticipated.

Many people have also been concerned about false alarm rates associated with UNHS programs. At the time of the NIH Consensus Conference, the most extensive evaluation of TEOAE-based screening had been done at the Rhode Island Hearing Assessment Project.[17] At that time, a 27% refer rate was reported after the first-stage screen. Because the results of that project have been so widely cited, many people have incorrectly assumed that any TEOAE-based program would have similarly high referral rates from the first-stage screen. It is interesting to note, however, as shown in Table 11–3, that the percentage of babies who pass the initial screen is substantially higher than it was at the time of the NIH Consensus Conference. OAE-based programs report nearly 92% of the infants passing prior to hospital discharge, while ABR-based programs report an even higher pass rate at discharge.

It is important to remember that all UNHS programs do their best to legitimately pass as many babies as possible prior to discharge. By so doing, they substantially reduce the time and effort needed to follow babies with additional

Table 11–3.   Reported Percentage of Babies Screened and Referral Rates for Universal
Newborn Hearing Screening Programs

	No. of Hospitals	Percent Babies Screened Before Discharge	Reported Pass Rate at Discharge (%)
OAE-Based Programs	64	94.9	91.6
ABR-Based Programs	56	96.2	96.0
All Programs	120	95.5	93.7

screening or diagnostic procedures. Additionally, they reduce the burden on parents for bringing babies back for additional evaluation. Thus, most of the OAE- and ABR-based programs attempt to screen babies several times before discharge if the baby does not pass at the first attempt. In addition, as shown earlier in Figure 11–2, a number of hospitals have implemented two-stage screening protocols prior to discharge using OAE and ABR.

It is also important to note that the referral rate at discharge reported in Table 11–3 is not necessarily synonymous with the percentage of babies referred for a diagnostic evaluation. Most of the OAE-based programs and about half of the ABR-based programs do a second-stage screening after the baby is discharged from the hospital before recommending a diagnostic evaluation. As an example of how this substantially reduces the number of babies referred for diagnostic evaluations, consider the following. In TEOAE-based programs, about 8% do not pass prior to discharge. However, about 90% of those babies will pass at the rescreen following discharge. Thus, only about 1% of the babies in a TEOAE-based program are referred for a diagnostic evaluation. However, in AABR-based programs that refer babies directly for a diagnostic evaluation if they do not pass the first-stage screen, about 4% of the babies would be referred for a diagnostic evaluation.

Where, When, and By Whom is Screening Done?

Hospitals also report substantial variation in who does the screening and where and when it is done. As shown in Table 11–4, screening in UNHS programs is frequently done by technicians, audiologists, nurses, volunteers, and others. Technicians and audiologists conduct the screening more frequently in OAE-based programs, and nurses conduct it most frequently in ABR-based programs. However, these numbers are changing as programs become better established. Specifically, fewer audiologists and nurses, and more technicians or other nursery personnel (e.g., licensed practical nurses, health-care assistants, and clerical staff) are screening babies, regardless of the technology used for screening. The main message from Table 11–4 is that virtually anyone who is given brief training and is adequately supervised can successfully implement any of the newborn hearing screening protocols that are currently being used.

In the same way that hospitals have implemented a variety of different screening protocols, there is similar heterogeneity with respect to where screening is

Table 11–4.   Who Does the Screening in Universal Newborn Hearing Screening Programs?

	No. of Hospitals	Technicians %	Audiologists %	Nurses %	Volunteers %	Others %
OAE-Based Programs	64	42	41	34	2	8
ABR-Based Programs	56	21	14	56	23	11
All Programs	120	32	28	45	12	9

done and when it is done. Given the shorter and shorter stays in the hospital, more and more screening is being done right in the nursery, although some programs still screen in specially designated rooms or in the mother's room. Where the screening is done is more a function of the hospital policies with regard to where babies are located for most of the time or the availability of extra space. However, it is clear that screening can be done successfully in many different locations, regardless of the technique used.

Similarly, screening is done at different times of the day or night, depending on which personnel are used. Some hospitals find that the night shift is a particularly good time because there are not as many competing activities and babies tend to be more available while their mothers are sleeping. Most programs try to avoid the time in the morning when doctors usually do their rounds and need to have access to the babies.

Financial Issues

As shown in Table 11–5, only about two-thirds of the hospitals who had UNHS programs at the beginning of 1996 were billing third-party payers as a way of financing the program. In a few cases this was because state or federal grant money was being used to operate the program during an initial evaluation period. In most cases where billing was not being done, however, hospitals were simply offering hearing screening as a service to patients without trying to bill, or the programs were so recently implemented that they had not yet worked out the billing procedures.

It is clear, however, that financial reimbursement continues to be a major issue as administrators consider the implementation of newborn hearing screening. In most cases, hospital administrators want to make sure that the screening program will at least cover its cost. However, the cost of implementing a UNHS program (as is discussed in more detail later in this chapter) is so reasonable that financing has not been the major obstacle that many feared.

Many hospitals have been able to secure funding for the purchase of equipment from service organizations or other foundations. However, the costs for the ongoing screening program either have to be covered by existing hospital budgets or the program has to pay for itself as a result of third-party payments. The degree to which hospitals have been successful in obtaining third-party pay-

Table 11–5.   Third-Party Billing for Newborn Hearing Screening

	No. of Hospitals	Billing for Screening? (%)	Average Amount Billed for Screening
OAE-Based Programs	64	63	$43.26 (n = 40)
ABR-Based Programs	56	66	$62.65 (n = 37)
All Programs	120	64	$52.58 (n = 77)

ments depends on a variety of factors that vary from state to state and oftentimes within states. Although it was true 2 or 3 years ago that ABR programs tended to have an easier time getting reimbursed, that trend has changed substantially in the last year, and the reported rate of reimbursement is similar now, regardless of the technology being used. As shown in Table 11–5, ABR programs tend to charge about 50% more than OAE programs, which is consistent with the differences in costs between the two kinds of programs. However, the cost per baby depends more on the protocol being used and the personnel who do the screening than it does on the type of equipment being used.

Summary

It is clear from the foregoing data that most of the concerns about the feasibility of newborn hearing screening that were raised following the NIH Consensus Conference (See Gravel and Tocci, Chapter 1) are no longer an issue. As more and more hospitals have implemented UNHS programs, evidence continues to accumulate that a wide variety of protocols and procedures can be used successfully and that the issues of practicability, cost, and disruption of family functioning are not the serious issues or obstacles that some people thought they would be. There is, however, a great deal of variability in how programs are operated. This variability seems to be related to personal preferences, as well as local circumstance.

Implementing Statewide Newborn Hearing Screening Programs

With the current interest in the implementation of UNHS programs, it is important to remember that some states have been involved in efforts to screen for hearing loss at an early age for the past three decades. For example, in a survey conducted in 1990, Blake and Hall[18] showed that 30 of the 50 states were involved in some way in newborn hearing screening. At that time, 16 states had legislative mandates related to newborn hearing, and an additional 14 were reported as having a program or policy in place without a state mandate.

As reported by Johnson et al.,[19] however, a careful analysis of those data revealed alarming gaps and deficiencies. Of the 16 states that had a legislative mandate to do newborn hearing screening, only 9 were actually operating regional or statewide screening programs, and all but one of those focused only on infants who exhibited one of the risk criteria delineated by the Joint Committee on Infant Hearing[20] or who were in a NICU. Consequently, the majority of the babies, even in those states with legislative mandates, were not being screened for hearing loss. Furthermore, most of the programs were limited to large population centers, and the relationship between screening programs and early intervention systems was frequently weak. For example, although federal law at that time required all State Departments of Education to provide services to young children with hearing loss, Johnson et al.[19] reported that a telephone survey of Department of Education officials in those 16 states with legislative mandates found people in only six of these states who were even aware there was a newborn hearing screening mandate in their own state. In those states that Blake and Hall[18] reported as having a program or policy in place without a state mandate, the situation was about the same. Only 6 of the 14 had an operational program, and all of those focused only on high-risk or NICU babies. The other eight states encouraged screening or provided technical support and training on request.

With regard to the provision of services to young children identified as having hearing impairments, the picture was not much better. Most children with severe to profound bilateral sensorineural hearing disabilities received fairly good services, but those with less severe losses usually did not receive adequate services. As noted by Blake and Hall[18] (p. 73), even in those states with legislative mandates, "a system for identification and referral is lacking."

Similar findings were reported by Welch and Slater[21] in a survey conducted several years later under the auspices of ASHA on the status of infant hearing impairment identification programs as of December 1992. At that time, 19 states reported having some sort of legislatively mandated program, but all but 2 of them focused only on high-risk infants, and all of them reported that the legislative mandate did not require any type of systematic "follow-up care."

Fortunately, as shown earlier in Figure 11–2, there has been a rapid expansion of UNHS programs since the NIH Consensus Conference in March 1993. Unfortunately, most of this progress is limited to individual hospitals and not to statewide programs. There are, however, a few exceptions. Rhode Island and Hawaii now have coordinated statewide programs in place in which at least 90% of the babies in the state are being screened. Utah and Colorado (even without the benefit of a legislative mandate) are screening more than half of the births in their respective states, and Louisiana, Iowa, Kentucky, and New York each have multiple hospitals with UNHS programs that are screening thousands of newborns each year and are systematically moving forward with state-supported efforts to establish newborn hearing screening as the standard of care. However, a great deal of work remains to be done.

A key to continuing the progress of the last few years is for advocates of newborn hearing screening to understand the process by which public policy can be affected. Baumeister[22] has offered the following 14 general recommendations for people who wish to influence public service policies, such as programs to support early identification and intervention:

1. Develop a clear consensus statement about what must be done, by whom, when, and where.
2. Identify several well-respected individuals who have the interest, time, and energy to analyze the political environment, major players, and obstacles to implementation of the policy.
3. Generate an action plan that includes ongoing lobbying efforts, collection and packaging of supportive scientific data, and coordination among the various professional organizations and disciplines who have a stake in the outcome.
4. Enlist the involvement of various advocacy groups who have similar goals.
5. Identify legislators and agency officials who, by reason of personal circumstances, are likely to be sympathetic and supportive of the agenda.
6. Use the media and other public awareness events to elicit public support and awareness of the issue.
7. Cooperate, instead of competing, with other organizations also interested in affecting public policy, such as groups who advocate for individuals with special needs.
8. Make sure all materials and public awareness information avoids the use of jargon and is communicated in terms that people outside of any particular profession can understand.
9. Present scientific data in the context of children's and families' lives, instead of faceless numbers.
10. Develop a timeline with specific goals, always requesting a little more than appears to be possible at the moment.
11. Accept the need for compromise, given that other needs and interests must also be addressed within an already overloaded system.
12. Establish mechanisms for information exchange within your own professional groups, as well as those groups with comparable interests.
13. Be prepared and develop mechanisms for financial support. Efforts that depend solely on voluntary resources will often not be able to engage in the type of sustained efforts necessary to affect policy.
14. Do not become discouraged. Setbacks and redirection of efforts are almost always a part of any significant change in human services policies.

Any change as substantial as implementing UNHS will require sustained effort of many people over an extended period of time. The general guidelines for such activities outlined by Baumeister[22] provide a context for discussing the specific types of activities implemented by states that have been most successful in establishing statewide systems for UNHS programs. A description of those activities with examples from states that have made substantial progress is discussed below.

Documenting the Need

The first step in building a coalition for developing and implementing coordinated UNHS programs within a state is to convince various constituency groups of the existence of a need that has a feasible and practical solution. Inadequate fiscal resources in virtually all sectors of state government make this a difficult time for policymakers to mandate additional services. Furthermore, there is reluctance to identify infants with any type of disability unless policymakers can be convinced that the infrastructure exists to provide adequate services to those children. Although these are real obstacles in most cases, they can be overcome if appropriate information is used. Citing evidence from other states that have successfully implemented programs or referencing the conclusions of national groups, such as the NIH Consensus Conference[36] or the Joint Committee on Infant Hearing (JCIH) Position Statement,[20] is helpful but is often not enough. Similarly, although substantial data are available demonstrating that congenital hearing loss is usually not identified until 2–3 years of age if UNHS programs are not in place,[5,23] data from one's own state are often necessary to generate support, especially among physicians and legislators.[24] Gathering such data requires a considerable commitment of resources. If it is done well, however, it can be an effective mechanism for generating support, as well as enabling the state to tailor the program more specifically to meet local needs.

For example, following the NIH Consensus Conference in 1993,[36] an ad hoc group of people in Utah, who were concerned about early identification of hearing loss, began meeting informally to decide what could be done to improve upon the existing birth-certificate-based, high-risk registry program. This group included representatives from the State Department of Health, hospitals, early intervention programs, private practice audiologists, pediatricians, nurses, and university faculty. As a first step, data concerning the performance of the long-established, high-risk registry program in the state was assembled. This was possible in part because of the existence of an excellent database, which documented the performance of the birth-certificate-based, high-risk registry program over the previous 15 years. By comparing those data to known information about prevalence and also examining what was happening in other states, it became clear that many infants were being missed and much more was possible. Officials at the State Department of Health who were responsible for the high-risk registry program led the way in concluding that although many young children were being identified as a result of the program, many other young children were being missed or identified far too late. As a result, the ad hoc group was established as a Task Force, and the Department of Health incorporated specific goals as a part of their annual planning process to reduce the age of identification of hearing loss within the state. As a result of these activities, the percentage of babies born at hospitals in Utah with UNHS programs has increased from less than 10% to more than 60% during the last 3 years.

Although the situation in Hawaii was similar, efforts to implement statewide UNHS began there prior to the NIH Consensus Development Conference. Initial efforts to convince legislators and agency administrators of the need for UNHS using data collected in other states or countries were largely unsuccessful. Consequently, the people responsible for serving birth to 3-year-old children in Hawaii conducted a study and found that the average age of identification for children with sensorineural hearing loss in Hawaii was actually much higher than that reported by other states. Children in Hawaii were not being identified until an average of 4.1 years of age, and the age of identification varied according to whether the child's family had health insurance or lived in rural or urban areas. To make the data more meaningful and personal, they were presented using case studies and individual accounts of people who had experienced the consequences of late identification. As a result, legislators and agency administrators became convinced of the critical need for earlier identification of hearing loss.

Although Rhode Island was one of the leaders in demonstrating that TEOAE-based newborn hearing screening programs were feasible to implement on a statewide basis, it was only when local data were collected that state legislators and policymakers became convinced they could design a comprehensive statewide program that would be responsive to the multilingual, multicultural population within the state. Furthermore, having data specific to Rhode Island allowed the program to document more adequately the benefits of early identification by being able to compare the situation before and after the UNHS program was implemented. These data were instrumental in establishing the fledgling program as an ongoing part of the state's health-care system and linking it to other efforts to provide comprehensive, community-based, family-centered services to children with special health-care needs and their families.

Generating Constituency Support

Although data demonstrating the importance of early identification of hearing loss are critical for convincing legislators and public officials of the need for such programs, broad-based constituency support from a variety of groups is usually necessary to make newborn hearing screening a reality. Many different people have a vested interest in the population to be served via statewide UNHS programs. If their support is not obtained at the beginning, later opposition (often resulting from simple misunderstandings) can seriously impede and delay the implementation of an effective UNHS program. It is especially important that those with competing financial needs become committed to the development of a UNHS system. Several of the most important groups are discussed briefly below.

CONSUMERS

Persons with hearing disabilities (particularly those who were not identified early) are often excellent advocates for establishing UNHS programs. As referred to briefly above in describing the efforts to establish a program in Hawaii, personal experiences of the effects of late identification have strong impact on legislators, agency administrators, and hospital staff who are considering the implementation of UNHS programs. Newspaper stories and television special reports can be used to help people become aware of the feasibility of implementing UNHS programs and the associated benefits. Such stories have strong public interest appeal and are eagerly sought by television stations and newspapers. People who have personally benefitted from newborn hearing screening programs can also be excellent witnesses at legislative hearings and can be instrumental in convincing local hospital administrators to implement a program.

AUDIOLOGISTS

In most cases, audiologists will be leading the effort to establish a statewide UNHS program. In some cases, however, successful programs have been started with relatively little audiological involvement. For example, the statewide program in Rhode Island became operational with little support from community-based audiologists. When the time arrived to move the program from the first hospital to a statewide program, however, there was some opposition by the community-based audiologists that could have been prevented had they been more extensively involved from the beginning. In contrast, audiologists in Hawaii were the force behind developing and implementing the system. Their unified voice during legislative hearings was a significant factor in the passage of legislation mandating UNHS in the state.

PHYSICIANS

Although pediatricians, family practice physicians, and otolaryngologists are supportive of early identification of hearing loss, they often have appropriate concerns about unnecessarily alarming parents because of false-positives during the initial screen, the cost to families of screening and diagnosis, and the way in which a UNHS program will affect their relationship with their patients.[25] Our experience suggests that even though physicians are sometimes criticized for their "wait and see" attitude,[26,27] most are supportive of newborn hearing screening programs that provide a realistic potential for early identification linked with effective intervention services.[28,29] Although considerable effort may be necessary to enlist their support, the benefits are worth it. In Rhode Island, not only have the primary-care physicians been supportive, but the frequent contact between the screening programs and the physicians in the course of following patients through the referral and diagnostic process produced an unanticipated "halo effect" in the early years of the program. For example, as shown in Figure 11–3, the number of children referred to the early intervention program for children with hearing loss in Rhode Island dramatically increased following the implementation of the newborn hearing screening program in 1991 at the state's largest hospital. The vast majority of the children referred to and accepted into services for young children with hearing loss did not come directly from the screening program, since at that point only about 20% of the children in the state were being screened. Instead, most of these children came from the increased number of referrals from physicians who had become more aware of the importance and benefits associated with early identification of hearing loss as a result of their contacts with the existing pilot project.

NURSES

In most cases, UNHS programs will function under the auspices of the hospital nursery. Particularly because babies are being discharged from hospitals at earlier and earlier ages, it is absolutely essential to coordinate with nursing staff to have a successful program. Unless nursery staff understand the purpose of the

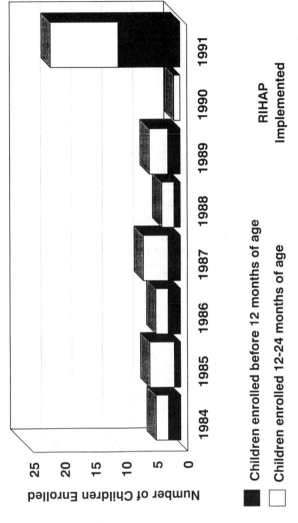

Figure 11–3. Children under 24 months enrolled in early intervention programs for hearing-impaired children in Rhode Island.

newborn hearing screening program and are committed to its success, the program is unlikely to achieve its goals. It is not unusual to have newborn hearing screening programs approved by the hospital administration and established as a standing order by the medical committee at the hospital and still fail miserably because nurses were not brought on board in a way that would lead them to be supportive of the program.

Obtaining a Legislative Mandate

Although some states have been quite successful without legislation that requires newborn hearing screening, an appropriate legislative mandate for newborn hearing screening can be extremely helpful, and the only states that have achieved statewide status have had such mandates prior to establishing statewide programs.

WRITING THE BILL

Each state should approach this task somewhat differently according to the state's demographics, organization of health and education services, and the key players who are involved in writing and supporting the effort to secure legislation. In every case, the various constituencies whose support has been acquired should be involved in the process of developing the legislation. A good first step is to secure copies of legislation from other states. Although 19 different states currently have some type of legislative mandate related to newborn hearing screening, 17 of these focus only on children who exhibit one or more of the high-risk indicators. Thus, Rhode Island and Hawaii are still the only two states with legislative mandates for universal newborn hearing screening. However, several other states (Utah, Minnesota, Pennsylvania, Colorado, New York, and Connecticut) are currently considering legislation that would mandate UNHS programs.

Those states that have already passed legislation (Hawaii and Rhode Island) approached the task in substantially different ways. In Hawaii, legislation was proposed and passed before any hospitals had implemented UNHS programs. In contrast, the majority of the births in Rhode Island were already being screened prior to the passage of the legislative mandate. Consequently, much more data were available in Rhode Island to demonstrate the feasibility and benefits of such a program. In fact, a significant factor in passing the Rhode Island legislation was having key members of the legislative committees observe some of the UNHS programs in operation.

In both cases, the legislation is simple and concise and does not specify a specific screening methodology or protocol. Given how rapidly the technology for newborn hearing screening continues to evolve, this is certainly the best approach. The key provision is to make sure that "every newborn infant" is to be screened, instead of focusing only on a specific subpopulation. Copies of previously passed legislation, as well as bills currently being considered by state legislatures, are available from the National Center for Hearing Assessment and Management at Utah State University.

NEGOTIATING THE LEGISLATIVE PROCESS

The legislative process can easily become a quagmire, but there are several ways to increase the probability of getting a bill passed. First, it is essential to have someone familiar with the process who can continually monitor the status of the legislation and be prepared to provide additional information, support, and advocacy as it is needed. The bill is more likely to be passed if influential legislators can introduce the bill and are willing and able to educate other committee members about the merits of having a mandate for newborn hearing screening. It is even more effective if the bill already has the support of key executive agencies. For example, the ideal situation, as was done in Rhode Island, is to work with the governor's office early enough so that the bill can be introduced as a part of a package of initiatives that the governor sends to the legislature. If key committee members are already supportive of the bill, and if the bill has the support of the executive branch, then the likelihood of passage is substantially increased.

The importance of constituency support as a part of the legislative process cannot be overstated. As a part of the legislative hearings in Rhode Island and Hawaii, testimony was presented by pediatricians, otolaryngologists, audiologists, and various professional organizations. However, the most effective advocates were the parents of young children with hearing loss and adults with significant congenital hearing loss who spoke eloquently about the need for earlier identification of hearing disability. This broad-based support from a variety of constituency groups was the key to quick passage of the legislation.

Successful passage and signing of legislation is only the beginning of implementing a successful UNHS program. A mandate is of limited value unless it is followed by a strategic plan to implement its provisions within a reasonable time frame throughout the state. In most cases, rules and regulations that describe the way in which hospitals will do the screening, how follow-up and tracking of referred infants will be accomplished, and how the screening program will be coordinated with early intervention efforts will need to be negotiated and written. This is an essential step to make sure that a UNHS program is the foundation of early detection of hearing loss and successful intervention.

Implementing the Program

Even if a legislative mandate is obtained, community commitment must be nurtured and sustained to have a successful statewide UNHS program. A statewide task force representing the various groups to be involved in early identification and intervention is often helpful to develop the necessary components for a comprehensive, coordinated, family-centered system. Because it is unlikely that universal screening can begin simultaneously for all birthing facilities, the various constituencies need to agree on a strategy that phases in a UNHS program within a reasonable time. During this phase-in period, extensive coordination will be necessary between the various groups that have an interest in the outcomes, such as the state's Title V, Part H, and Medicaid programs.

Based on the data referred to earlier in this chapter about how existing UNHS programs have been implemented, it is clear that most states will have a fair amount of heterogeneity with respect to the specific protocol being followed in various hospitals, the way in which the screening program is organized within the hospital, and the procedures to follow and assist infants referred from the screening program. Thus, it is important that there be a mechanism to coordinate this process and to provide assistance to hospitals as they define the various roles and responsibilities to make newborn hearing screening successful at their institution. Procedures will also need to be created for monitoring the implementation of the program so that data can be available on how well the system has been implemented, as well as demonstrating that the goals of the program are being accomplished.

One of the issues that needs to be addressed in designing a statewide system is to make sure that the small birthing hospitals or hospitals located in rural and remote areas are also able to implement the system. Although there are a few exceptions, most of the newborn hearing screening programs currently in operation are located in hospitals in metropolitan areas with at least 1000 births per year. Interestingly, however, almost 50% of the more than 4200 birthing hospitals in this country have fewer than 400 births per year, and 18% of all birthing hospitals have less than 100 births per year. Although a relatively small number of babies are born in these small hospitals (for example, less than 2% of all babies are born in hospitals with less than 100 births per year), there are legal and ethical problems with having a statewide UNHS program that does not address the needs of these hospitals. The most important issues that need to be addressed relate to providing appropriate training to the hospitals as they implement programs and then making sure that they have support for audiological input, follow-up, and intervention services.

In a state like Rhode Island where all hospitals in the state are within 40 miles of each other, the issues are different from a state like Montana where hospitals are often separated by hundreds of miles from the types of support services that people in larger cities have available on a routine basis. In Utah, these issues are being addressed by having hospitals linked together so that data from the screening program can be electronically transferred, having itinerant audiologists available for providing support to those programs, and by coordinating with the state's parent–infant program for providing services to families who have a child with a hearing loss. Most states have already dealt with these kinds of issues to some degree as a result of providing services to other children with special health-care needs. Thus, the issues are not completely new, but they do need to be addressed as a part of the implementation process.

Financing the System

One of the first questions that hospital administrators have when confronted with the possibility of implementing a UNHS program is how much such programs cost. The next question is whether third-party payers will reimburse for newborn hearing screening services. Because newborn hearing screening is a relatively new procedure, there are still many unanswered questions in this area, but more and more answers are becoming available as the number of hospitals with UNHS programs expands.

Unfortunately, there are few systematic studies about the actual costs of operating UNHS programs. This lack of information about costs is exacerbated by the fact that there are many different approaches to doing UNHS: Who does the screening (e.g., nurses, technicians, audiologists, volunteers, heath-care aides); where it is done (directly in the nursery, in an adjacent room, as an outpatient); when it is done (prior to or following discharge); and what equipment is used (TEOAE, DPOAE, AABR, or conventional ABR). How such questions are answered will have a significant effect on the cost of operating a UNHS program. The most complete economic analyses about the costs of operating a UNHS program are available for programs that use a two-stage TEOAE screening protocol. For example, using Levin's[30] ingredients approach to cost analysis, the Rhode Island Hearing Assessment Program (RIHAP) calculated that screening could be done for approximately $25 per baby (see Table 11–6, which has been adapted from Maxon, White, Behrens, and Vohr.[31]

Depending on how the screening program is organized, however, costs can be substantially more or less than those reported for Rhode Island. For example, a recent study conducted at Logan Regional Hospital in northern Utah[32] showed an average cost per baby of only $7.42 (see Table 11–7). Because the same basic cost analysis strategy and procedures were used in the two studies and because both hospitals included all of the costs for doing the two-stage screening, tracking the babies through the referral and diagnostic process, and included costs for fringe benefits, overhead, supplies, and equipment, an obvious question is why there is such a big difference in the costs. Analyzing that question reveals four factors:

1. The average salary at Logan Regional Hospital for people doing the screening was about 20% lower than the average salary in Rhode Island. This accounted for approximately $2 of the cost differential.

Table 11–6.   Actual Costs of Operating a Universal Newborn Hearing Screening Program at Women & Infants Hospital of Rhode Island

	Cost ($)
Personnel Screening Technicians (avg. 103 h/week) Clerical (avg. 60 h/week) Audiologist (avg. 18 h/week) Coordinator (avg. 20 h/week)	60,654
Fringe Benefits (28% of Salaries)	16,983
Supplies, Telephone, Postage	12,006
Equipment	5,575
Hospital Overhead (24% of Salaries)	14,557
Total Costs	$110,775

Cost per infant screened = $110,775: 4,253 = $26.05.

Table 11–7.   Costs of Operating a TEOAE-based Universal Newborn Hearing Screening Program at Logan Regional Hospital (Utah)

	Hours Worked	Average Rate/hour ($)	Cost ($)
Personnel	118.07	9.90	1,168.63
Screening	65.40	9.45	617.84
Rescreening	9.48	10.72	101.65
Screening Management	15.32	8.94	136.95
Program Management	5.23	10.15	53.12
Patient Management	12.90	11.05	142.54
Scoring	9.73	11.97	116.54
Fringe Benefits (30% of salaries)			350.59
Supplies			416.97
Equipment			446.00
Overhead (20% of costs)			476.44
Total Costs			2,858.62

Cost per baby = $7.42.
Number of initial screens = 385.

2. At Logan Regional Hospital, newborn hearing screening was done by unit clerical staff who fit screening in around their other job responsibilities. At RI-HAP, screening technicians were hired whose only job was to screen babies. By having someone do the screening who is already working at the hospital, the screening program is only paying for the time actually spent with tasks associated with the UNHS program. If people are hired who have no other job responsibilities, the screening program is paying for some time associated with staff meetings, down time because of the necessity of staffing for high volume times, waiting time, and so forth.

3. If it is possible, it is much more efficient to operate a screening program directly in the nursery (as was the case at Logan Regional Hospital) rather than having a separate room where babies are brought for screening, as was the case at RIHAP when the data reported by Maxon et al.[31] were collected. Not only is transportation time eliminated, but when the program is conducted right in the nursery, screeners can focus their attention on those babies who are in the best behavioral state to be screened.

4. The screening and patient management at Logan Regional Hospital was substantially more efficient because of the use of a computerized data and patient information management software (HI*SCREEN 96). This data management software integrated all of the data entry for screening and tracking, allowed scoring to be done online, generated reports necessary for tracking and referral, and automatically printed letters to parents and pediatricians informing them about the results of various screening and diagnostic tests. Thus, the use of the HI*SCREEN 96 software not only increased the accuracy of the screening program, but substantially reduced the personnel time associated with

these tasks. Furthermore, by having all of the data related to the screening program electronically stored, the need for time-consuming and cumbersome filing and tracking of information was largely eliminated.

Obviously, the cost per baby in a newborn hearing screening program will depend on factors that vary from hospital to hospital and region to region. Salary levels, overhead and fringe benefit rates, and who is doing the different screening tasks will all have a substantial impact on the cost per baby. In addition, these costs will fluctuate from month to month depending on birth rate. However, it is clear from available data that newborn hearing screening can be done economically. Depending on how the program is organized, the cost figures reported by Maxon et al.[31] are a good estimate of what average programs will cost. Some programs can be operated much more efficiently, and others will cost more.

There is even less concrete information available about how likely insurance companies are to pay for newborn hearing screening. Of course, in states like Rhode Island where the legislation requires newborn hearing screening to be a covered benefit of all insurance policies, the issue is clear cut. In other states, there is no guarantee that insurance companies will reimburse for newborn hearing screening. However, hospitals in most states have had moderate to excellent success in obtaining payment for newborn hearing screening. Working out the details of how this will be accomplished often requires negotiation between individual hospitals and the third-party payers with whom they normally deal.

Refining the Early Intervention Services System

The early identification of a hearing disability will only be beneficial if there are early intervention services available to provide appropriate habilitation. Without adequate follow-up services, hearing screening programs will continue to fall short of the objective of identifying all significant hearing disabilities before 12 months of age because the people responsible for implementing UNHS programs will lose interest if infants and families are not receiving the assistance they need once they are identified. To provide the intervention and management strategies necessary to enable infants and toddlers with significant hearing loss to make optimal developmental progress, a combination of strategies is needed, including effective neonatal hearing screening based on sound and effective technology and criteria, parent education and involvement, appropriate diagnostic testing, aggressive follow-up, and education of health-care professionals.

SERVICE COORDINATION

Whenever an infant fails the screening test, there should be a coordinated effort to help the family obtain diagnostic services as soon as possible. In states where infants and toddlers with hearing loss qualify for the Part H program, completion of the diagnostic testing and the implementation of an individualized family-service plan is required by federal law within 45 days of the initial referral. Such a system can provide an ideal mechanism for the follow-up and monitoring of those children who are identified by the hearing screening program.

MEDICAL HOME

Just as constituency support from physicians is a critical factor in developing a program, the continuing coordination of services with their medical home is a key component of a successful intervention system for infants and toddlers with a hearing disability. Service coordination should continually provide opportunities for input from the pediatrician or primary health-care provider. This coordination would include referrals for diagnostic services, ear, nose, and throat consultations, and participation in the individualized family-service plan.

Identifying Gaps in the System

The identification of increasing numbers of newborns and infants with hearing disabilities will multiply the stresses on any state system of services, which must be prepared to provide services to an ever younger clientele, as well as infants and toddlers with types and severities of hearing disability that are different from those that have traditionally been served in many states. Diagnostic services may need to be bolstered to assure that clinicians can provide diagnostic and therapeutic management for the young infant. Many audiologists and speech pathologists may have limited experience with this population. Home-based mother–infant education, parent support groups, and center-based service systems will need to be expanded to assure the appropriate provision of educational intervention and parental support to families with a newborn or infant with a hearing disability. The Part H system requires that the services needed by the child and family be made available, regardless of whether the child lives in a rural or urban area, and that those services be delivered in a culturally appropriate manner and in the "natural environment" whenever possible. Transportation and interpreter services must also be provided whenever necessary.

Is Newborn Hearing Screening Becoming the Standard of Care?

As more and more newborn hearing screening programs are implemented throughout the country, an obvious question is whether screening newborns for hearing loss is becoming accepted by health-care providers as the "standard of care." In other words, has newborn hearing screening been accepted by the medical and legal community as such a routine and obvious part of reasonable health care that every hospital would be expected to provide it as a part of its services? Clearly, whether or not UNHS is viewed as being a "standard of care" has important ramifications for how rapidly such programs are implemented. Once the legal and medical communities recognize a practice as being the standard of care, hospitals would have almost no alternative but to implement that practice as a normal part of their services. Unfortunately, as noted by Marlowe,[33] determining whether a practice has achieved "standard of care" status is often not a straightforward and easily-defined matter.

> Every medical and allied health practitioner and every hospital administrator should be keenly aware that they are held to a hypothetical standard of care whenever their professional conduct is being evaluated legally. . . . Definition of a standard of care is

complicated by the fact that it is not usually articulated in a specific, identifiable form and may be subject to clarification on a case-by-case basis should legal actions arise. (See also Ginsburg[34] and Hoffman[35].)

Even though the determination of when a particular practice has become the standard of care is subject to debate, the decision is usually based on information and evidence related to the following three questions:

- What are the typical expectations for a "reasonable practitioner" under similar circumstances?
- Are there guidelines or standards from authoritative groups that recommend the practice?
- Is there appropriate and generally available technology or procedures to implement the practice?

The current situation regarding newborn hearing screening as it relates to each of these questions is discussed briefly below.

Expectations for a Reasonable Practitioner Under Similar Circumstances

According to Hoffman,[35] an oft-cited case in determining what constitutes the standard of care in a particular situation was the 1898 *Pike v. Honsinger* case, in which the Court of Appeals decision stated that:

> A physician . . . impliedly represents that he possesses . . . that reasonable degree of learning and skill . . . ordinarily possessed by physicians in his locality. . . . [It is the physician's] duty to use reasonable care and diligence in the exercise of his skill and learning . . . [he must] keep abreast of the times . . . departure from approved methods and general use, if it injures the patient, will render him liable.

In addition to the obvious ramifications of this decision, there are at least two components of the *Pike v. Honsinger* case that are important for deciding whether newborn hearing screening has become the standard of care. First, what is considered acceptable is determined in part by what happens in your locality. However, with improved communication, greater mobility, and broader availability of continuing education, regional and even national practices are often being used by the courts to determine what constitutes "local" practice. Thus, the fact that successful hospital-based universal newborn hearing screening programs are being operated in at least 31 states from New York to Hawaii and from Michigan to Texas means that there is no part of the country in which hospital administrators can be confident that they will be able to successfully argue that no one in their area is doing universal newborn hearing screening. Second, health-care providers are expected to keep "abreast of the times." The fact that successful UNHS programs have been operating for almost 10 years makes it difficult to argue that UNHS programs are still so new that they should be viewed as experimental or unproven.

Guidelines and Standards

Pronouncements of accreditation bodies, expert panels, professional groups, and governmental advisory committees are another important factor in determining what constitutes the standard of care. The support for universal newborn hearing screening in this area is particularly strong. Indeed, it is difficult to think of health-care procedures that are not yet routinely implemented that have been endorsed by such authoritative groups as the NIH Consensus Panel, the American Academy of Pediatrics, the American Academy of Otolaryngology Head and Neck Surgery, the American Speech-Language-Hearing Association, and the American Academy of Audiology. The recommendations of these professional groups are further buttressed by the fact that several state legislatures (RI and HI) have mandated UNHS, and similar legislation has been proposed in at least five other states (UT, MN, PA, CO, and CT). There is clearly no shortage of expert opinion in favor of UNHS programs.

Availability of Technology

In writing about how a standard of care is established, Ginsburg[34] asked, "when does a guideline become a standard?" The question was answered as follows:

> The answer is when an inexpensive, reliable device comes onto the market, the technology and concept of which have already been adopted by a group who specializes in the concept . . . . A guideline becomes a standard of care when the device behind the guideline is available and readily useable. (p. 125)

Given the widespread and long-standing agreement about how important it is to identify hearing loss as early as possible, newborn hearing screening would have become the standard of care many years ago had there been an "available and readily useable" device for doing such screening. Unfortunately, until just recently, the only effective technique for detecting infant hearing loss, ABR, was too expensive, time-consuming, and difficult to be feasible for UNHS. The technological developments of the past few years, however, have resulted in a number of feasible and cost-effective options. As noted earlier, TEOE, DPOE, and AABR are all being used successfully in many different UNHS programs. There are at least eight different manufacturers of newborn hearing screening equipment, and the cost of equipment remains relatively inexpensive. Most importantly, the equipment is continually improving (i.e., becoming faster and easier to use). Thus, there is no doubt that newborn hearing screening equipment is "available and readily useable."

Summary

The prospects for a child born in the United States with congenital hearing loss of being identified before his or her first birthday are better than they have ever been and are likely to improve dramatically over the next several years. Given the progress that has been made so far this decade, it is realistic to expect that we will have nationwide UNHS by the year 2000. Activities now underway to improve statewide tracking and referral of infants referred from such programs, and improvements in diagnosis and intervention for children under 6 months of age, make it plausible that all newborns with hearing losses will be identified and involved in appropriate intervention programs by the time they are 6 months old.

The fact that more than half of all babies in Rhode Island, Hawaii, Utah, and Colorado are now born in hospitals with UNHS programs, coupled with the availability of appropriate technology and the recommendations from the National Institutes of Health, the Joint Committee on Infant Hearing, and the American Academy of Pediatrics suggests that newborn hearing screening has already become the standard of care in some states. Implementing programs in the remaining states will still require a lot of effort. However, the progress that has already been made provides a solid foundation for UNHS to become a reality throughout the country.

References

1. Berg FS. *Educational Audiology: Hearing and Speech Management.* New York, Grune & Stratton, 1976
2. Downs MP. The rationale for neonatal hearing screening. In Swigart ET (ed): *Neonatal Hearing Screening.* San Diego, College-Hill Press, 1986, pp. 3–19
3. Ewing IR, Ewing AWG. The ascertainment of deafness in infancy and early childhood. J Laryng Otol 1944;59:309–33
4. Babbidge H. *Education of the Deaf in the United States: Report of the Advisory Committee on Education of the Deaf.* Washington, DC, U.S. Government Printing Office, 1965
5. Commission on Education of the Deaf. *Toward Equality: Education of the Deaf.* Washington, DC: Author, 1988
6. U.S. Department of Health, Education, and Welfare. *Education of the Deaf: The Challenge and the Charge. A Report of the National Conference on Education of the Deaf.* Washington, DC, Author, 1967
7. Goldstein R, Tait C. Critique of neonatal hearing evaluation. J Speech Hearing Disord 1971; 26:3–18
8. Ruben RJ, Levine R, Fishman G, Baldinger E, Feldman W, Silver M, Stein M, Umano H, Kruger B. Moderate to severe sensorineural hearing impaired child: Analysis of etiology, intervention, and outcome. Laryngoscope 1982;92:38–46
9. Stewart IF. After early identification: A study of some aspects of deaf education from an otolaryngological viewpoint. Laryngoscope 1984;94:784–99
10. Department of Health and Human Services. *Healthy People 2000: National Health Promotion and Disease Prevention Objectives.* Washington, DC, Public Health Service, 1990
11. Coscarelli-Buchanan JE. Finding ears that do not hear. Health Environ Rep 1986;39
12. Lyon DJ, Lyon ME. Early detection of hearing loss. Can J Public Health 1982;73:410–15
13. Riko K, Hyde ML, Alberti PW. Hearing loss in early infancy: Incidence, detection and assessment. Laryngoscope 1985;95:137–145
14. Riko K, Hyde ML, Corgin H, Fitzhardinge PM. Issues in early identification of hearing loss. Laryngoscope 1985;95:373–81
15. Clark TC. *Language Development Through Home Intervention for Infant Hearing Impaired Children.* Chapel Hill, NC, University of North Carolina, 1979 (University Microfilms International, 8013924)
16. Northern JL, Downs MP. *Hearing in Children,* 3rd ed. Baltimore, Williams & Wilkins, 1984
17. White KR., Behrens TR. (Eds.) The Rhode Island Hearing Assessment Project: Implications for universal newborn hearing screening. Semin Hear 1993;14:1–119
18. Blake PE, Hall JW. The status of state-wide policies for neonatal hearing screening. J Am Acad Audiol 1990;1:67–74
19. Johnson JL, Mauk GW, Takekawa KM, Simon PR, Sia CCJ, Blackwell PM. Implementing a statewide system of services for infants and toddlers with hearing disabilities. Semin Hear 1993;14:105–19
20. Joint Committee on Infant Hearing. 1990 Position statement. ASHA 1991;33 (Suppl. 5):3–6
21. Welch R, Slater S. The state of infant hearing impairment identification programs. ASHA 1993; 35:49–52
22. Baumeister AA. Policy formulation: A real world view. In Bess FH, Hall JW III (eds): *Screening Children for Auditory Function.* Nashville, TN, Bill Wilkerson Center Press, 1992, pp. 111–123

23. Mace AL, Wallace KL, Whan MQ, Stelmachowicz PG. Relevant factors in the identification of hearing loss. Ear Hear 1991;12:287–93
24. Moore WG, Josephson JA, Mauk GW. Identification of children with hearing impairments: A baseline survey. The Volta Rev 1991;93:187–96
25. Clayton E. *Legal/ethical issues associated with newborn hearing screening.* Paper presented at the Fourth International Symposium on Childhood Deafness, Kiawah Island, SC, 1996
26. Coplan J. Deafness: Ever heard of it? Delayed recognition of permanent hearing loss. Pediatrics 1987;79:206–13
27. Epstein S, Reilly JS. Sensorineural hearing loss. Pediatr Clin North Am 1989;36:1501–20
28. Herrmann BS. Audiometry primer. In Eavey RD, Klein JO (eds): *Hearing Loss in Childhood: A Primer. Report of the 102nd Ross Conference on Pediatric Research.* Columbus, OH. Ross Laboratories, 1992, pp. 55–61
29. Thornton A. Neonatal screening. In Eavey RD, Klein JO (eds): *Hearing Loss in Childhood: A Primer. Report of the 102nd Ross Conference on Pediatric Research* Columbus, OH, Ross Laboratories, 1992, pp.55–61
30. Levin HM. *Cost-effectiveness: A primer.* Beverly Hills, CA, Sage, 1983
31. Maxon AB, White KR, Behrens TR, Vohr BR. Referral rates and cost efficiency in a universal newborn hearing screening program using transient evoked otoacoustic emissions (TEOAE). J Am Acad Audiol 1995;6:271–77
32. Weirather Y, Korth N, White KR, Downs D, Woods-Kershner N. Cost analysis of TEOAE-based universal newborn hearing screening. J Commun Disord (in press)
33. Marlowe JA. Legal and risk management issues in newborn hearing screening. Semin Hear 1996;17:153–64
34. Ginsburg WH Jr. When does a guideline become a standard? The new American Society of Anesthesiologists guidelines give us a clue. Ann Emer Med 1993;22:1891–96
35. Hoffman AC. Medical malpractice. In Sanbar SS, Gibofsky A, Firestone MH, LeBlang TR (eds): *Legal medicine* St. Louis, Mosby, 1995, pp. 129–140
35. National Institutes of Health (NIH): Early identification of hearing impairment in infants and young children. NIH Consensus Statement 1993;11:1–24

APPENDIX
SUMMARY OF STATES' LEGISLATIVE MANDATES FOR NEONATAL HEARING SCREENING

Summary of States' Legislative Mandates for Neonatal Hearing Screening

State	Date of Mandate	Specifics of Mandate
Arizona	1987	Establishes a central register of infants who are at high risk for hearing loss. Requires implementation of a comprehensive child hearing loss education program for the general public, the medical community, child-care providers, and other professional groups. Establishes a Hearing Impaired Children Advisory Committee.
Arkansas	1995	All hospitals required to complete a questionnaire for all newborns indicating the presence of high-risk indicators. Information is sent to the Department of Health, which must notify parents, provide them with educational information and a list of places where the parents can obtain additional information about the infant's auditory functioning.
California	1983	Establishes a system to screen newborn infants at high risk for deafness and create and maintain a system of follow-up and assessment for infants identified by such screening in neonatal intensive care units (NICUs).
Connecticut	1981	Requires development of a plan to implement and operate a program of early identification of infant hearing impairment based on risk factors. Parents are to be notified of such infants at risk, informed about resources available for further testing and treatment, and given information about financial assistance available through the Department of Health Services.
Florida	1983, 1992	1983 legislation: A statewide coordinated program created to screen, diagnose, and manage high-risk infants identified as hearing impaired. Requires development of risk criteria and provision to parents of materials regarding hearing impairments prior to discharge of such infants from the hospital. Creates a Council for the Infant Hearing Impairment Program and establishes five pilot sites for implementation of the program plan. 1992 Amendments: References to pilot sites and pilot programs were deleted. The Council for the Infant Hearing Impairment Program was eliminated.
Georgia	1978	Requires State Department of Health to develop guidelines for the detection of hearing impairment in infants determined to be at risk and to develop rules and regulations to ensure that all such high-risk infants are evaluated within one year of their birth.

State	Date of Mandate	Specifics of Mandate
Hawaii	1990	The Department of Health is to provide a statewide comprehensive and coordinated interdisciplinary program of early hearing impairment screening, identification, and follow-up for children from birth to 36 months of age and their families. The Department of Health is responsible for developing: (a) appropriate methodology to establish, implement, and evaluate the program; (b) guidelines for screening, identification, diagnosis, and monitoring of infants with hearing impairment and infants at risk for delayed onset of hearing impairment; (c) a plan, in conjunction with the State Department of Education, to involve the parents or guardians with the medical and educational follow-up and management; and (d) a plan for the collection of data and evaluation of the program.
Kansas	1990	Newborn infant hearing-impaired risk criteria and a questionnaire to identify high-risk infants to be developed. Each medical care facility must provide risk screening of newborn infants and promptly notify the infant's parents or guardian, primary-care physician, and the Secretary of Health and Environment that the infant is high risk Parents/guardians must be given information on the developmental and language effects of hearing loss and a listing of medical care facilities which provide follow-up hearing evaluations. Establishes a system to gather and maintain data and a statewide registry.
Kentucky	1986	Requires the development of a system for identifying newborns who have higher risk than normal of being hearing impaired. Also mandates a program to provide medical and educational information to the families, assist families in securing screening, diagnostic, and medical services at minimal cost, conduct timely review of risk factors, and involve other agencies which provide services to deaf and hearing-impaired children.
Louisiana	1992	Requires the State Department of Health to develop criteria to identify infants at-risk for hearing impairment and to create a high-risk registry. Hospitals are required to administer a high-risk questionnaire for all newborns prior to discharge and do follow-up screening by ABR or other screening devices. Written materials regarding hearing impairment must be disseminated to parents and an advisory council for the hearing detection program must be established.
Maryland	1985	Establishes a program for the early identification and follow-up of infants who have a risk factor for developing a hearing impairment. The program is operated under the auspices of the Advisory for Hearing-Impaired Infants and Children.

State	Date of Mandate	Specifics of Mandate
Massachusetts	1971	Revised in 1985. Establishes high-risk factors for hearing impairment in infants. Parents or guardians must be provided with literature describing conditions that cause children to be at high risk for hearing impairment. The Department of Health is required to offer parents of high-risk children complete diagnostic evaluations at approved centers.
Mississippi	1974	Establishes a central registry within the State Department of Education for hearing and visually impaired persons under age 12. In 1979, a section of the Mississippi Code was amended to place responsibility for the registry under the State Department of Health.
New Jersey	1977	Requires Department of Health to appoint a Hearing Evaluation Council responsible for ensuring that (a) all parents of newborns are provided with literature describing the normal development of auditory function; and (b) all hospitals complete a high-risk questionnaire for each newborn, and (c) information about infants with risk factors is sent to the Department of Health. A registry of high-risk infants is to be maintained to remind parents of the need for auditory screening when the child is 6 months old.
Ohio	1988	Infants who are at risk of hearing impairment are to be identified using a high-risk questionnaire developed by the Department of Health. Each hospital is to provide risk screening of newborns and notify primary-care physicians and the Department of Health of infants at risk for hearing impairment. Hospitals must provide a hearing assessment of at-risk infants or provide the infant's parent/guardian with a list of facilities that provide hearing assessment. Establishes a registry of infants at risk for hearing impairment.
Oklahoma	1982	Directs State Board of Health to develop a screening procedure and guidelines for the detection of hearing impairments. Annual publication of the results of the infant screening procedures is required.
Rhode Island	1988, 1992	1988 legislation: Every newborn infant must be screened for hearing impairment based on high-risk guidelines established by the director of the Department of Health. Cost of audiological evaluation of high-risk infants borne by the state in the absence of third-party payment. 1992 amendment: Requires *every* newborn infant to be evaluated for the detection of hearing impairment and specifies that the testing shall be a covered benefit reimbursable by all health insurers. Establishes a Hearing Impairments Testing Advisory Council.

State	Date of Mandate	Specifics of Mandate
Virginia	1986	Requires the State Department of Health to maintain a system for the purpose of identifying and monitoring infants who are at risk for hearing impairment. A high-risk registry approach is to be used for well babies and in-hospital hearing screening for infants in the NICU. Using data from the hospital-based screening, a registry is to be maintained by the Department of Health of those children diagnosed with hearing impairment and a list of those for whom no response has been received on follow-up. Information packets on hearing and speech–language development are to be given to the parent/guardian of each infant transferred or discharged from the newborn nursery. Families and primary care providers of those infants reported "at risk" and those who failed the hearing screening must be notified.
West Virginia	1991	Establishes a Commission for the Hearing Impaired, which maintains a registry of all hearing-impaired persons and a clearinghouse of information and provides training and outreach programs.

States with Pending Legislation

Minnesota	Creates an advisory committee for identification of infant hearing loss under the Department of Health. Requires every newborn to be screened for hearing loss using ABR, EOAE, or other technology approved by advisory committee. Such screening shall be a covered benefit of all health plan companies or paid for by the hospital in the absence of a third-party payer.
New York	Requires the Department of Health to promulgate standards for all hospitals caring for newborn infants to test every newborn infant for hearing prior to discharge.
Pennsylvania	Requires the Department of Health to establish a program for universal testing of newborn children for hearing impairment prior to hospital discharge (but no later than 3 months of age) with ABR, OAE, or other approved technology. Follow-up services related to diagnosis must also be provided. Health insurance policies or the Department of Public Welfare to pay for newborn hearing impairment testing. Establishes a Newborn Child Hearing Testing Advisory Committee.
Utah	Creates an Advisory Committee for Identification of Infant Hearing Loss and requires hospitals to evaluate every newborn infant for detection of hearing loss using ABR, EOAE, or other appropriate technology approved by the advisory committee. The hearing evaluation is a covered benefit of all health plan companies or will be paid by the hospital in the absence of a third-party payor. The Department of Health shall establish rules and regulations for the program and coordinates a central data management system.

Index

Accuracy of screening programs, 6, 10, 17–20

Acoustic reflex screening, 19

Acquired hearing loss
communication development in, 3
risk factors for, 146, 152

Administrative concerns in planning screening program, 31–34
consent issues in, 34
enhancement of hospital mission, 31
financial issues in, 31–32, 33
public relations and publicity, 33
risk management and standard of care, 33–34

Age
in detection of hearing loss, 3, 4–6, 145, 225–226
degree of hearing loss affecting, 4–5
goals on, 6
information for physicians on, 221
risk status affecting, 5
in follow-up program, 189, 191, 192, 193
of infant at discharge, 56, 60, 157, 159
in interventions for hearing loss, 145, 246
and communication development, 3–4

in late onset and progressive hearing loss, 155–156, 157
in otoacoustic emissions screening, 53, 159
and readiness for testing, 56, 158–159

ALGO systems (Natus), 20, 59, 88, 104–106
in noisy conditions, 90
in office-based screening, 162

Aminoglycoside antibiotics, ototoxicity of, 151, 153

Animal studies on neonatal hearing loss, 2, 3

Antibiotics, ototoxicity of, 151, 153

Apgar score, and risk for hearing loss, 152

Apnea in premature infants, 139

Arizona, legislation on newborn hearing screening in, 251

Arkansas, legislation on newborn hearing screening in, 251

Arms of newborn, appearance and characteristics of, 124

Arousal screening techniques, sensitivity and specificity of, 17–18

Attachment process of newborn and parents, 128

Attire of personnel, and infection control, 131, 141

Audiologists, 29–30, 44
  as advocates in legislative process,
      238
  as coordinator of program, 68–69
  as director of program, 68
  report for hospital record at time of
      screening, 214
  report to parents on test results, 200
  as screeners, 70, 77, 89
Audiology coordinator,
      responsibilities of, 68–69
  supervisory, 72–80
Auditory brainstem response
      screening, 3, 7–8, 50, 51–52
  automated procedures, 20, 51
    equipment and instruments in,
        20, 59, 88, 102–106
    model of, 59
    in office-based screening, 162
    time required for, 36
  combined with otoacoustic
      emissions screening, 53–54, 88
    equipment and instruments in,
        100, 102, 104, 107–109
    model of, 62
  compared to behavioral responses,
      18–19, 51–52
  configuration of hearing loss
      identified in, 55
  cost considerations in, 233
  equipment and instruments in, 20,
      59, 88, 102–109
    comparison of, 109
    computer systems, 90
    electrical interference affecting, 90
    with otoacoustic emissions
        screening, 100, 102, 104,
        107–109
  false-positive results in, 74, 75
  flow chart on, 60
  follow-up evaluation in, 59, 188,
      189
  in follow-up rescreening, 189, 192
    chloral hydrate order in, 219
    parent information on, 207–209
  in two-stage programs, 16, 53, 88,
      228

  in intensive care unit nursery, 57, 62
    documentation of, 140, 141, 171
  model of, 59
  in New York screening program, 22
  in noisy conditions, 57, 90
  nonautomated procedures, 51
    equipment and instruments in,
        106–107
  number of programs using, 226–227
  percentage of infants evaluated
      with, 230, 231
  personnel in, 51, 55, 59
    hospital variations in, 231–232
    with otoacoustic emissions
        screening, 62
  philosophy of program in, 54
  prior experience affecting use of, 55
  referral rates in, 59, 62, 231
  in Rhode Island screening program,
      20, 171
  sensitivity and specificity of, 19–20,
      51
    compared to behavioral
        screening techniques, 18–19
  severity of hearing loss detected in,
      54–55, 188, 189
  size of hospitals using, 227
  technique in, 51
Auditory neuropathy, 7, 52
Automated screening procedures
  auditory brainstem responses in.
      See Auditory brainstem
      response screening, automated
      procedures
  behavioral tests in, sensitivity and
      specificity of, 18–19

Bacterial meningitis of neonate, risk
      for hearing loss in, 151–152
Battery-powered equipment, 90
  in auditory brainstem response
      screening, 106
  in distortion product otoacoustic
      emissions screening, 96, 100,
      101
  in transient otoacoustic emissions
      screening, 92–93

Behavior of newborn, 124–125
    evaluation of, as screening
        technique, 17–19, 51–52
    in fatigue, 137
    in intensive care unit nursery,
        136–138
    in overstimulation, 137
    in periods of reactivity, 125
    reflexes in, 124–125
    in stress, 137
Behavioral screening techniques
    compared to auditory brainstem
        responses, 18–19, 51–52
    sensitivity and specificity of,
        17–19
        in automated tests, 18–19
        in observation of arousal, 17–18
Bilateral hearing loss, 3
    follow-up program in, 188, 189
    screening for, 54
Bilirubin serum levels
    and auditory brainstem response
        screening, 52, 151
    in intensive care unit nursery, 140
    as risk factor for hearing loss,
        150–151
Billing practices, 32, 232–233
    data management in, 176–177
    quality indicators on, 182
Bio-logic Systems Corporation, 118
    Scout, Ranger, and Sport systems
        from, 100–101, 109
    Traveler Express and Navigator E
        systems from, 109
Birth weight, and risk for hearing
    loss, 150
Birthing rooms, 120–121
Bonding of newborn and parents,
    127–128
Branchio-oto-renal syndrome, 153
Brochures for parents, 196–199
Budget proposal, in planning of
    screening program, 31–32

Calibration of equipment
    in distortion product otoacoustic
        emissions screening, 98, 99
    in transient otoacoustic emissions
        screening, 93
California, legislation on newborn
    hearing screening in, 251
Cardiovascular response audiometry,
    19
CareMap, 157–158
Celesta 503 Cochlear Emissions
    Analyzer (Madsen), 98–99
CHARGE association, risk for hearing
    loss in, 153
Charts and records in well-baby
    nursery, 130
Chemotherapy agents, ototoxicity of,
    151
Chloral hydrate order, 219
Choanal atresia, and risk for hearing
    loss in CHARGE association,
    153
Cisplatin, ototoxicity of, 151
Clarity system (SonaMed
    Corporation), 102–104
Cleft defects
    branchial, 153
    of lip and palate, 149–150
Clinic, as site of screening, 161–162
Clothing of personnel, and infection
    control, 131, 141
Cold stress of newborn, 121
    in intensive care unit nursery, 139
Coloboma, and risk for hearing loss
    in CHARGE association, 153
Colorado, newborn hearing screening
    program in, 21, 234, 240, 249
Community involvement in screening
    programs
    in educational measures, 163
    in generation of constituency
        support, 237–238
    in implementation, 241
    in planning, 29, 237–238
Compass system (Nicolet
    Biomedical), 107–108
Compliance rate with follow-up
    services, 184
Computer systems in screening
    programs, 90, 91

database management software of,
169, 171, 172
  entry of data in, 173
  reports and correspondence
    generated with, 173, 174, 175
  transfer of files in, 172–173
Conferences on hearing loss in
  infants, 13–17
  National Institutes of Health
    Consensus Conference of 1993,
    15–17
    growth of hearing screening
      programs after, 226, 227
    recommendation on two-stage
      screening procedure, 16, 53, 88,
      227–228
  Nova Scotia Conference of 1974,
    14
  Saskatoon Conference of 1978,
    14–15
Confidentiality issues, 176
  training of personnel on, 77, 176
Congenital hearing loss
  risk factors for, 146
  speech and language development
    in, 1–2, 3
Connecticut, newborn hearing
  screening in, 240, 251
Consensus statements on hearing loss
  in infants, 13–17
Consent to hearing screening, 34
Coordinator of screening program,
  68–69
  supervisory responsibilities of,
    72–80
Cost considerations, 6–7, 10
  affecting availability of screening
    programs, 156, 157
  and billing practices, 32, 232–233
    data management in, 176–177
    quality indicators on, 182
  in budget proposal to hospital
    administration, 31–32
  compared to cost of not screening,
    33
  in data collection and management,
    244–245

in equipment for screening, 89,
  90–91, 112, 117
  hospital funding of, 232–233
in follow-up program, 188, 192, 193
  parent information on, 208
  revenue generated in, 32
in high-risk register, 17
and insurance reimbursement. See
  Insurance reimbursement
pediatrician concerns on, 36–37
personnel factors in, 243–244
in quality management, 178
in statewide screening programs,
  242–245
  in Rhode Island, 36–37, 52–53,
    243–244
Cough reflex of newborn, 124
Craniofacial abnormalities, 3
  risk for hearing loss in, 149–150
Crib-o-gram screening, 18–19
Critical period of development
  effects of sound deprivation in, 2
  for language acquisition, 4, 156
Crying of newborn, 127
  and problems in hearing screening,
    160
Cube Dis system (Mimosa Acoustics),
  97–98
Cytomegalovirus infection in
  pregnancy, and risk for hearing
  loss in infant, 148

Data collection and management,
  167–177
  billing and reimbursement based
    on, 176–177
  computer software in, 169, 171, 172
    entry of data in, 173
    reports and correspondence
      generated with, 173, 174, 175
  confidentiality issues in, 77, 176
  cost of, 244–245
  defining objectives of, 169–170
  entry of data in, 173
  identification of eligible infants in,
    171–172
  interpretation of test results in, 173

on need for universal newborn hearing screening program, 235–237
personnel required for, 72
planning for, 44, 169
quality control in, 173, 178
on quality indicators, 180–181
retention and storage of information in, 175–176
on risk factors, 154, 172
security of data in, 176
Sound Beginnings form in, 170–171, 172, 173
in tracking system, 174–175
transfer of computer files in, 172–173
Database manager, 72
Diagnostic testing, 191–192
referral rates for, 58
scheduling of appointments for, 205–206
Director of screening program, 68
in planning process, 30–31
with hospital administrators, 31, 32
with obstetricians, 42, 43
with pediatricians, 35, 36, 37
responsibilities of, 46, 68
Discharge from hospital
age of infant at time of, 56, 60, 157, 159
and length of hospital stay. *See* Length of hospital stay
percentage of infants screened prior to, 230–231
Distortion product otoacoustic emissions screening, 52, 53, 59
equipment used in, 94–102, 227
number of programs using, 227
Documentation. *See* Record keeping
Drug therapy, ototoxicity of, 151, 153

EarCare Products, 118
disposable earphone covers from, 110
Ears of newborn
appearance and characteristics of, 123

fluid and debris in, 56, 123
affecting otoacoustic emissions scanning, 53, 158–159
Echoport ILO88 system (Otodynamics), 92–93
Education and training
community outreach in, 163
groups targeted for, 162–163
of intensive care unit nursery staff, 134, 142–143
of nurses
in intensive care unit nursery, 134
as screeners, 40
on universal newborn hearing screening, 38–39, 40, 238–240
of obstetricians, on universal newborn hearing screening, 43
of parents, 162–163
on auditory brainstem response screening, 207–209
brochures for, 196–199
in notification of test results, 163, 190
of pediatricians, on universal newborn hearing screening, 35–36
reference materials for, 35–36, 48–49
of primary-care physicians, on newborn hearing screening, 212, 221, 238
responsibilities of program director in, 46
of screeners, 40, 70, 73–77
on common problems in intensive care unit nursery, 139, 140
on confidentiality and privacy rights, 77
curriculum in, 82–83
on equipment, 89, 112, 136
evaluation of, 79–80
on handling of newborns, 40
on interactions with other personnel, 76
on interactions with parents, 74–76

on interpretation of test results,
73–74
on security procedures, 76–77
on stress reactions of newborn,
137
Electrical interference affecting
screening equipment, 90
Embryonic development, craniofacial
abnormalities in, 149–150
Environment of screening, 56–57,
160–162
in dedicated hospital site, 56–57,
161
electrical interference in, 90
in hospital room of mother, 57, 161
hospital variations in, 231–232
in intensive care unit nursery, 57,
161
noise in. See Noise in screening
environment
in office or clinic, 37, 161–162
and selection of screening
equipment, 89–90
and selection of screening protocol,
56–57
in well-baby nursery, 57, 160–161
Equipment and instruments, 87–119
in auditory brainstem response
screening, 20, 59, 88, 90,
102–109
with otoacoustic emissions
screening, 100, 102, 104,
107–109
availability of, 33, 248
computer systems. See Computer
systems in screening programs
cost of, 89, 90–91, 112, 117
hospital funding of, 232–233
electrical interference affecting, 90
factors considered in selection of,
88–91, 112–117
in intensive care unit nursery, 136,
159
safety of, 142
in noisy conditions, 33, 90, 118
in otoacoustic emissions screening,
88, 90, 92–102, 227

with auditory brainstem
response screening, 100, 102,
104, 107–109
comparison of, 103
portable, 90, 96, 100
power source of, 90
quality indicators on utilization of,
182–183
sources of, 118–119
training of screeners on, 89, 112,
136
in well-baby nursery, and infection
control, 130
Europe, universal neonatal hearing
screening programs in, 23
Evaluation of screening personnel,
79–80
form used in, 83–86
Evoked otoacoustic emissions
screening. See Otoacoustic
emissions screening
Eyes of newborn
appearance and characteristics of,
123
and eye contact with parents, 128
in Usher syndrome, 153

Face of newborn, appearance and
characteristics of, 123–124
Failure rates, 8
learning curve affecting, 37
in New York screening program,
22, 37, 88
quality indicators on, 182
and referral rates, 58
False-negative screening results,
117
False-positive screening results
in auditory brainstem response
screening, 74, 75
impact on family, 4
in otoacoustic emissions screening,
53, 74, 75
pediatrician concerns on, 37
screener training on, 74
Family. See also Parents
in birthing rooms, 120–121

in false-positive screening results, 4
history of hearing loss in, 146–147,
    154
Fatigue of newborn, behavioral signs
    of, 137
Feeding of newborn in intensive care
    unit nursery, 135, 136, 140
Fees charged for services, 32
    billing for, 32, 232–233
        data management in, 176–177
        quality indicators on, 182
    insurance reimbursement of. *See*
        Insurance reimbursement
    and revenue generated in follow-
        up program, 32
Florida, legislation on newborn
    hearing screening in, 251
Follow-up services, 187–224
    age of infants in, 189, 191, 192, 193
    auditory brainstem response
        rescreening in, 189, 192
        chloral hydrate order in, 219
        parent information on, 207–209
        in two-stage programs, 16, 53, 88,
            228
    in auditory brainstem response
        screening, 59, 188, 189
    compliance rate in, 184
    coordination of, 245–246
    cost considerations in, 188, 192, 193
        parent information on, 208
    diagnostic testing in, 58, 191–192
        scheduling of appointments for,
            205–206
    identifying gaps in, 246
    indications for, 188–189
    insurance coverage for, 192, 208
    legislation on, 234
    otoacoustic emissions rescreening
        in, 59–60, 62, 189, 192
    parent notification in, 41, 42, 190,
        195–211
    physician notification in, 190–191,
        211–221
    planning for, 44–45, 187
    priority groups in, 188–189, 193
    quality management in, 184, 220

referral rates for, 58. *See also*
    Referral rates
revenue generated in, 32
sample report forms in, 213–217,
    219, 224
    on diagnostic data, 192, 224
    scheduling of, 189–190, 193
        appointment arrangements in,
            203–206, 209
    in statewide programs, 245–246
    tracking system in, 191, 193
        in difficult-to-contact parents, 210
        Infant Child Health Assessment
            Program assistance in, 191, 223
    in urban areas, 45, 46
    in urban areas, 45, 46
Furosemide therapy, risk for hearing
    loss in, 151, 153

Gag reflex of newborn, 124
Genetic factors in hearing loss,
    146–147
Genital abnormalities, and risk for
    hearing loss in CHARGE
    association, 153
Georgia, legislation on newborn
    hearing screening in, 251
Goldenhar syndrome, risk for hearing
    loss in, 153–154
Grason Associates, 118
    single-use eartips from, 109
Grason-Stadler, Inc., 118
    GSI 55 auditory brainstem response
        screener from, 106–107
    GSI 60 distortion product
        otoacoustic emission system
        from, 95–96
Grasp reflex of newborn, 125
Growth retardation, and risk for
    hearing loss in CHARGE
    association, 153

Hand washing for infection control,
    130, 141
Hawaii, newborn hearing screening
    program in, 234, 236–237, 238,
    249

legislation on, 240, 241, 252
Head of newborn, appearance and
    characteristics of, 123–124
Healthy People 2000 report of the
    Health and Human Services
    Department, 15
Heart disorders, and risk for hearing
    loss in CHARGE association,
    153
Heart rate
    in apnea of prematurity, 139
    in response to auditory stimulation,
    19
Herpes simplex virus infection in
    pregnancy, and risk for hearing
    loss in infant, 148
High-risk register, 17
    compared to behavioral
        observation screening
        techniques, 18
    Joint Committee on Infant hearing
        statement on, 12–13
    sensitivity and specificity of, 17
Historical development of newborn
    screening, 10–17
    conferences and consensus
        statements in, 13–17
    Joint Committee on Infant Hearing
        in, 11–13
History of family, and risk for hearing
    loss, 146–147, 154
HIV infection in infants, risk for
    hearing loss in, 148–149
Home visit, hearing screen in, 162
Hyperbilirubinemia
    auditory brainstem response
        screening in, 52, 151
    in intensive care unit nursery, 140
    risk for hearing loss in, 150–151
Hyperthermia of newborn, 122
Hypothermia of newborn, 121

Identification of newborn
    in intensive care unit nursery, 79,
    142
    in well-baby nursery, 121, 129

ILO88 otoacoustic emissions
    equipment (Otodynamics)
    distortion product, 94–95
    transient, 53, 92–94, 95
        board kit, 92
        cleaning ear canal with, 53, 159
        Echoport configuration, 92–93
        probes used in, 93
        recent version of, 93
Indications for hearing screening,
    145–157
Infant Child Health Assessment
    Program referral form, 191, 223
Infections
    in intensive care unit nursery,
        prevention of, 141–142
    meningitis, 3
        risk for hearing loss in, 151–152
    otitis media, 3, 55
        recurrent or persistent, 156
    in pregnancy, and risk for hearing
        loss in infant, 148–149
    in well-baby nursery, prevention of,
        130–131
Instruments and equipment. *See*
    Equipment and instruments
Insurance reimbursement
    for follow-up services, 192, 208
    and length of hospital stay, 55–56
    for screening, 32, 245
        data management for, 176–177
        program variations in, 232–233
Intelligent Hearing Systems, 118
    Smart EP device from, 104, 107
    Smart Screen device from, 104, 107
Intensive care unit nursery, 132–144
    auditory brainstem response
        screening in, 57, 62
    documentation of, 140, 141,
        171
    developmental behaviors of
        newborn in, 136–138
    equipment in, 136, 159
        safety of, 142
    feeding of newborn in, 135, 136, 140
    infection control in, 141–142

levels of care provided in, 132–134
noise in, 57, 62, 79, 135
    reduction for screening, 161
nursing staff in, 134–135, 142,
        143–144
otoacoustic emissions screening in,
        57, 62, 160
    documentation of, 140, 141
parent notification on hearing test
        results in, 201–202
prevalence of hearing loss in, 6–9
record keeping in, 140–141
    and data management
        procedures, 171, 172
respiratory problems in, 139, 140
risk-based screening programs in,
        17, 156–157
routines in, 78–79, 135–136
safety concerns in, 142
scheduling of screening in, 56,
        78–79, 135
    readiness of infant in, 56, 159–160
selection of screening protocols in,
        56, 57
as site of screening, 57, 161
temperature regulation in, 136,
        139–140
transportation of infants in, 41, 142
Internal Review Board requirements
        on informed consent, 34
Interpretation of test results
    ease of, as factor in equipment
        selection, 115
    initial report on, 173
    quality control in, 173
    screener training on, 73–74
Iowa, newborn hearing screening
        program in, 234
Israel, behavioral observation
        screening techniques in, 18

Jaundice of newborn, 140
    phototherapy in, 140
        and hearing screening, 161
    risk for hearing loss in, 150–151
    transfusions in, 150–151

Joint Committee on Infant Hearing,
        11–13, 50
    on risk for hearing loss, 12–13,
        145–146

Kansas, legislation on newborn
        hearing screening in, 252
Kentucky, newborn hearing screening
        in, 234, 252

Language. See Speech and language
Legal issues
    in failure to identify hearing
        impairment, 33–34
    in length of hospital stay for
        mothers and infants, 55–56
    in liability of obstetrician for
        hearing impairment, 42–43
    in medical record retention and
        confidentiality, 176
    in standard of care, 33–34, 246–247
    in state mandates for newborn
        hearing screening programs,
        20, 233–234, 240–241
        documentation of need for,
            235–237
        generation of constituency
            support for, 237–240
        summary listing on, 251–255
    in volunteer screeners, 71–72
Legs of newborn, appearance and
        characteristics of, 124
Length of hospital stay
    affecting screening protocol
        decisions, 55–56
    and age of infant at discharge, 56,
        60, 157, 159
    and readiness of infant for
        screening, 56, 158–160
Letters
    computer generation of, 174, 175
    to parents
        on appointment confirmation,
            204, 209
        on diagnostic testing, 206
        difficult-to-contact, 210

on test results, 201–202
to physicians
    in quality assurance activities, 220
    on recall of infant for diagnostic
        testing, 218
Lip, cleft, 150
Log book in well-baby nursery, 130
Long Island Jewish Medical Center
        newborn hearing screening
        program
    evaluation of screeners in, 86
    failure rate in, 88
    medical records on, 44
    notification procedures in, 38, 42
    pediatrician reactions to, 47
    scheduling of, 36
    training of screeners in, 40, 73,
        82–83
Louisiana, newborn hearing
        screening in, 234, 252

Madsen Electronics, 118
    Celesta 503 Cochlear Emissions
        Analyzer from, 98–99
Maico Hearing Instruments, Inc., 99,
        118
Malpractice concerns in detection of
        hearing impairment, 42–43
Maryland, legislation on newborn
        hearing screening in, 252
Massachusetts, legislation on
        newborn hearing screening in,
        253
Mechanical ventilation, risk for
        hearing loss in, 152–153
Meningitis, 3
    risk for hearing loss in, 151–152
Milia, 124
Mimosa Acoustics, 118
    Cube Dis system from, 97–98
Minnesota, newborn hearing
        screening in, 240, 255
Mississippi, legislation on newborn
        hearing screening in, 253
Models for universal newborn
        hearing screening programs,
        50–64

Multidisciplinary cooperation in
        planning hearing screening
        program, 30

National Association of Special
        Instrument Distributors, 118
National Center for Hearing
        Assessment and Management
        nationwide survey, 226
National Institutes of Health
        Consensus Conference of 1993,
        15–17
    growth of hearing screening
        programs after, 226, 227
    recommendation on two-stage
        screening procedure, 16, 53, 88,
        227–228
Natus Medical Inc., 118
    ALGO systems from, 20, 59, 88,
        104–106
        in noisy conditions, 90
        in office-based screening, 162
Navigator E system (Biologic
        Systems), 109
Neonatologists as program director,
        68
Neurofibromatosis, risk for hearing
        loss in, 153
Neurologic development, neonatal
        hearing loss affecting, 2
Neuropathy, auditory, 7, 52
New Jersey, legislation on newborn
        hearing screening in, 253
New York, newborn hearing
        screening in, 21–23, 234, 240
    failure rates in, 22, 37, 88
    legislation on, 255
    in Long Island Jewish Medical
        Center. *See* Long Island Jewish
        Medical Center newborn
        hearing screening program
Nicolet Biomedical Inc., 119
    Compass system from, 107–108
    Spirit system from, 108–109
Noise in screening environment
    and equipment selection, 53, 90,
        116

in intensive care unit nursery, 57,
    62, 79, 135
  reduction of, 161
  and protocol selection, 56, 57, 62
Normal newborn nursery, 120–131.
    See also Well-baby nursery
Nose of newborn, appearance and
    characteristics of, 124
Nosocomial infections in newborn,
    141–142
Notification procedures
  computer generation of letters in,
    174, 175
  for parents
    audiologist report in, 200
    on diagnostic testing, 205–206
    educational measures in, 163, 190
    in follow-up program, 41, 42, 190,
      195–211
    of infant in intensive care unit,
      201–202
    nurse concerns on, 41
    obstetrician concerns on, 42
    pediatrician concerns on, 38
    on rescreening appointments,
      203–204
    screener training on, 74–76
    in urban areas, 45
  for physicians, 38
    in follow-up program, 190–191,
      211–221
    sample reports in, 215–217
Nova Scotia Conference of 1974, 14
Nurse practitioners, as screeners, 40,
    70
Nurses
  concerns in planning newborn
    hearing screening program,
    38–41, 238–240
    on handling of newborns by
      technicians, 40
    on notification procedures, 41
    on transport of newborns, 40–41
    on work load, 39–40
  education and training of, 38–39,
    40, 238–240
    in intensive care unit nursery, 134

in intensive care unit nursery,
    134–135, 142, 143–144
  as screeners, 39–40, 70
  schedules of, 77–78
  work load of, 39–40
    in intensive care unit nursery, 143

Obstetrician concerns in planning
    newborn hearing screening
    program, 41–43
  on malpractice claims, 42–43
  on notification of parents, 42
Oculo-auriculo-vertebral syndrome,
    risk for hearing loss in, 153–154
Office-based screening, 161–162
  pediatrician concerns in, 37
Ohio, legislation on newborn hearing
    screening in, 253
Oklahoma, legislation on newborn
    hearing screening in, 253
Otitis media, 3, 55
  recurrent or persistent, 156
Otoacoustic emissions screening, 7–8,
    20, 50, 52–54
  age at time of, 53, 159
  combined with auditory brainstem
    response screening, 53–54, 88
    equipment used in, 100–104,
      107–109
    model of, 62
  configuration of hearing loss
    detected in, 55
  cost considerations in, 233
  data collection and management in,
    170–171
    transfer of computer files in,
      172–173
  distortion product, 52, 53, 59
    equipment used in, 94–102, 227
    number of programs using, 227
  equipment and instruments in, 88,
    92–102, 227
    with auditory brainstem
      response screening, 100, 102,
      104, 107–109
    comparison of, 103
    computer systems, 90

electrical interference affecting, 90
false-positive results in, 53, 74, 75
flow chart on, 61
fluid and debris in ear affecting, 53, 158–159
in follow-up rescreening, 59–60, 62, 189, 192
in intensive care unit nursery, 57, 62, 160
   crying affecting, 160
   documentation of, 140, 141
model of, 59–62
in New York screening program, 22
in noisy conditions, 57, 90
number of programs using, 226–227
in office setting, 162
percentage of infants evaluated with, 230, 231
personnel in, 55, 60–62
   with auditory brainstem response screening, 62
   hospital variations in, 231–232
philosophy of program in, 54
prior experience affecting use of, 55
readiness of infant for, 158–159
referral rates in, 58, 62, 230, 231
in Rhode Island, 20–21, 52–53, 58
   data collection and management in, 171, 172–173
sensitivity and specificity of, 52
severity of hearing loss measured in, 54, 188
size of hospitals using, 227
time required for, 36, 94
   in distortion product systems, 95, 98, 99, 100, 102
in two-stage program, 16, 53, 88, 227–228
Otodynamics, Ltd., 119
   otoacoustic emissions equipment from, 53, 92–95
Otolaryngologists in planning newborn hearing screening program, 40–44, 200
Ototoxic drug therapy, risk for hearing loss in, 151, 153

Overstimulation of newborn, behavioral signs of, 137

Palate, cleft, 149–150
Parents
   bonding with newborn, 127–128
   consent obtained from, 34
   difficult to contact, sample letter to, 210
   education and training of. See Education and training, of parents
   length of hospital stay for mothers affecting screening protocol decisions, 55–56
   notification of. See Notification procedures, for parents
   refusal of hearing screening, 34, 59
   quality indicators on, 182
   reporting concerns on hearing status of child, 155
   rooming-in with newborn, 128–129, 161
   screening of newborn hearing in hospital room of, 57, 161
   training of screeners on interactions with, 74–76
Pass-fail criteria
   in auditory brainstem response screening, 106–107
   in distortion product otoacoustic emissions screening, 95, 99, 100
   and referral rates, 58
   in transient otoacoustic emissions screening, 94
Pediatricians
   concerns in planning newborn hearing screening program, 34–38, 238
      on cost effectiveness, 36–37
      on false-positive results, 37
      on notification procedures, 38
      in office-based screening, 37
      on schedule conflicts, 36
      on testing procedures, 34–35
      on time required for testing, 36
   reference materials for, 35–36, 48–49

screening in office, 37, 161–162
survey on reactions to newborn
    hearing screening program, 47
Pendred syndrome, 153
Pennsylvania, newborn hearing
    screening in, 240, 255
Personnel, 67–86
    administrative, 31–34
    audiologists. *See* Audiologists
    audiology coordinator, 68–69
    in auditory brainstem response
        screening, 51, 55, 59
        hospital variations in, 231–232
        with otoacoustic emissions
            screening, 62
    and cost of screening program,
        243–244
    hospital variations in, 231–232
    in intensive care unit nursery,
        134–135
        and infection control, 141
    multidisciplinary cooperation of, 30
    nurses. *See* Nurses
    obstetricians, 41–43
    in otoacoustic emissions screening,
        55, 60–62
        with auditory brainstem
            response screening, 62
        hospital variations in, 231–232
    otolaryngologists, 43–44, 238
    pediatricians, 34–38, 238
    in planning of screening program,
        29–44
    program director. *See* Director of
        screening program
    in quality improvement program,
        184–185
    in Rhode Island hearing screening
        program, 70, 168, 243–244
        in data collection and
            management, 171, 172
    screeners. *See* Screeners
    in support positions, 72
    in well-baby nursery, and infection
        control, 131
Philosophy of screening program
    affecting protocol decisions, 54
Phototherapy in jaundice of newborn,
    140
    and hearing screening, 161
Pike v. Honsinger case, 247
Planning newborn hearing screening
    program, 28–46
    administrative concerns in, 31–34
    audiologists in, 29–30, 44, 238
    community involvement in, 29,
        237–238
    on data collection and management
        procedures, 44, 169
    documentation of need in, 235–237
    on follow-up procedures, 44–45,
        187
    legislative process in, 240–241
    multidisciplinary cooperation in, 30
    nurses in, 38–41, 238–240
    obstetrician concerns in, 41–43
    otolaryngologists in, 43–44, 238
    pediatrician concerns in, 34–38, 238
    on quality improvement, 185
    selection of screening protocol in,
        50–51
        factors affecting, 54–58
    in urban areas, 45–46
Portable equipment, 90
    in distortion product otoacoustic
        emissions screening, 96, 100
Posture of newborn, 124
Pregnancy, infections in, and risk for
    hearing loss in infant, 148–149
Premature infants, 138
    feeding of, 140
    respiratory problems of, 139, 140
        and risk for hearing loss, 152
    temperature control in, 139
Prevalence of hearing loss in infants,
    6–9
    and cost effectiveness of screening
        programs, 6–7
Primary-care physicians, education
    on newborn hearing screening,
    212, 221, 238
Principles of screening programs,
    9–10
Privacy rights, 77

Probes
  in Biologic Systems Scout and
    Ranger devices, 100
  in Grason Stadler GSI 60 system, 95
  in Mimosa Acoustics Cube Dis
    system, 97, 98
  in Otodynamics IL088 system, 93
  quality indicators on use of, 182
  in Virtual model 330 system, 99
Program director. *See* Director of
  screening program
Protocols in newborn hearing
  screening programs, 50–51,
  227–230
  factors affecting selection of, 7–8,
    54–58, 228
  hospital variations in, 227–228,
    241–242
  two-stage process in, 16, 53, 88,
    227–228
Public relations and publicity in
  newborn hearing screening, 33

Quality management, 167, 177–185
  benefits of, 178
  classification of indicators in, 181
  in follow-up program, 184, 220
  in interpretation of test results, 173
  measurement system in, 178,
    179–180
  plan on, 185
  referral indicators in, 183–184
  screening indicators in, 181–183
  selection of indicators in, 179
  sources of data in, 180–181
  staff participation in, 184–185
  validity of indicators in, 179

Ranger system (Biologic Systems),
  100–101, 109
Reactivity periods of newborn, 125
Record keeping
  CareMap in, 157–158
  data collection and management
    procedures in, 167–177
  in intensive care unit nursery,
    140–141, 171, 172

on need for universal newborn
  hearing screening program,
  235–237
planning for, 44
sample report forms in, 213–217,
  219, 224
  on diagnostic data, 192, 224
  Infant Child Health Assessment
    Program referral form, 191,
    223
  on screener evaluation, 83–86
  Sound Beginnings form, 170–171,
    172, 173
training of screeners on, 77
in well-baby nursery, 130
Recruitment of screeners, 73
Referral rates, 58, 230–231
  in auditory brainstem response
    screening, 59, 62, 231
  equipment selection affecting, 116
  in otoacoustic emissions screening,
    58, 62, 230, 231
  quality indicators on, 183–184
  in Rhode Island program, 58, 230,
    238
Reflexes of newborn, 124–125
  acoustic, 19
Refusal rate
  in auditory brainstem response
    screening, 59
  consent procedures affecting, 34
  quality indicators on, 182
Register of high-risk infants, 17, 18
  Joint Committee on Infant hearing
    statement on, 12–13
Respiratory disorders
  Apgar score and risk for hearing
    loss in, 152
  in intensive care unit nursery, 139,
    140
  mechanical ventilation and risk for
    hearing loss in, 152–153
Respiratory distress syndrome of
  neonate, risk for hearing loss
  in, 152
Response Cradle screening method,
  18

Rhode Island newborn hearing
      screening program, 20–21, 234
   audiologists in, 238
   cost of, 36–37, 52–53, 243–244
   data collection and management in,
      167–177
   documentation of need for, 237
   education of parents in, 163
   equipment used in, 92
   identification of eligible infants in,
      171–172
   legislation on, 20–21, 240, 241, 245,
      253
   notification procedures in, 174
   organization of personnel in, 168
   otoacoustic emissions screening in,
      20–21, 52–53, 58
      data collection and management
         in, 171, 172–173
   physician support of, 238
   quality management in, 167,
      179–185
   referral rates in, 58, 230, 238
   screening personnel in, 70, 171, 172
Risk factors for hearing loss, 145–157
   and age of detection, 5
   Apgar score, 152
   birth weight, 150
   craniofacial abnormalities, 149–150
   data collection on, 154, 172
   family history, 146–147
   in follow-up decisions, 188
   hyperbilirubinemia, 150–151
   in-utero infection, 148–149
   Joint Committee on Infant Hearing
      statements on, 12–13, 145–146
   in late onset and progressive
      hearing loss, 155–156, 157
   limitations of screening program
      based on, 154–155
   mechanical ventilation, 152–153
   meningitis, 151–152
   ototoxic drug therapy, 151
   populations served in screening
      program based on, 156–157
   and register of high-risk infants,
      12–13, 17, 18

and selection of screening protocol,
      7–8
   syndromes associated with, 153–154
RITRACK software, 169, 171, 172
   data entry in, 173
   reports and correspondence
      generated with, 173, 174, 175
Rooming-in of newborn with mother,
      128–129
   site of screening in, 161
Rooting reflex of newborn, 125
Rubella in pregnancy, and risk for
      hearing loss in infant, 148

Safety of newborn
   in intensive care unit nursery, 142
   nurse concerns about, 40–41
   training of screeners on, 40, 76–77,
      129–130
   in transport of newborns, 40–41,
      129–130, 142
   in well-baby nursery, 129–130
Saskatoon Conference of 1978, 14–15
Scheduling concerns
   in follow-up program, 189–190, 193
      appointment arrangements in,
         203–206, 209
   hospital variations in, 232
   in intensive care unit nursery, 56,
      78–79, 135–136
      readiness of infant in, 56, 159–160
   length of hospital stay issues in,
      55–56, 77, 157
   of pediatricians, in planning of
      screening program, 36
   of screeners, 77–78
   in well-baby nursery, 78, 126
      readiness of infant in, 158–159
Scout system (Biologic Systems),
      100–101, 109
Screeners, 69–72
   audiologists as, 70, 77, 89
   education and training of, 40, 70,
      73–77. *See also* Education and
      training, of screeners
   evaluation of, 79–80
      form used in, 83–86

nurse practitioners as, 40, 70
nurses as, 39–40, 70, 77–78
recruitment of, 73
schedule arrangements for, 77–78
technicians as, 40, 72, 77, 89, 213
volunteers as, 70–72, 78
Secretarial personnel, 72
Security issues
in data storage, 176
training of screeners on, 76–77,
129–130
in transport of newborns for
screening, 40–41, 129–130, 142
in well-baby nursery, 129–130
Sensitivity and specificity of
screening tests, 6, 10, 17–20
in auditory brainstem response
screening, 19–20, 51
compared to behavioral
techniques, 18–19
in behavioral techniques, 17–19
equipment selection affecting, 117
in otoacoustic emissions screening,
52
and referral rates, 58
Sensorineural hearing loss risk
factors, 145–146, 157
Apgar score, 152
associated syndromes, 153–154
family history, 146–147
HIV infection, 149
hyperbilirubinemia, 150–151
mechanical ventilation, 152–153
ototoxic medications, 151
Severity of hearing loss detected
affecting age of detection, 4–5
in auditory brainstem response
screening, 54–55, 188, 189
equipment selection affecting, 89,
113–114
and follow-up decisions, 188, 189
in otoacoustic emissions screening,
54, 188
protocol decisions on, 54–55
Sleep cycles of newborn, 125–127
in intensive care unit, 135, 137, 160
scheduling of hearing screening
during, 126, 135, 160

Smart EP device (Intelligent Hearing
Systems), 104, 107
Smart Screen device (Intelligent
Hearing Systems), 104, 107
Smell sense of newborn, 124
SonaMed Corporation, 119
Clarity system from, 102–104
Sound Beginnings form, 170–171,
172
transfer of computer files on, 173
Specificity of screening tests. See
Sensitivity and specificity of
screening tests
Speech and language development,
1–4, 225
after brief period of normal
hearing, 3
critical period in, 4, 156
in early intervention, 3
follow-up on, 188
in otitis media, 156
parent reports on, 155
Spirit system (Nicolet Biomedical),
108–109
Sport system (Biologic Systems),
100–101
Staff. See Personnel
Standard of care, universal newborn
hearing screening as, 33–34,
246–248
consent issues in, 34
equipment and technology issues
in, 33, 248
expert opinions supporting, 33,
247–248
legal issues in, 33–34, 246–247
Statewide newborn hearing screening
programs, 233–246
cost of, 242–245
in Rhode Island, 36–37, 52–53,
243–244
follow-up services in, 245–246
implementation of, 241–242
recent efforts in, 20–23
legislative mandates on, 20,
233–234, 240–241
documentation of need for,
235–237

generation of constituency
support for, 237–240
summary listing on, 251–255
in Rhode Island. *See* Rhode Island
newborn hearing screening
program
Stress reactions of newborn, 137
Student screeners, 71
schedules of, 78
Sucking reflex of newborn, 125, 138
Supervisory responsibilities in
screening program, 72–80
Support personnel, 72
Syphilis in pregnancy, and risk for
hearing loss in infant, 148, 149

Technician screeners, 40, 72
nurse concerns about, 40
report for hospital record at time of
screening, 213
schedules of, 77
selection of screening equipment
for, 89
Telephone calls to parents, in follow-
up program, 203–205
Temperature regulation
in intensive care unit nursery, 136,
139–140
in well-baby nursery, 121–122
Thyroid disorders, and risk for
hearing loss in Pendred
syndrome, 153
Time required for hearing screening,
36
coordination with nursery routines,
36, 78, 122–123, 126
in intensive care unit, 78–79,
135–136
equipment selection affecting, 113
in otoacoustic emissions systems,
36, 94
distortion product, 95, 98, 99, 100,
102
scheduling of. *See* Scheduling
concerns
TORCH infections in pregnancy, and
risk for hearing loss in infant,
148–149

Touching and handling of newborn
hand washing prior to, 130, 141
by parents, 128
by technicians, nurse concerns on,
40
Toxoplasmosis in pregnancy, and risk
for hearing loss in infant, 148,
149
Tracking system
data collection and management in,
174–175
in follow-up program, 191, 193
in difficult-to-contact parents,
210
Infant Child Health Assessment
Program assistance in, 191, 223
in urban areas, 45, 46
in intensive care unit nursery, 79,
159
quality indicators on, 184
in well-baby nursery, 129
Transient evoked otoacoustic
emissions screening, 7–8,
52–53. *See also* Otoacoustic
emissions screening
Transport of newborns for screening
nurse concerns about, 40–41
safety and security in, 40–41,
129–130, 142
training of screeners on, 76–77,
129–130
Traveler Express system (Biologic
Systems), 109

Unilateral hearing loss, 3
follow-up program in, 188, 189
screening for, 54
Urban newborn hearing screening
programs, 45–46
Usher syndrome, risk for hearing loss
in, 153
Utah, newborn hearing screening in,
234, 236, 240, 249
cost of, 243–244
legislation on, 255

Ventilatory support, risk for hearing
loss in, 152–153

Viral infections in pregnancy, and risk
    for hearing loss in infant,
    148–149
Virginia, legislation on newborn
    hearing screening in, 254
Virtual Corporation model 330
    otoacoustic emission system,
    99–100
Vision of newborn, 123
    and eye contact with parents, 128
Volunteer screeners, 70–72
    schedules of, 78

Waardenburg syndrome, risk for
    hearing loss in, 154
Weight at birth, and risk for hearing
    loss, 150
Well-baby nursery, 120–131
    acoustic reflex screening in, 19
    appearance and characteristics of
        newborn in, 123–125
    bonding of newborn and parents
        in, 127–128
    infection control in, 130–131

initial procedures in, immediately
    after birth, 121–122
noise in, 57
periods of reactivity in, 125
prevalence of hearing loss in, 6–9
record keeping in, 130
    charts in, 130
    log book in, 130
risk-based screening programs in,
    17, 157
    limitations of, 154
routines in, 78, 122–123
safety and security concerns in,
    129–130
scheduling of screening in, 78, 126
    readiness of infant in, 158–159
as site for hearing screening, 57,
    160–161
sleep cycles in, 125–127
temperature regulation in, 121–122
West Virginia, legislation on newborn
    hearing screening in, 254
Work load of nurses, 39–40
    in intensive care unit nursery, 143